The Microbiome
and the Brain

The Microbiome and the Brain

Edited by
David Perlmutter, M.D.

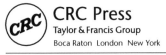

CRC Press
Taylor & Francis Group
Boca Raton London New York

CRC Press is an imprint of the
Taylor & Francis Group, an **informa** business

CRC Press
Taylor & Francis Group
6000 Broken Sound Parkway NW, Suite 300
Boca Raton, FL 33487-2742

First issued in paperback 2021

© 2020 by Taylor & Francis Group, LLC
CRC Press is an imprint of Taylor & Francis Group, an Informa business

ISBN-13: 978-0-8153-7672-9 (hbk)
ISBN-13: 978-1-03-217630-7 (pbk)
DOI: 10.1201/9781351235709

Contents

Editor

Dr. David Perlmutter is a Board-Certified Neurologist and four-time *New York Times* bestselling author. He serves on the Board of Directors and is a *Fellow* of the American College of Nutrition. Dr. Perlmutter received his M.D. degree from the University of Miami School of Medicine where he was awarded the *Leonard G. Rowntree Research Award.* He serves as a member of the Editorial Board for the *Journal of Alzheimer's Disease* and has published extensively in peer-reviewed scientific journals including *Archives of Neurology, Neurosurgery,* and *The Journal of Applied Nutrition.* He is a frequent lecturer at symposia sponsored by institutions such as the World Bank and IMF, Columbia University, Scripps Institute, New York University, and Harvard University and serves as an Associate Professor at the University of Miami Miller School of Medicine. Dr. Perlmutter is a recipient of the *Linus Pauling Award* for his innovative approaches to neurological disorders.

List of Contributors

Kirsten Berding
APC Microbiome Ireland
University College
Cork, Ireland

John Bienenstock
Institute of Nutritional Medicine
University of Hohenheim
Stuttgart, Germany

Jeffrey Bland
Personalized Lifestyle Medicine
    Institute
Bainbridge Island, Washington, USA

Thomas Borody
Medical Director, Centre for Digestive
    Diseases
Five Dock, NSW, Australia

Dale Bredesen
Department of Molecular and Medical
    Pharmacology
University of California, Los Angeles
Founding President and Professor
    Emeritus
Buck Institute for Research on Aging

Shrish Budree
University of Cape Town
Cape Town, South Africa
OpenBiome
Somerville, Massachusetts, USA

Sharon Donovan
Department of Food Science and
    Human Nutrition
University of Illinois
Urbana, Illinois, USA

Alessio Fasano
Department of Pediatric
    Gastroenterology and Nutrition
Mucosal Immunology and Biology
    Research Center
Massachusetts General Hospital
Boston, Massachusetts, USA
Department of Pediatrics
Harvard Medical School
Harvard University,
    Massachusetts, USA

Maria R. Fiorentino
Department of Pediatric
    Gastroenterology and Nutrition
Mucosal Immunology and Biology
    Research Center
Massachusetts General Hospital
Boston, Massachusetts, USA
Department of Pediatrics
Harvard Medical School
Harvard University,
    Massachusetts, USA

Leo Galland
Foundation for Integrated Medicine
New York, New York, USA

Arpana Gupta
Oppenheimer Center for Neurobiology
    of Stress and Resilience
Division of Integrative Medicine
Greater Los Angeles VA Healthcare
    System

Thomas Gurry
MIT Center for Microbiome
    Informatics and Therapeutics
Cambridge, Massachusetts, USA

Zain Kassam
Massachusetts Institute of Technology
Cambridge, Massachusetts, USA
OpenBiome
Somerville, Massachusetts, USA

Alim Ladha
Department of Biological Engineering
Massachusetts Institute of Technology
Cambridge, Massachusetts, USA

Bharat Ramakrishna
OpenBiome
Cambridge, Massachusetts, USA

George Tetz
Chief Scientific Director, Human
    Microbiology Institute
New York, New York, USA
Tetz Laboratories,
New York, New York, USA

Victor Tetz
Chief Scientific Director, Human
    Microbiology Institute
New York, New York, USA

Kirsten Tillisch
Oppenheimer Center for Neurobiology
    of Stress and Resilience
Division of Digestive Diseases,
    Department of Medicine
David Geffen School of Medicine at
    University of California
Division of Integrative Medicine
Greater Los Angeles VA Healthcare
    System

Helen Tremlett
Medicine (Neurology) and the Djavad
    Mowafaghian Centre for Brain
    Health
University of British Columbia
Vancouver, BC, Canada

Aristo Vojdani
Immunosciences Lab., Inc.
Los Angeles, California, USA
Department of Preventive Medicine,
Loma Linda University School of
    Medicine
Loma Linda, California, USA

Elroy Vojdani
Regenera Medical
Los Angeles, California, USA

Emmanuelle Waubant
University of California, San Francisco
San Francisco, California, USA

Can (Martin) Zhang
Harvard Medical School
Genetics and Aging Research Unit
Mass General Institute for
    Neurodegenerative Disease
Massachusetts General Hospital
Charlestown, Massachusetts, USA

Introduction

David Perlmutter, MD, FACN

Ignaz Philipp Semmelweis was a German Hungarian physician who received his doctoral degree in Vienna in 1844. He was then appointed to serve as an assistant at the obstetrics clinic in the city's General Hospital.

Soon thereafter, Semmelweis gained a keen interest in the problem of puerperal infection. At that time, most women delivered their babies at home. However, for various reasons including poverty or obstetrical complication, hospitalization was an infrequently used option. Semmelweis observed that mortality for mothers delivering in a hospital was dramatically increased in comparison to home deliveries, with death occurring in a staggering 25 to 30% of hospitalized women. And many of these deaths were a consequence of puerperal infection.

Vienna's general hospital had two obstetrical wards that provided virtually identical facilities for its patients. There was, however, one important difference. While one ward was under the care of midwives and their students, the other was manned by medical students. Dr. Semmelweis and his colleagues were aware of a striking fact: the patients in the ward overseen by the medical students had a markedly higher mortality rate—threefold higher—compared to the ward overseen by the midwives.

One popular explanation for this disparity centered on the idea that aggressive physical handling of the obstetrical patients by the male medical students somehow increased a woman's risk for puerperal fever. Semmelweis believed that some other mechanism was involved.

In 1847, a close colleague of Semmelweis died quite quickly of a disease that looked remarkably like puerperal fever. Semmelweis learned that his friend had accidentally cut his hand while performing an autopsy on a woman who had died of this disease. It is then that Semmelweis began to ponder the idea that doctors and medical students who were working with cadavers might somehow be transmitting "cadaverous particles" which manifested disease. Indeed, at that time, it was common practice for doctors and students alike to go directly from dissecting cadavers to assisting women with their deliveries.

Semmelweis believed that puerperal fever might well be caused by "infective material" in dead bodies. As such, he mandated that all students, prior to assisting in the obstetrics ward, wash their hands in a solution of chlorinated lime. He then went about carefully recording mortality rates in the obstetrics ward managed by the medical students. In April 1847, the mortality rate was 18.3%. Following the handwashing protocol, mortality rates plummeted to 2.2% in June, 1.2% in July, and 1.9% in August. In fact, in March and August 1848, there was not a single death of a woman related to childbirth in this obstetrics ward.

Despite these results, Semmelweis was highly criticized by his superiors, likely because they lacked a mechanistic framework by which they could understand his results. In 1861, Semmelweis published a book, *Die Ätiologie, der Begriff und die Prophylaxis des Kindbettfiebers* (*The Etiology, Concept, and Prophylaxis of Childbed Fever*) that clearly challenged accepted obstetrical methods of the time. Ultimately, the consensus opinion rejected his doctrine—a doctrine based on the idea that infection was somehow transmitted by living particles.

The rejection and castigation Semmelweis endured proved to be a tipping point in the life of this courageous researcher. Though he tried to defend his findings and recommendations, he ultimately suffered a mental breakdown and was eventually confined to a mental institution where ironically, he died as a consequence of an infected wound on his hand.

Semmelweis was by no means alone in challenging the prevailing miasma theory of infection in favor of a contagion-based etiology. Additionally, the work of Louis Pasteur was important in advancing the understanding of contagions as disease messengers. In 1859, he conducted an experiment using beef broth that had been sterilized by boiling. Pasteur then placed the broth two different styles of swan neck flasks. One was open at the top while the second was S-shaped so as to prevent the entrance of any dust or particles. Soon thereafter, the beef broth in the flask open to the environment was teeming with microbes while the material in the S-shaped flask remained virtually sterile. This simple but elegant experiment roundly challenged the notion of "spontaneous generation" that held that living organisms developed from nonliving matter—the same ideology that helped support the ridicule of Dr. Semmelweis. And to be sure, Pasteur himself sustained aggressive criticism by those adherent to the doctrine of spontaneous generation as evidenced by the damning sentiment expressed toward him in the well-respected scientific journal, La Presse in 1860: "I am afraid that the experiment you quote, M. Pasteur, will turn against you. The world into which you wish to take us is really too fantastic."

But rejection of Pasteur's theory that living "germs" were the agents of infectious disease was not universal. Pasteur's work came to the attention of British surgeon Joseph Lister, who had already concluded that living particles were somehow responsible for wound infections. As such, Lister focused his attention on finding an innocuous way of killing germs without further traumatizing wounds. Reflecting on Pasteur's work, Lister stated, "When I read Pasteur's article, I said to myself: just as we can destroy lice on the nit-filled head of a child by applying a poison that causes no lesion to the scalp, so I believe that we can apply to a patient's wounds toxic products that will destroy the bacteria without harming the soft parts of the tissue."

Ultimately, Lister identified carbolic acid as an antiseptic for both sterilizing surgical instruments and dressings. With time, the implementation of Lister's antiseptic technique proved undeniably effective in reducing surgical wound infections. The adoption of Lister's antiseptic system was, according to author Lindsey Fitzharris, "…the most prominent outward sign of the medical community's acceptance of a germ theory, and it marked the epochal moment when medicine and science merged."

By the mid-1870s, the awareness of the underlying role of germs as agents of disease had become widespread in the scientific community, spreading shortly thereafter to the general population. This understanding amplified the presumed importance of cleanliness and hygiene. Antiseptic products playing upon the public's fear of "dangerous germs" flooded the marketplace. With time, any use of the term "germ," or even "microbe" always carried a threatening connotation.

Until only recently, the terms bacteria, microbe, and germ almost always represented adversarial entities. And to this day, playing upon our fear, antimicrobial "hand-sanitizers" are still found on the end caps of our grocery store aisles, right next to the "antibacterial soaps."

Nonetheless, a paradigmatic change as dramatic as the shift from spontaneous generation to germ theory is at hand. In the past two decades the focus on bacteria primarily as agents of disease has been virtually upended. The multitude of diverse bacteria along with archaea, fungi, viruses and bacteriophages, helminths and protozoa living upon and within us, known collectively along with their genetic material and their metabolic products as the microbiome, are fundamental to our survival, influencing diverse aspects of physiology from immune function to metabolism, cognitive function, mood, sleep, exercise tolerance, appetite, and even our genetic expression. Indeed, the blossoming importance of the microbiome is well positioned in the current zeitgeist with Google Trends revealing that searches for the term "microbiome" have increased by more than 30-fold in just the last 11 years.

Western medicine is centered on a reductionist approach to understanding human physiology and pathology. Many have credited the 16th-century French philosopher René Descartes with codifying this paradigm. Descartes, in part V of his Discourses, described the natural world as nothing more than a clockwork machine that could be understood in its entirety through an exploration of its individual components. This philosophy ultimately made its way to the field of medicine where, to a significant degree, it remains influential. Segregating the human body into individual components and systems manifests the creation of "specialists" involved in their study. And the ever-increasing complexity of this specialty nomenclature is regarded as a metric of our scientific sophistication and advancement. Through this lens, the idea of the body as a highly integrated system, fully dependent on interplay between seemingly disparate components has been, until quite recently, the subject of derogation.

But integrated the human body is. And as explored in this text, the level of integration between the gut and the brain is profound and mysterious. Exploration of this fascinating new research is providing us with powerful and unanticipated tools for understanding and treating some of the most challenging maladies of our time.

The Microbiome and the Brain begins by exploring the various technologies and strategies used in microbiome research. Recent advances in microbiome sequencing technologies have supported an astonishing rate of data acquisition, facilitating incredible breakthroughs in our understanding of the relationship between the gut microbiome and the human host. This data provides us with a better understanding of disease and fuels interventional clinical applications.

Commonly used sequencing methods are described in terms of their utility as well as the information they provide. Data accumulated through these various sequencing techniques must undergo aggressive analysis, and a review of this analytic process that evaluates not only the meaning of the data, but its quality as well, is described.

In Chapter 2, The Microbiome and the Brain explores the interface between the microbiome and its human host. The microbiome directly or indirectly influences virtually every cell in the human body, and the manifestations of this dynamic interaction are a reflection of the uniqueness of both the microbial components and their metabolites and that of the human host.

We recognize that each of us is blessed by a vast array of characteristics that ultimately define us as individuals. And targeting these nuances for the maintenance of health and even treatment of disease is a central tenet in the application of a personalized medicine approach. This chapter pursues traditional areas of interest in personalized medicine including host genetics, diet, exposure to xenobiotics, detoxification function, medication, and others, in terms of how these variables manifest either health or disease. But it does so through the lens of the microbiome–host interface.

Clearly, the uniqueness of an individual's microbiome has been a fairly central theme in microbiome research over at least the past decade. And over this same time span there's been a surge in interest in a more personalized approach to medical care. As such, this chapter presents the convergence of two highly validated paradigms for understanding human health and disease.

Inflammation and altered immune responses are highly influential underpinnings for neurodegenerative conditions. Chapter 3 provides an in-depth understanding of the genesis of these two processes and their role in conditions including Alzheimer's disease and Parkinson's disease as well as in various inflammatory bowel diseases. Mechanistic correlations between brain and bowel inflammatory diseases are described in relation to degradation of barrier function, amplification of inflammatory mediators, and molecular mimicry. And the study of how the microbiome relates to these mechanisms is reviewed—with an emphasis on laboratory investigations.

Chapter 4 further explores the fundamental connection between inflammation and neurodegenerative disease. The chapter begins by focusing on the functional, bidirectional communication involving hormonal secretion and the engagement of the autonomic nervous system. Pathologic conditions such as hepatic encephalopathy, epilepsy, and celiac disease are reviewed to further establish an understanding of the gut's role in brain function.

This chapter then explores current research that demonstrates, through a variety of mechanisms, how changes in the array of gut microbiota influence the brain. These mechanisms include alterations in gut, blood–brain-barrier, and blood–spinal cord barrier permeability, variations in short-chain fatty acids and other metabolic products, and the possible role of these mechanisms in diverse neurological conditions including Alzheimer's disease, autism spectrum disorder (ASD), Parkinson's disease, attention-deficit disorder, amyotrophic lateral sclerosis, and multiple sclerosis.

The chapter concludes with a discussion of autism as a prototypic representation of a gut–brain disease process, exploring both the depths of research confirming significant and consistent gut dysbiosis in this condition and its possible relevance to neurological impairment. Research describing a novel intervention—fecal microbial transplantation (FMT)—for children with autism spectrum disorder and gastrointestinal problems is presented. The improvement in the treated children with respect to both their gastrointestinal and their autism spectrum disorder-related behavioral symptoms is examined, lending support to the role of the microbiota in the pathogenesis of this condition.

Chapter 5 continues the discussion of autism spectrum disorder with an in-depth presentation of the changes in the gut microbiota and mycobiota characteristic of this condition. Beyond these correlations, differences in various bacterial metabolites, including short-chain fatty acids, taurocholenate sulfate, 3-(3-hydroxyphenyl)-3-hydroxypropionic acid (HPHPA), 5-aminovalerate, and serotonin, characteristic of autism spectrum disorder, are presented in the context of how these differences might ultimately influence neurological function.

Next, this chapter details the role of nutrition in autism spectrum disorder. It approaches this topic from several perspectives, including the nutritional challenges posed by the almost universal feeding-related symptomatology characteristic of this disorder, the effectiveness of various dietary interventions on symptomatology, the effect of dietary interventions on microbiota composition, and finally, the potential influence of nutritional interventions on the microbiota-brain communication.

Chapter 6 begins the discussion of the role of the microbiome in the global pandemic of Alzheimer's disease. Expanding upon the impact of inflammation in this and other neurodegenerative conditions, Chapter 6 presents a subtyping of Alzheimer's disease based on pathological and clinical findings and describes how various downstream effects from disturbances of the microbiome may be uniquely influential in each of these subtypes. Mechanisms explored include: upregulation of inflammatory pathways as a consequence of increased gut permeability or as a consequence of overrepresentation of organisms including *Porphyromonas gingivalis* or *Fusobacterium nucleatum* from the oral microbiome, activation of NF-κB leading to up-regulation of the β-secretase and γ-secretase complex, and a shift toward a more amyloidogenic pathway, compromise of detoxification function, and importantly, the highly relevant role of the microbiome in regulating glucose metabolism.

Additionally, in recognizing the important potential role of dysbiosis in Alzheimer's disease, this chapter makes it clear that a variety of often overlooked issues should be considered as potentially playing a role in terms of etiology including various medications, stress, Cesarean birth, aging, inflammation, and xenobiotics.

Chapter 7 continues the discussion of Alzheimer's disease with a comprehensive review of pertinent animal research. Of particular interest are the studies demonstrating how a deficiency in the microbiome (using germ-free animals) directly impacts hippocampus-dependent memory formation. The fact that memory function could be restored by probiotics highlights the importance of gut microbiota in this fundamental brain function. Further, gut-administered antibiotics have been shown to reduce Alzheimer's pathology in the transgenic mouse model of Alzheimer's disease. In this research, not only was there reduction in Alzheimer's signature pathology, but significant changes in circulating cytokine levels were observed as well, again emphasizing the role of the gut microbiota in regulating the setpoint of inflammation.

The discussion then turns from gut-related organisms to the newly described brain microbiome and the possible pathogenic role of specific microbes related to Alzheimer's disease including Borrelia spirochetes, Chlamydia pneumonia, and herpes simplex virus type 1.

Thereafter, this chapter focuses on how modifiable lifestyle factors including use of nonsteroidal anti-inflammatory drugs, restorative sleep, consumption of folate, vitamin E, vitamin C, and coffee, bring about changes in the microbiome that may explain the association of these factors with reduced Alzheimer's risk. This is followed by a specific discussion of the role of diet, including probiotics, ketogenesis, and fiber and their influence on the make-up and functionality of the gut microbiota in the context of Alzheimer's disease.

The relationship between the microbiome and mood is explored in Chapter 8. The morbidity and mortality that result as consequences of mood disorders are clearly under-recognized. Further, pharmaceutical and non-pharmaceutical interventions targeting these disorders by and large provide less than significant improvement. As such, the potential for developing therapies based on modulation of the powerful relationship between the microbiome and the brain, specifically as this relationship influences mood, provides researchers opportunities to explore an entirely new venue that may well have the potential to ameliorate these pernicious but disabling disorders.

Chapter 9 is dedicated to clarifying the relationship between alterations in the microbiome and multiple sclerosis. As multiple sclerosis is characterized as both an inflammatory and autoimmune condition, correlation with intestinal dysbiosis should not be surprising. Nonetheless, the depth and scope of the emerging research in this area, as summarized in this chapter, is profound.

The chapter begins by presenting the challenges faced in dealing with multiple sclerosis (MS) from both societal and clinical perspectives. Current pharmaceutical inventions are only modestly effective for this disease. As such, it is important to recognize the implications for translating the emerging animal research relating variations in the microbiome to disease pathogenesis. Indeed, using the time-tested animal model for multiple sclerosis, experimental autoimmune encephalomyelitis (EAE) in which a brain demyelinating condition is created that mimics multiple sclerosis in humans, researchers now demonstrate that the production of the pathological hallmarks of this disease is significantly dependent on the microbiome. Further, EAE is noted to be more severe in mice that received transplant and stool from a person with multiple sclerosis. These observations are explained along with both circumstantial and somewhat more direct evidence linking changes in the gut microbiome to MS.

Finally, Chapter 9 tackles the question of the potential role of direct microbiome manipulation in MS, providing a state-of-the-art overview of our current status in this pursuit, as well as considering where we may be going.

Chapter 10, Bacteriophage Involvement in Neurodegenerative Diseases, provides an entrée to a relationship between neurodegenerative conditions and microbes that has received very little attention. Specifically, the chapter recognizes the importance of protein misfolding as an underlying mechanism in Alzheimer's disease, Parkinson's disease, as well as amyotrophic lateral sclerosis. The aggregates of these misfolded proteins ultimately induce neuronal death and synapse loss. As one might expect, therefore, the research dedicated to deciphering the mechanisms underlying protein misfolding is extensive.

As will be revealed in Chapter 6, a relationship exists between alterations in gut microbiota, the production of systemic inflammation, and protein misfolding. But a specific mechanism relating alterations in microbiota to protein misfolding in neurodegenerative diseases has remained elusive. This chapter explores the possibility that bacteriophages may be involved in this mechanism. Further, actual infection of eukaryotic cells is described along with possible implications of this finding. In addition, phages are described as activating NF-κB which is known to suppress TREM2 expression, and as such, inhibit amyloid clearance by microglia.

Finally, the text turns to the research indicating that phage infection may alter bacterial populations and diversity, creating patterns that have been established as correlating with neurological conditions. Further, since phages can spread between humans, the chapter includes a discussion that speculates as to the transmissibility of Alzheimer's, Parkinson's, or ALS between humans.

Without question, one of the most aggressive and certainly controversial interventions implemented with the goal of establishing a more eubiotic microbiome is fecal microbial transplant. FMT is the subject of Chapter 11 which begins with an overview of the various constituents of the gut's inhabitants including viruses, fungi, archaea, and bacteria, as well as their potential contribution to human health and disease.

Thereafter, the discussion centers more specifically on bacteria, with an overview of various mechanisms by which bacteria may influence brain function, as well as risk for disease. FMT is then introduced, first in the context of the substantial data demonstrating the effective use of this therapy for the treatment of *Clostridium difficile* infection.

Clinical application of FMT in neurological disorders is then explored in the context of hepatic encephalopathy, epilepsy, Parkinson's disease, Tourette syndrome, and autism spectrum disorder.

The Microbiome and the Brain concludes with Chapter 12, Lifestyle Influences on the Microbiome. This important chapter provides an in-depth understanding of the influence of dietary choices, including both macronutrient and micronutrient components, on microbial diversity and metabolic function. Additionally, it covers other extrinsic influences known to be potentially disruptive to the microbiome including stress, inflammation, alcohol, tobacco, and various medications including proton pump inhibitors, now used by millions of Americans. In this context, the chapter concludes with a recommendation for clinicians to consider the possible detrimental effects upon the microbiome when implementing medical interventions.

Conclusion

The challenges confronting us today posed by neurodevelopmental and neurodegenerative conditions are daunting. But they are no less daunting than the rampant infectious diseases that galvanized the efforts of Lister and Semmelweis toward a paradigm-shifting resolution. With our new understanding of the influence of the microbiome on brain health, functionality, and disease predilection, it is intriguing that once again our attention is drawn to the world of microbes.

It is hard to imagine two more seemingly disparate functions in human physiology than those subserved by the nervous and digestive systems. And yet, the term gut–brain axis is now solidly entrenched in our lexicon. Although the physical connection between the brain and gut has been long described, along with a more recent discovery of chemical communication involving neurotransmitters, it is truly the role of the microbiome in terms of its influence upon all manner of brain function that has fully validated the importance of the discussion of the intimate bidirectional connection between the gut and the brain.

The pages that follow investigate many aspects of our current understanding of this fascinating relationship. Undoubtedly, this text, while portraying our most current knowledge of the science in this area, will be supplanted by exciting upcoming developments in the field. Nonetheless, these chapters stand as important benchmark resources for researchers and clinicians moving forward with a perspective that more fully understanding, embracing, and exploiting the relationship between the microbiome and the brain may well offer up effective resources in our efforts to impact many of our most pernicious neurological conditions.

1 Assessing the Microbiome—Current and Future Technologies and Applications

Thomas Gurry, Shrish Budree, Alim Ladha, Bharat Ramakrishna and Zain Kassam

CONTENTS

Andrew is an energetic 7-year-old, but his parents suspect something isn't quite right. His eyes always dart away, never quite meeting their gaze. He watches the same repeating eight seconds of a bright red monster truck squashing the shells of abandoned cars. He dutifully watches every day for exactly three hours. Andrew's parents are worried, and bring him to see his pediatrician, Dr. Sara McDonald, who suspects that Andrew has autism spectrum disorder (ASD), a complex neuro-developmental disorder. In the past, Dr. McDonald would have had to perform an in-depth, time-consuming evaluation of diagnostic criteria because there were no laboratory or diagnostic tests for ASD. But today, in 2040, the world is different. Dr. McDonald sends Andrew's stool sample off to a lab for microbiome sequencing, and the microbial profile comes back with decreased Lachnospiracea and Dialister bacteria, a finding which supports a diagnosis of ASD. Crazy as it may seem, a world where a patient's microbial signature deeply impacts their care is not far from real-ity. The goal of this chapter is to highlight the current methods for sequencing the microbiome, including common analyses, to understand potential future advances in the field, and to arm clinicians with practical knowledge for critically appraising extant and future literature surrounding the microbiome.

Recent advances in microbiome sequencing technology have led to an explosion of intestinal microbiome research (Lloyd-Price et al. 2016 and Jovel et al. 2016). Innovation in bacterial DNA sequencing methods has allowed researchers to describe the intestinal microbial community with unparalleled ease and precision. Previously, the identification of intestinal microbes was performed using culture-based techniques, which were limited both in resolution and throughput. Furthermore, bacterial sequencing has led to the identification of many bacterial species that were previously unculturable (Knight et al. 2017). These technological breakthroughs have opened new avenues through which to explore the relationship between the gut microbiome and the human host, including the role of gut bacteria in the pathogenesis of disease.

Although multiple sequencing technologies were at the forefront of this developing field, the Illumina sequencing platform has undoubtedly outperformed all others in terms of cost, reliability, user interface, and data quality. Illumina is now considered the gold standard technology for performing the two most common methods of bacterial DNA sequencing: 16S rRNA sequencing and shotgun metagenomic sequencing (Knight et al. 2017).

METHODS FOR SEQUENCING THE MICROBIOME

The term "sequencing" describes the scientific technique of determining the order of nucleotides in a given sample's genomic material (e.g. bacterial DNA/RNA). This genetic information can, in turn, be used to describe the identity, population distribution, and, as discussed later in this chapter, the complex functional characteristics of the host microbiome. 16S rRNA sequencing and shotgun metagenomic sequencing differ significantly in cost, resolution, and difficulty. Therefore, investigators deciding which technique to use must consider numerous factors, including the experimental question being explored, the samples being analyzed, and the total budget.

16S rRNA Sequencing

In bacteria and archaea, the 16S rRNA gene contains both highly conserved and variable regions. Although this domain is always present in bacteria, differences in the variable regions of the gene correlate with specific bacterial species. 16S rRNA sequencing works by leveraging the known sequence of highly conserved regions of the 16S rRNA gene to amplify and sequence the variable regions (often regions V3, V4, and V5) in order to accurately characterize a sample's microbial community (Knight et al. 2017 and Olsen 2016).

16S rRNA sequencing is a relatively simple technique with many advantages over more complex sequencing strategies, including its low cost, standardized protocols—including sample preparation, sequencing, and downstream analysis—and high-quality reference databases against which to map obtained sequence data. However, limiting the scope of sequenced DNA to the 16S gene only allows identification at the level of bacteria *genera*, excluding *species*-level resolution. For example, a sequence read of the V4 region may include hits to multiple species in a reference database, restricting an investigator's ability to draw conclusions about the specific species associated with the sequence read (Jovel et al. 2016 and Olsen 2016).

SHOTGUN METAGENOMIC SEQUENCING

Shotgun metagenomic sequencing, commonly referred to as whole-genome sequencing, determines the nucleotide sequence of all the genomic materials present in a sample. The DNA in a sample is too lengthy to amplify and sequence in one piece, so sample DNA is typically fragmented before being sequenced. The process of piecing sequence fragments back together requires both deep expertise and significant computational power. Once the fragments are realigned, the whole-genome sequence reads can be mapped against a reference database of known bacterial sequences to determine the microbial community. Marker genes, specific genes that are well characterized and sequenced across multiple bacterial strains and species, are mapped to a reference database to identify microbes. Given that this method sequences the entire bacterial genome, it enables much higher-resolution characterization of the microbial community, allowing investigators to make definitive conclusions about the species, and in some cases, the specific strains, present in a sample (Franzosa et al. 2016).

While shotgun metagenomics can increase the sequence resolution, it also generates vast amounts of "noisy" data. Therefore, significant computational expertise is required to clean and filter the resulting data into a more usable form. Furthermore, the added complexity of analysis means that significant variation can be introduced into the results by divergent analysis techniques. Shotgun metagenomics is also relatively expensive, often limiting study size, and, consequently, the statistical power of studies employing this sequencing technique.

GENERATING DATA FROM SAMPLES

Processing biological samples (e.g. stool, skin, etc.) for sequencing begins with the extraction of DNA from bacterial cells. This can be achieved by chemically dissolving the bacterial membrane, bursting the membrane using physical force, or a combination of the two (Olsen 2016). This process is commonly referred to as bacterial cell lysis. Cell lysis is also often accompanied by methods aimed at separating DNA from other components inside the cell membranes, including proteins, lipids, and other cell lysates. It is important to note that one of the main sources of variation in sequencing data stems from the different approaches to DNA extraction, as this step is a primary determinant of DNA purity and integrity (Debelius et al. 2016).

DNA extraction is followed by polymerase chain reaction (PCR) amplification. In the case of 16S rRNA sequencing, primers first bind to the constant region of the 16S gene and are subsequently extended into the 16S variable regions using a specifically engineered DNA polymerase enzyme. This process creates amplified sequences of the variable 16S regions, referred to as amplicons. In shotgun metagenomics, PCR is used to amplify the fragmented DNA sequences from the sample. Amplified sequences are then tagged with sample-specific barcodes, which facilitate multiplexing—a process in which multiple samples are run in a single Illumina sequencing lane, significantly increasing the sequencing throughput and reducing the overall cost of analysis. In the final preparatory step, adapters, which are required for binding the Illumina flow cell, are added to the amplicon sequences. Once this is completed, the sample is ready for sequencing. In a process similar to PCR, the Illumina platform is able to identify the exact nucleotide sequence of amplicons and amplified fragments by monitoring fluorescent output. Barcoded and adapter-modified nucleotide sequences are amplified using fluorescently labeled nucleotides, emitting a unique fluorescent pattern that can be directly translated into a sequence readout. The Illumina sequencing platform outputs FASTQ files which contain the "raw" data comprised of both sequence reads and accompanying quality control scores. Finally, using open-source computational pipelines, the raw data can be quality trimmed and filtered.

In 16S rRNA sequencing, characterization of the microbial community using the sequence data begins by either clustering the 16S reads or comparing individual reads to a reference database. Clustering can be done using various computational methods, but the output is generally the same: groups of sequences (called operational taxonomic units or OTUs) that meet a threshold criterion for similarity (usually 97%). The defined OTUs are then mapped to a reference database to assign a taxonomic classification (Jovel et al. 2016 and Olsen 2016). In contrast, sequence reads can be directly mapped to a reference database without previous clustering to identify groups of OTUs and their most likely taxonomic classifications. Both methods are valid but often produce divergent results. The final product, in either case, is referred to as an OTU table, which contains the abundance of each identified OTU and its corresponding taxonomic classification. Using common descriptive analysis techniques, which are described later, the processed data is analyzed to answer experimental questions. More advanced comparative statistics, beyond the scope of this discussion, including linear modeling, may also be performed to identify statistically significant differences in microbial communities between samples or clinical covariates.

COMMON DESCRIPTIVE ANALYSIS TECHNIQUES FOR MICROBIOME DATA

DIVERSITY ANALYSIS

Diversity measures provide information about the composition of a microbial community. Diversity analysis, in the context of the intestinal microbiome, is classified into alpha diversity and beta diversity. Alpha diversity is a metric used to quantify microbial diversity within a single sample (Jovel et al. 2016 and Olsen 2016). It may refer to the richness, or a number of different species present, the abundance of different species, or distribution of different species in the sample. The most common method of reporting alpha diversity is the Shannon Diversity Index, which is the sum of the proportion of each species relative to the total number of species in the community; therefore, it is a measure of both microbial abundance and distribution. Typically, studies will compare the alpha diversity between covariates under investigation, such as a comparison of the alpha diversity between the diseased and healthy control group. Numerous studies have correlated low alpha diversity with poorer health outcomes (Jovel et al. 2016 and Knight et al. 2017).

On the other hand, beta diversity is an analysis technique used to compare diversity between samples (Jovel et al. 2016 and Olsen 2016). It is typically used to determine "how different" samples are from each other by effectively measuring the distance between samples because similar samples are "closer" together. This technique can be done with the supervision of phylogenetic data (e.g., UniFrac) or without it (e.g., Bray–Curtis dissimilarity). Once the beta diversity is computed, it is often displayed graphically by reducing the dimensionality of the dataset using either non-metric multidimensional scaling or principal coordinate analysis. These methods are extremely useful for both data visualization and clustering based on the covariates under investigation, but both rely on the assumption that variation in beta diversity can be explained by a few independent factors.

RELATIVE ABUNDANCE PLOTS

The processed OTU table contains the absolute abundance of the individual OTUs and accompanying taxonomic classification in the sequenced sample. It is a common practice for researchers to normalize the OTU count and report the relative abundance of organisms present in samples at various taxonomic levels, including the phylum level to genus level, with 16S data and species level with shotgun metagenomic data (Jovel et al. 2016 and Olsen 2016). Relative abundances are usually represented using graphical plots, including heat maps, bar-plots, and circular phylogenetic trees. Heatmaps utilize color-coding to represent numerical values, like OTU abundance, and are particularly common and a useful method of representing large-scale data graphically as they are visually appealing.

FUNCTIONAL GENOMICS

As the field of microbiome sequencing progresses, investigators are striving to unearth the mechanisms underlying host–microbiome interactions. This requires researchers to study the function of a host's microbiome and not just its identity. Using both 16S and, more reliably, shotgun metagenomics, researchers can now determine the functional capacity of a microbial community. This type of analysis is facilitated by a computational software package like PICRUSt. Metagenomic data can be mapped against a reference database called the Kyoto Encyclopedia of Genes and Genomes (KEGG) Orthology (KO) to determine representative metabolic pathways present in a given sample. With 16S data, OTUs must be mapped to phylogenetic trees and reference databases containing information on their broader genetic code, a method which is only moderately reliable (Langille et al. 2013). Therefore, shotgun metagenomics provides a significantly more reliable method for determining functional profiles of the microbiome.

However, while this type of functional analysis can identify whether the gene for a metabolic pathway is present, it cannot determine whether these genetic pathways are active. Techniques such as transcriptomics and metabolomics measure actual gene transcription or microbial metabolites, which can significantly deepen our understanding of the microbiome's functionality when combined with genomics data (Franzosa et al. 2016 and Franzosa and Abu-Ali 2015).

CRITICAL APPRAISAL OF MICROBIOME DATA

As the number of clinical microbiome studies continues to increase, it is of paramount important that clinical researchers and practitioners are confident in their ability to assess the scientific validity and the clinical and statistical significance of their results. Evaluating microbiome data involves several levels of scrutiny, which can be grouped into two categories: assessing the methodologies used to generate the data and assessing the extent to which the data supports the conclusions of the authors. Moreover, as previously discussed, microbiome data comes from two primary sequencing methodologies: 16S rRNA sequencing and shotgun metagenomic sequencing. The questions that each of these approaches can answer differ. Generally speaking, 16S rRNA sequencing data is used for community-level characterization of the microbiota, whereas shotgun metagenomic sequencing is used for functional genomic analyses or a greater degree of taxonomic resolution—including strain tracking. The first step in appraising a microbiome study is to understand which type of sequencing data is being considered, and how this choice fits with the study design and results. We consider the two cases separately, along with some examples, and present a set of key points for consideration when critically appraising both the methodologies and the results of a clinical study involving microbiome data.

SIMPLE, COMMUNITY-LEVEL ANALYSES—16S rRNA SEQUENCING

16S rRNA sequencing is best suited to providing a quantitative description of the composition of the microbiota in a given sample. As previously stated, 16S rRNA sequencing is frequently used to quantify alpha diversity, beta diversity, and the relative abundance of different microorganisms in a sample. Processed 16S rRNA sequencing data and OTU tables are relatively simple in nature. There are, however, several aspects in the process of generating and analyzing this data that merit particular consideration from a reader or reviewer.

a. *Methodological considerations*
   1. **Were all samples treated in the same facilities using the same protocols?** 16S rRNA data is particularly sensitive to batch effects, which can arise at the level of DNA extraction, sequence preparation, or sequencing. If the methods of the paper describe clearly distinct batches of samples that could confound the results, then the results of the paper could be called into question.
   2. **Which amplicon (i.e. which specific region of the 16S rRNA) was used to generate the data?** Each amplicon can generate different organism-specific biases. Therefore, if a clinically or statistically significant result is reported, then comparisons made with results from distinct but similar studies are stronger if both studies used the same amplicon.

3. **What sequencing depth was achieved across samples?** Typically, researchers will exclude any samples that have fewer than a previously specified number of reads from downstream analyses. This impacts the detection of signals in lower abundance organisms. For example, a commonly used filter is 10,000 reads: in practice, the organism with the lowest relative abundance that can be detected from a sample with 10,000 sequencing reads is 0.01% (1 out of 10,000 reads). If a more permissive filter of 1,000 reads is used, fewer samples may be excluded, but the detection limit falls to 0.1%. Therefore, detection and accurate quantification of signals in lower abundance organisms require deeper sequencing. If the signals reported in a paper involve low abundance organisms close to the detection threshold, interpretation of the results should remain conservative.

b. *Interpretation and analysis*

1. **Are analyses conducted at the appropriate taxonomic resolution?** 16S rRNA sequencing data can provide quantitative information about the *relative* abundance of different bacterial genera and their associations with various clinical outcomes (Duvallet et al. 2017). However, it does not provide accurate subgenus-level annotation (Cole et al. 2005). In fact, strains with the same 16S rRNA gene sequence can have dramatically different genomic contents (Boucher et al. 2011). Conversely, analyses conducted at a taxonomic level that is too high may be limited in clinical significance. For example, phylum-level descriptions (e.g., ratio of *Bacteroidetes* to *Firmicutes*) are mechanistically uninformative, difficult to translate into novel therapeutic strategies, and possibly limited as diagnostic tools.

2. **If associations between the relative abundance of a particular microorganism and a given clinical outcome are reported, were multiple test corrections performed?** Computing associations between clinical outcomes and microbiome data usually involves performing independent statistical tests on a large number of bacterial taxa or OTUs, sometimes over 1,000. When statistical tests are performed on samples with more than 1,000 OTUs, an uncorrected threshold for significance of $p = 0.05$ will lead to dozens of erroneous inferences (false positives), simply by chance alone. Examples of statistical procedures used to correct for this discrepancy include the Bonferroni correction, or the less conservative and more commonly used false discovery rate (Benjamini and Hochberg 1995).

3. **If alpha- and beta-diversity calculations are presented, was rarefaction of read depth performed across all samples prior to these calculations?** Rarefaction is the process of down-sampling read counts to the lowest read count across all samples and is critical in obtaining accurate measures of diversity.

4. **If correlations between bacterial taxa are presented, was the compositionality of the data taken into account?** 16S rRNA data is referred to as "compositional", which means that calculated abundances are *relative*,

not absolute. As a result, an increase in the relative abundance of one organism may yield a decrease in the relative abundance of all other organisms in the sample, without necessarily changing their *absolute* abundance. This can result in spurious correlations between the abundances of different bacteria. There are a number of methods, including SparCC (Friedman and Alm 2012) and SPIEC-EASI (Kurtz et al. 2015), to correct for compositionality of data, and readers should be aware of the issue and be prepared to assess for the above-named corrective methods.

5. **Were associations with clinical outcomes performed at the level of composition?** Most analyses are conducted at this level. However, distinct microbiome compositions can have the same function, and the association with disease may frequently be at a functional level. Accordingly, an absence of association at the compositional level does not exclude an association at the functional level.

6. **Were functional interpretations included with the 16S rRNA analysis?** As previously mentioned, 16S rRNA sequencing selectively sequences the 16S rRNA gene and therefore does not provide data about the rest of the metagenome. Functional or mechanistic interpretations built on top of associations between the relative abundance of specific bacteria and clinical outcomes are, therefore, at best, suggestive.

DETAILED METAGENOMIC ANALYSES—SHOTGUN METAGENOMIC SEQUENCING

In contrast to 16S rRNA sequencing, sufficiently deep metagenomic sequencing can provide information about gene content, the abundance of specific strains and even non-bacterial (e.g., fungal or viral) microorganisms. However, they require a greater degree of expertise to analyze, and they contain more pitfalls. Some of the considerations that the critical reader should account for when analyzing studies using shotgun metagenomic sequencing include the following:

a. *Methodological considerations*
   1. **Was the sequencing depth sufficient?** Sequencing depth is particularly important in shotgun metagenomic sequencing because the number of reads per sample greatly influences the detectability of any signals. The typical sequencing depth required for metagenomic analyses is approximately 10,000,000 reads per sample on average.
   2. **Was the appropriate bioinformatics quality control implemented in the data processing steps?** This is particularly important in analyses examining specific single nucleotide polymorphisms (SNPs), either as markers associated with a particular clinical outcome or as markers of specific strains (e.g. to track engraftment of a strain into the host microbiota). Key points to examine include appropriate quality filtering of sequencing reads (typically, a quality score Q of 20 or greater is sufficient) and the use of stringent parameters in the alignment of sequencing reads to reference databases or reference genomes (e.g. >95% identity requirement).

3. **If virome or bacteriophage results are presented, were the samples appropriately processed to enrich for viral-like particles?** Specific mention of this should be found in the Methods.

b. *Interpretation and analysis*

1. **How many samples were sequenced?** Due to higher costs associated with shotgun metagenomic sequencing, the number of samples actually included in the analysis is frequently lower than the total number of samples collected for the study. Frequently, low sample numbers (compared to 16S studies) result in insufficient statistical power to detect small effect sizes. Therefore, an absence of signal should be considered in the context of the total number of samples used for the analysis.

2. **If living organisms, in the form of fecal slurry, probiotics or synbiotics (probiotics + prebiotics) were used, was their engraftment measured and reported?** Ideally, a study should have whole-genome or metagenomic sequencing data from the treatment (e.g., the strain being administered as a probiotic) and conduct bioinformatics analyses at the level of individual genomic markers or SNPs to demonstrate the absence of the organism in patients prior to treatment, and its presence following treatment. This allows for the tracking of engraftment of the organisms in question into the host microbiota (Li et al. 2016 and Smillie et al. 2018). More generally, this provides a framework analogous to Koch's postulates for identifying organisms associated with the clinical outcome in question.

3. **If bacteriophage analyses are conducted, are phage abundances presented as relative abundances?** Phage loads can vary significantly over time and relative abundances do not capture these dynamics.

Returning to Andrew, after Dr. McDonald used his microbiome profile to make the diagnosis of autism spectrum disorder, a treatment plan was initiated that transformed the lives of Andrew and his parents. He started a microbiome therapy and, after ten weeks, the results were remarkable. Andrew hugged his Mother and began making friends for the first time in his life. While this vision of the future is still a few years away, the idea that the microbiome is a driver of health and disease has already emerged and has the potential to revolutionize the diagnostics and therapeutics for a variety of common diseases.

REFERENCES

Benjamini Y & Hochberg Y 1995. Controlling the false discovery rate: A practical and powerful approach to multiple testing. *J R Stat Soc Ser B Methodol* 57(1).

Boucher Y et al. 2011. Local mobile gene pools rapidly cross species boundaries to create endemicity within global *Vibrio cholerae* populations. *mBio* 2(2).

Cole JR et al. 2005. The Ribosomal Database Project (RDP-II): Sequences and tools for high-throughput rRNA analysis. *Nucleic Acids Res* 33(Database issue):D294–D296.

Debelius J, Song SJ, Vazquez-Baeza Y, Xu ZZ, Gonzalez A & Knight R 2016. Tiny microbes, enormous impacts: What matters in gut microbiome studies? *Genome Biol* 17(1):1–12. http://dx.doi.org/10.1186/s13059-016-1086-x.

Duvallet C, Gibbons SM, Gurry T, Irizarry RA & Alm EJ 2017. Meta-analysis of gut microbiome studies identifies disease-specific and shared responses. *Nat Commun* 8(1):1784.

Franzosa EA & Abu-Ali G 2015. Introduction to shotgun meta'omic analysis. Harvard CFAR Workshop on Metagenomics. http://evomicsorg.wpengine.netdna-cdn.com/wp-content/uploads/2015/07/CFAR2015_METAGENOMICS.pdf.

Franzosa EA, Hsu T, Sirota-madi A, Shafquat A, Abu-Ali G, Morgan XC & Huttenhower C 2016. Sequencing and beyond: Integrating molecular 'omics' for microbial community profiling. *Nat Rev Microbiol* 13(6):360–372.

Friedman J & Alm EJ 2012. Inferring correlation networks from genomic survey data. *PLOS Comput Biol* 8(9).

Jovel J et al. 2016. Characterization of the gut microbiome using 16S or shotgun metagenomics. *Front Microbiol* 7(Apr):1–17.

Knight R, Callewaert C, Marotz C, Hyde ER, Debelius JW, McDonald D & Sogin ML 2017. The microbiome and human biology. *Annu Rev Genomics Hum Genet* 18(1):65–86. http://www.annualreviews.org/doi/10.1146/annurev-genom-083115-022438.

Kurtz ZD, Müller CL, Miraldi ER, Littman DR, Blaser MJ & Bonneau RA 2015. Sparse and compositionally robust inference of microbial ecological networks. *PLOS Comput Biol* 11(5):e1004226.

Langille MGI et al. 2013. Predictive functional profiling of microbial communities using 16S rRNA marker gene sequences. *Nat Biotechnol* 31(9):814–821. http://dx.doi.org/10.1038/nbt.2676.

Li SS et al. 2016. Durable coexistence of donor and recipient strains after fecal microbiota transplantation. *Science* 352(6285):586–589.

Lloyd-Price J, Abu-Ali G & Huttenhower C 2016. The healthy human microbiome. *Genome Med* 8(1):1–11. http://dx.doi.org/10.1186/s13073-016-0307-y.

Olesen SW 2016. 16S processing for fun and profit. MIT/Alm lab. https://leanpub.com/primer16s/.

Smillie CS et al. 2018. Strain tracking reveals the determinants of bacterial engraftment in the human gut following fecal microbiota transplantation. *Cell Host Microbe* 23:229.e5–240.e5.

2 The Microbiome – Role in Personalized Medicine

Jeffrey Bland

CONTENTS

INTRODUCTION

One of the greatest challenges in human biology is the quest to decipher the underpinnings of health and disease in the individual. It seems every discovery only further complicates our understanding of the complex organisms human beings truly are. Every individual is composed of approximately 100 trillion cells, nearly 70% of which are the microorganisms located in the gut. In addition, there are approximately 30,000 genes within each cell that code for more than ten million proteins, including antibodies and nearly 3,000 metabolites.

Research conducted over the past decade has helped us further understand the complexity and importance of the microbiome. We now know that the function of nearly every cell in the body is influenced either directly or indirectly by the microbiome – its speciation, number, and activity. The relationship between an individual and their microbiome is the relationship between an individual and their function, a personal, unique, and significant dynamic that has ramifications across the entire body. Is it any wonder then that the microbiome has taken center stage in the revolution to make medicine more personalized?[1]

It has taken decades of research to drive medicine to the threshold of a new era of personalization. Studying the uniqueness of the individual requires a systems approach to human biology, and contained within this systems approach is the incorporation of concepts surrounding our understanding of the interaction between microbiome and host. Leroy Hood, MD, PhD is one of the pioneers of this movement and has been instrumental in developing an integrated approach to health care that incorporates vast amounts of information derived from both eukaryotic and prokaryotic cell types. Dr. Hood is a co-founder of the renowned Institute for Systems

Biology (ISB) in Seattle, WA. The work done there and by other co-investigators around the world is considered to be at the forefront of medical development.[2]

An excellent example of systems biology is the ongoing work being done to understand the unique factors that connect insulin resistance to cognitive decline with aging.[3] Numerous studies have demonstrated that the Mediterranean diet – which involves a substantial intake of fruits, vegetables, and fish, while consumption of dairy, red meat, and limited sugar – is associated with improved insulin sensitivity and reduced cognitive decline in apparently healthy older adults.[4] In a collaborative work published in the *American Journal of Clinical Nutrition* in 2019, researchers reported that, on average, individuals with higher self-reported adherence scores to the Mediterranean diet exhibited larger bilateral dentate gyrus volumes in their brains, as well as better learning and memory test scores.[5] Although observations like this are groundbreaking, the mechanism(s) through which the Mediterranean diet positively impacts insulin resistance and its association with obesity, hypertension, systemic inflammation, and cognitive function in some – but not all – individuals is still unknown. Is it because a Mediterranean diet has direct effects on eukaryotic cellular metabolism? Or could it be due to the impact the diet has on the prokaryotic cells of the microbiome, which in turn has an impact on eukaryotic cellular metabolism? Clearly the questions only multiply the longer one peruses the research. In terms of microbial uniqueness, what might the differences in composition be among individuals who respond to the diet? How can intervention be personalized to improve outcome? There is now clear evidence that our diet has direct and indirect impacts on signaling molecules that regulate cognition, linking diet to both the microbiome and overall brain function.[6] Understanding this unique and dynamic relationship represents a major opportunity for the clinical application of personalized medicine.

THE MICROBIOME AND ITS IMPACT ON CELLULAR MODULATION

Interrogating the impact of the human gut microbiome on physiological function is a rapidly evolving field of study. It is widely accepted that a variety of host- and microbiome-associated intrinsic and extrinsic factors influence the relationship.[7] These include, among other things, composition of the diet, uniqueness of the host adaptive and innate immune systems, the speciation and activity of the microbiome, the integrity of the intestinal mucosal barrier function, medications, xenobiotics, intestinal and hepatic detoxification functions, and lifestyle factors. These elements can influence – through the microbiome – a wide range of disease states, including obesity, inflammatory diseases, type 2 diabetes, cardiovascular diseases, renal diseases, neurological diseases, and cancer.[8]

It turns out that the architecture of the microbiome can be an etiological agent for many diseases, but at the same time it can also be altered by disease states.[9] In order to fully appreciate the role the microbiome plays in health and disease, it is necessary to consider multiple areas of uniqueness; for instance, the genotype of the individual, their physiological state, and the composition and metabolic activity of their intestinal flora.[10] Furthermore, data from a variety of tools can be used in a complementary fashion to determine the functional status of an individual, including genomic analysis of the host, metagenomic analysis of the microbiome, biomarker, and metabolite evaluation, and a detailed clinical assessment.

The intestinal mucosa houses specific receptors throughout the gut that respond to dietary inputs and changes in the composition of the microbial community. Many of these receptors belong to the G-protein coupled receptor family (GPCRs), which is the largest family of signaling molecules in the human genome and are known to demonstrate genomic and functional diversity.[11] These receptors influence the enteric nervous system function and its communication with the central nervous system, the enteric immune system, and enterochromaffin cells of the gut, all of which exert significant influence on systemic multiorgan function.

The intestinal signaling system is highly complex and sophisticated, highlighting both how and why responses to diet and microbiome changes are unique to each individual.[12,13] We can look to recent advances in the understanding of gut pharmacogenomics as an example of the complex relationship between the microbiome and intestinal mucosal function. Pharmacogenomics is a field that has recently emerged to define the important role the microbiome plays in the metabolism and effect of orally administered drugs and dietary phytochemicals.[14] Some of the drugs that are known to be influenced by the composition of an individual's microbiome and its activity include acetaminophen, chloramphenicol, digoxin, flucytosine, metronidazole, sulfasalazine, sulfinpyrazone, sulindac, sonvudine, and zonisamide.

THE UNIQUENESS OF THE MICROBIOME-BRAIN CONNECTION

We have come a long way towards recognizing the connection between central nervous system function and the composition and activity of the intestinal microbiome.[15] Two decades ago, when Michael Gershon, MD wrote *The Second Brain: A Groundbreaking New Understanding of Nervous Disorders of the Stomach and Intestine,* the relationship was not widely understood. This book was an early resource that laid out important discoveries related to the communication flow between the intestinal system and the brain through the nervous system and the release of neurotransmitter substances.[16] As it turns out, the gut communicates with the brain in a variety of situations, including anxiety, depression, impaired cognition, and even autistic spectrum disorders. The cues for this gut-brain connection largely track to the composition and activity of the intestinal microbiome. Clearly, the gut microbiome is an integral player in the development and function of the nervous system and it is highly relevant to mental health and disease.[17] There is also evidence that the composition of the gut microbiome influences the function of the hypothalamic/pituitary/adrenal-mediated stress response, and therefore has an important influence on the body's physiological response to stress.[18]

In animal models, researchers have made important progress in demonstrating a connection between microbiome composition and the behavioral and physiological abnormalities associated with neurodevelopmental and neurodegenerative conditions, including autistic spectrum disorders and Parkinson's disease.[19,20] Recently, Dr. Elaine Hsiao and her colleagues at the University of California, Los Angeles, demonstrated that the antiseizure effects attributed to the administration of the ketogenic diet are mediated through the intestinal microbiome.[21] This discovery may help explain why we see wide variation in outcomes in individuals suffering from seizure disorders when the ketogenic diet is used as a therapeutic intervention.[22] If the body's response to a ketogenic diet is mediated by the microbiome, which is highly individualized, it makes sense that we would see a correspondingly wide range of outcomes.

It has been clinically reported that fecal microbial transplant (FMT) using stool microbiota from a healthy donor is capable of achieving remission of the seizures associated with epilepsy in a girl with a 17-year history of epilepsy and Crohn's disease.[23] This case study follows other reports of the successful use of fecal microbial transplant for the treatment of conditions such as ulcerative colitis and intestinal *Clostridium difficile* infection.[24,25] One study involving 116 patients demonstrated that the administration of oral capsules containing fecal microbiota from healthy volunteers was as successful in treating recurrent *Clostridium difficile* infection as the administration of fecal microbial transplant by direct colonic exposure.[26,27] Furthermore, it may not be the case that the administration of a live fecal microbial transplant is necessary to achieve positive results as a report has been published showing that the administration of a sterile fecal filtrate transfer (FFT) was clinically successful in treating patients with *Clostridium difficile* infection. The researchers involved in this study stated the following: "This finding indicates that bacterial components, metabolites, or bacteriophages mediate many of the effects of FMT, and that FFT might be an alternative approach, particularly for immunocompromised patients."[28]

There is also evidence that oral supplementation with probiotics representing a variety of symbiotic and commensal microbial species may be of value in restoring a healthy microbiome in patients with antibiotic-associated *Clostridium difficile* infection.[29] It is interesting to note that the impairment of post-antibiotic gut mucosal microbiome reconstitution by probiotic administration can be improved by fecal microbial transplant.[30] When taken together, these studies suggest that the use of single-species probiotic supplementation after antibiotic treatment might result in exposure to soluble factors derived from the single probiotic organism, which in turn retard the restoration of the complex microbial ecosystem of the gut.

INFLUENCE OF THE MICROBIOME ON IMMUNOMETABOLISM

The understanding that the gut and the brain are in conversation with one another, and that this communication is influenced by the microbiome, has resulted in increasing interest in how this relationship affects the body's metabolism. Recent progress has been made towards identifying the signaling networks through which the brain and the gastrointestinal system communicate about the regulation of food intake. This has resulted in a deeper understanding of how these processes influence metabolic functions governing cellular bioenergetics.[31] This cross-talk among the gut, microbiome, and brain and the influence this network has on metabolism has been found to vary considerably between individuals.

Furthermore, the enteric immune system is yet another voice participating in the cross-talk. More than half of an individual's immune system is clustered around their gastrointestinal system in the form of the mucosal-associated lymphoid tissue

(MALT) and the gastrointestinal-associated lymphoid tissue (GALT). The contents of the gut, which includes the microbiome, has a significant impact on the functional status of the MALT and GALT. Cross-talk between the microbiome and these immune systems can result in immune activation of both the gut-associated innate and adaptive immune cells.[32] In this capacity, the microbiome is an immunomodulator that can have an impact on systemic metabolism. In 2018, Olefsky et al. published a paper in *Cell* describing an integrated view of immunometabolism and the important role that microbiota-produced metabolites have on influencing host inflammation and metabolism.[33] The release of metabolites such as lipopolysaccharides (LPS) from the cell wall of specific enteric bacteria can activate toll-like receptors, like TLR4, that initiate the inflammatory process. Other gastrointestinal receptors such as GPR41 and GPR43, as well as bile acid receptors TGR5 and farnesoid X receptor (FXR), modulate systemic inflammation and metabolism and have been shown to be influenced by the microbiome.

Activation of the toll-like receptors of the gastrointestinal tract by exposure to microbiome-derived LPS results in increased intestinal mucosal permeability, increased risk of translocation of gram-negative bacteria across the intestinal barrier, and increased systemic absorption of immune-activating substances. In animal models, it has been shown that the translocation of a specific gut pathobiont drives autoimmunity.[34] There is increasing evidence that the status of the microbiome and its relationship to the enteric immune system may play an important role in a variety of autoimmune diseases, including rheumatoid arthritis, systemic lupus erythematosus, type 1 diabetes, and multiple sclerosis.[35]

An exciting new field of inquiry among microbiome researchers relates to helminths and the role they may play in modulating the immune system in autoimmune disease. Several studies have been conducted to evaluate the ability of specific helminths to exert a protective effect against many autoimmune diseases.[36] Helminths have been shown to secrete substances like phosphorylcholine that serve as immunomodulatory agents. This work provides some rationale for the hygiene hypothesis of autoimmune disease, which has demonstrated that the lowest frequency of autoimmune disease is seen in countries with lower hygiene levels and increased incidence of enteric helminths infection.

It is now widely accepted that the status of the gut microbiome is linked to inflammatory cytokine production and alteration in metabolism. Disturbed gut microbiome composition is commonly referred to as dysbiosis and is linked to the increased production of inflammatory cytokines such as TNF-alpha, IFN-gamma, IL-1 beta, IL-6, and IL-17.[37] These inflammatory cytokines are produced in response to the presence of metabolites from a dysbiotic microbiome, including palmitoleic acid metabolism and tryptophan degradation to tryptophol. The bacterial metabolites associated with dysbiosis shape the intestinal immune environment in part by regulating the NLRP6 inflammasome.[38] One study of the immunomodulatory effect of 53 individual gut bacterial species found that most gut microbes exerted specialized, complementary, and redundant transcriptional effects. The research team behind this work concluded the following: "Microbial diversity in the gut ensures the robustness of the microbiota's ability to generate a consistent immunomodulatory impact, serving as a highly important epigenetic system."[39] Imbalances in the composition of the microbiome can result in dysbiosis that can shift the immunomodulatory status into a Th1 dominant state that favors inflammation.

In the intestinal mucosa, Th17 cells impart important immune-modulating effects. It has been found that the adherence of specific segmented filamentous bacteria to the gut epithelium results in the induction of Th17 producing cells.[40] Th17 cells provide protective immunity to fungi and extracellular bacterial infections and appear to have a role in protecting against gastric cancer, but are also involved in chronic inflammation. These cells produce IL-17, a cytokine that is associated with autoimmunity.[41] Th17 cells can remain dormant for long periods of time and may only be activated and become contributors to inflammation as a result of dysbiosis or exposure to a triggering agent. This example once again illustrates the importance of a complex, stable gut microbial ecosystem in establishing and maintaining the balance between pro and anti-inflammatory immunomodulatory effects.

It is very clear that intestinal permeability is one of the principal determinants of intestinal immune system status and its relationship to the microbiome. Intestinal permeability can be measured clinically in vivo through two types of challenge tests: lactulose-mannitol or Cr51-EDTA.[42] Clinical studies have shown a wide variation in intestinal permeability among patients with dysbiosis, and prognosis can be adversely affected by increases in permeability.[43] Research demonstrates that if a patient with Crohn's Disease had increased intestinal permeability when discharged, they had more than a 90% probability of relapse in the following year, whereas if they had low permeability they had less than a 10% probability of relapse. It appears that intestinal permeability might be one of the better surrogate markers for assessing dysbiosis and its impact on immunometabolism. One study that utilized the lactulose-mannitol challenge test found that increased permeability was associated with obesity, fatty liver disease, and insulin resistance in participants.[44] An editorial associated with this study suggested that an intestinal, microbiota-driven, increased-permeability pathway may be involved in the pathogenesis of immunometabolic diseases such as insulin resistance, type 2 diabetes, obesity, and fatty liver disease.[45]

TAKING IT PERSONALLY: DYNAMIC HUMAN EXPOSURE AND THE MICROBIOME

It is well recognized that environmental exposures can impact overall health. Such exposures can also have an impact on the composition and function of the microbiome. Noted quantified-self researcher Michael Synder, PhD and his team at the Stanford University School of Medicine have developed a sensitive method to monitor personal airborne biological and chemical exposures. They tested this wearable device by following the personal exposomes of 15 people for up to 890 days over 66 distinct geographical locations. Their work found that personal exposomes and their relationship to the composition of the metagenome are highly dynamic and vary in time and space, even for individuals who are located in the same general geographical area. Furthermore, these dynamic exposomes were determined to have the potential to impact health.[46]

The observation that the dynamic environment plays a role in modulating the metagenome is further evidenced by our understanding that the intestinal microbiota undergoes its own diurnal rhythmicity.[47] Alteration in the production of metabolites by the microbiome varies throughout the day, resulting in changes in its ability to impact immunometabolism.[48] This affects not only the function of the gastrointestinal system, but also distant sites such as the liver, beta cells of the pancreas, adipocytes, and immune cells. It is well established that the "microbiota clock" is regulated by a 24-hour cycle that is entrained by the light-dark cycle of the day. There is an intimate relationship between the light-dark cycle, the microbiota clock, eating times and metabolism. Disruption of the circadian clock results in an increased incidence of dysbiosis and alteration in immunometabolism that shifts the microbiome towards a state of chronic inflammation. This is documented in studies looking at the influence on cellular transcription throughout the day of the host and its relationship to diurnal rhythmicity of the microbiome. The host circadian clock appears to be the "master clock" from which the diurnal rhythmicity of the microbiome takes its lead.[49] There is clear evidence that altering an individual's circadian clock through sleep interruption, shift work, or stimulants alters intestinal microbiota and contributes to adverse immunometabolic outcomes, including insulin resistance, obesity, and chronic inflammation.[50]

Our thinking about the impact of the microbiome on human health is evolving. What was once considered an interesting area of investigation is now recognized as a critically important factor in personalizing a patient's treatment program.[51] Jeffrey Gordon, MD and the group he leads at Washington University School of Medicine have done pioneering work linking the microbiome with obesity, and these efforts have led to an explosion of interest in the personalized role the human microbiome plays in health and disease care.[52] At present, research on the microbiome is shifting from a descriptive focus on the microbiome structure and disease association to a more precise understanding of the contributions that components of the microbiome make to the molecular pathophysiology of specific complex chronic diseases. Furthermore, the interrelationship between the microbiome and diet is being recognized as an important component of the precision personalized medicine movement. Areas of focus include the development of new diagnostic methods for better defining the complexity of the microbiome and its relationship to immunometabolic disorders, early detection of shifts in biomarkers associated with immunometabolic disorders, and individualized food plans and prebiotic/probiotic supplementation that result in improvement in microbiome composition and activity. Although dietary intake has long been understood to influence immunometabolic disorders, general nutrition recommendations have had variable success when used therapeutically to manage these conditions. This is due to the high level of genetic variability, which affects how the microbiome is influenced by the specific components of a diet and how the microbiome influences immunity and metabolism of the individual.

If we take a closer look at certain dietary constituents, we can find a number of examples of the variability concept described in the previous paragraph. Stanley Hazen, MD, PhD leads a highly regarded research team at the Cleveland Clinic, whose work has shown that the gut microbiome converts L-carnitine (found in abundance in red meat) into the toxic metabolite trimethylamine-N-oxide (TMAO). TMAO has been implicated as an atherosclerosis-inducing substance.[53] In a 2019 study published in the *European Heart Journal*, this group demonstrated that introducing a vegetable protein-based diet in individuals with elevated TMAO production resulted in reduced TMAO levels.[54]

Other researchers have reported that the intestinal microbiome is responsible for the conversion of the soy isoflavone daidzein into equol, a weak estrogen receptor agonist/antagonist that has been shown to help stabilize estrogen activity in women. Only about 50% of people have a microbiome that is capable of converting daidzein into equol. Studies have shown that a higher consumption of fish, soy, and vegetables can positively affect microbiome production of equol, whereas a high intake of refined flour can result in lower equol production.[55]

These examples demonstrate our increased understanding of the role that the microbiome plays in metabolizing constituents of the diet, which is a process that results in the production of metabolites that in turn influence health and disease. The next step on the path ahead will require us to better analyze microbiome-related metabolites to understand their mechanisms of action. These discoveries, along with those that are yet to come, are creating an opportunity for the development of new therapeutic approaches and nutritional products that are derived from metabolites and how they are secreted, modulated, or degraded by the microbiome.[56]

Endocannabinoids are a family of bioactive molecules that bridge the interface between the gut microbiota and host metabolism.[57] Accumulating evidence indicates that the intestinal endocannabinoid system and its related bioactive lipid metabolites contribute to physiological processes that relate to obesity, type 2 diabetes, and inflammation. It has been suggested that the gut microbiome can control levels of endocannabinoids in the gut and adipose tissue. When dysbiosis is present, it can alter endocannabinoid signaling, which in turn can increase gut mucosal permeability, post-meal endotoxicity, and systemic inflammation. Various bioactive lipids derived from arachidonic acid and omega-3 fatty acids have endocannabinoid receptor agonist and antagonist activities, respectively.

The gut microbiota actively produces a variety of signals that influence the organs involved in the regulation of immunometabolism in health and disease.[58] These signals, which are generated by the metabolic activity of the microbiome, can impact adipocyte size and number, adipocyte thermogenesis and inflammation, hepatic bile acid metabolism and lipogenesis, insulin secretion and sensitivity, brain serotonin metabolism, and genetic expression in the lung related to pulmonary function. There is now evidence to suggest that asthma and chronic obstructive pulmonary disease may originate from signals derived from the gut microbiome.[59] There has also been considerable study of the role of gut microbial enterotypes (dominance of either *Prevotella* or *Bacteroides)* in the selection of an appropriate personalized diet for the management of obesity.[60] The connection between obesity and the microbiome is now recognized as an important factor in the delivery of personalized nutrition advice.[61] Increasing the intake of specific dietary fibers from vegetables and grains has been found to improve the gastrointestinal immune system through its impact on the diversity and activity of the microbiome.[62] In an animal study, fiber-deprived mice were found to have intestinal microbiota that degraded the colonic mucus barrier and enhanced susceptibility to pathogen infection.[63] Using a method called shotgun metagenomics, other researchers have shown that the administration of fiber into the diet has a favorable impact on the short-chain fatty acid-producing bacteria of the gut microbiome, and also results in the reduction of hemoglobin A1c in type 2 diabetes.[64] On the other hand, administration of an 11-strain probiotic combination was found to result in differing resistance to gut mucosal colonization by specific bacteria, which demonstrates the need for a personalized approach to probiotic supplementation.[65]

The Weizmann Institute of Science in Israel has produced groundbreaking research that has garnered international attention in recent years. By predicting glycemic response to foods using intestinal microbiome analysis, the team at Weizmann may be taking the concept of personalized nutrition to a whole new level. In a study published in *Cell* in 2015, they described how they continuously monitored week-long glucose levels in an 800-person cohort, measured responses to 46,898 meals, and found high variability in the response to identical meals, suggesting that universal dietary recommendations may have limited clinical utility. Data from this effort was used to create an algorithm that integrated blood parameters, anthropometrics, physical activity, and gut microbiota that accurately predicted postprandial glycemic responses to real-life meals. This algorithm was then used as the basis for a blinded randomized controlled dietary intervention study that resulted in significantly lower postprandial responses and consistent configuration of the intestinal microbiome among participants.[66] This assessment algorithm has been successfully applied in the United States to develop a personalized approach to predicting glycemic responses to food among individuals without diabetes.[67] A follow-up study published in 2017 by the original group reported the ability to predict the glycemic response to different bread types using microbiome analysis.[68]

PRECISION PERSONALIZED MEDICINE FROM THE MICROBIOME

Over the past five years, overwhelming evidence has been published outlining a strong connection between disturbances of the microbiome and various immuno-metabolic diseases.[69] In cancer therapy, it is now known that there are responders and non-responders to PD-1 targeted immunotherapy, and response status is influenced by the composition of an individual's microbiome. This finding suggests that the intestinal microbiota should be considered when assessing therapeutic intervention.[70,71] A 2018 study reported that the abundance of certain bacterial species in the microbiome – *Bifidobacterium longum*, *Collinsella aerofaciens*, and *Enterococcus faecium* – was found to be associated with responders to anti-PD-1 efficacy in metastatic melanoma patients.[72] Another recent publication stated that the bacterium *Fusobacterium nucleatum* is a chemoresistance mediator in colorectal cancer therapy.[73] In lung cancer, the commensal microbiota is closely correlated with chronic inflammation and lung adenocarcinoma through the activation of lung-resident gamma delta T cells.[74]

These studies and many more like them support the idea that we must consider the microbiome in the personalization of therapy for all immunometabolic diseases. This, despite the fact that there are still many questions yet to be answered about how to best harness this emergent information in the prevention and treatment of disease. New discoveries are uncovering the unique personalities of many of the organisms that make up the complex microbiome. One that has generated great attention in recent years is *Akkermansia muciniphila*, which has been found to influence fat mass and metabolic syndrome in mice with diet-induced obesity.[75] *A. muciniphila* is a gram-negative strict anaerobe and mucin-degrading bacterium that has been shown to blunt metabolic endotoxemia in high fat-fed mice, reduce proinflammatory lipopolysaccharides in the circulation, and alleviate insulin resistance and cardiometabolic disease indicators.[76] A recent report indicated that a purified membrane protein from *A. muciniphila* or the pasteurized bacterium was found to improve metabolism in obese and diabetic mice.[77] This finding once again highlights a significant question: is the activity of the microbiome a result of the living organism's association with the enteric immune system or is it an effect mediated through specific metabolites or chemical constituents of the microbiota? This same question has been raised about the role of the microbiome in non-alcoholic fatty liver disease (NAFLD) and non-alcoholic steatohepatitis (NASH). It is well known that NAFLD and NASH are the major hepatic manifestations of cardiometabolic syndrome, and, as such, are immunometabolic disorders that have a relationship to the composition and activity of the microbiome.[78] The question in this specific example is therefore "Is it the organisms within the microbiome that contribute directly to the pathogenesis of NAFLD/NASH or is it metabolites or chemical constituents of the microbiota?"

Harnessing of the power of the microbiome in personalized medicine has become a central focus of basic and clinical science studies.[79] The scientific literature exploring the relationship among the microbiome and health and disease has doubled in the space of two years. To those of us who are following this evolution closely, it is now clear that the most common chronic diseases of our age that relate to the field of immunometabolism are also connected to the composition and function of the intestinal microbiome. This research has led us to recognize that there is tremendous diversity among individual microbiomes, but that stability also plays an important role in signaling to distant organs, a process that in turn influences functional status. For practitioners who focus on nutrition and lifestyle medicine, there is an urgent need for tools to evaluate microbiome status and its contribution to immunometabolic function. This will be an important step forward in the clinical application of personalized lifestyle medicine.

NOTES

1. Naylor S, Chen JY. Unraveling human complexity and disease with systems biology and personalized medicine. *Per Med.* 2010 May;7(3):275–289.
2. Hood L. Systems biology and p4 medicine: past, present, and future. *Rambam Maimonides Med J.* 2013 Apr 30;4(2):e0012.
3. Alfaro FJ, Gavrieli A, Saade-Lemus P, et al. White matter microstructure and cognitive decline in metabolic syndrome: a review of diffusion tensor imaging. *Metabolism.* 2018 Jan;78:52-68.
4. Hardman RJ, Kennedy G, Macpherson H, et al. Adherence to a Mediterranean-style diet and effects on cognition in adults: a qualitative evaluation and systematic review of longitudinal and prospective trials. *Front Nutr.* 2016 Jul 22;3:22.
5. Karstens AJ, Tussing-Humphreys L, Zhan L, et al. Associations of the Mediterranean diet with cognitive and neuroimaging phenotypes of dementia in healthy older adults. *Am J Clin Nutr.* 2019 Feb 1;109(2):361–368.

6. Rodriguez RL, Albeck JG, Taha AY, et al. Impact of diet-derived signaling molecules on human cognition: exploring the food-brain axis. *npj Science of Food*. 2017;1:2.
7. Schmidt TSB, Raes J, Bork P. The human gut microbiome: from association to modulation. *Cell*. 2018 Mar 8;172(6):1198–1215.
8. Gilbert JA, Blaser MJ, Caporaso JG, et al. Current understanding of the human microbiome. *Nat Med*. 2018 Apr 10;24(4):392–400.
9. Fischbach MA. Microbiome: focus on causation and mechanism. *Cell*. 2018 Aug 9;174(4):785–790.
10. Lynch SV, Pedersen O. The human intestinal microbiome in health and disease. *N Engl J Med*. 2016 Dec 15;375(24):2369–2379.
11. Insel PA, Wilderman A, Zambon AC, et al. G protein-coupled receptor (GPCR) expression in native cells: "novel" endoGPCRs as physiologic regulators and therapeutic targets. *Mol Pharmacol*. 2015 Jul;88(1):181–187.
12. Beumer J, Clevers H. How the gut feels, smells, and talks. *Cell*. 2017 Jun 29;170(1):10–11.
13. Bellono NW, Bayrer JR, Leitch DB. Enterochromaffin cells are gut chemosensors that couple to sensory neural pathways. *Cell*. 2017 Jun 29;170(1):185.e16–198.e16.
14. Saad R, Rizkallah MR, Aziz RK. Gut pharmacomicrobiomics: the tip of an iceberg of complex interactions between drugs and gut-associated microbes. *Gut Pathog*. 2012 Nov 30;4(1):16.
15. Sharon G, Sampson TR, Geschwind DH, et al. The central nervous system and the gut microbiome. *Cell*. 2016 Nov 3;167(4):915–932.
16. Gershon, Michael D. *The Second Brain: A Groundbreaking New Understanding of Nervous Disorders of the Stomach and Intestine*. New York: Harper Perennial, 1999.
17. Wang HX, Wang YP. Gut microbiota-brain axis. *Chin Med J (Engl)*. 2016 Oct 5;129(19):2373–2380.
18. Galland L. The gut microbiome and the brain. *J Med Food*. 2014 Dec;17(12):1261–1272.
19. Hsiao EY, McBride SW, Hsien S, et al. Microbiota modulate behavioral and physiological abnormalities associated with neurodevelopmental disorders. *Cell*. 2013 Dec 19;155(7):1451–1463.
20. Sampson TR, Debelius JW, Thron T, et al. Gut microbiota regulate motor deficits and neuroinflammation in a model of Parkinson's disease. *Cell*. 2016 Dec 1;167(6):1469.e12–1480.e12.
21. Olson CA, Vuong HE, Yano JM, et al. The gut microbiota mediates the anti-seizure effects of the ketogenic diet. *Cell*. 2018 Jun 14;173(7):1728.e13–1741.e13.
22. Arya R, Peariso K, Gaínza-Lein M, et al. Efficacy and safety of ketogenic diet for treatment of pediatric convulsive refractory status epilepticus. *Epilepsy Res*. 2018 Aug;144:1–6.
23. He Z, Cui BT, Zhang T, et al. Fecal microbiota transplantation cured epilepsy in a case with Crohn's disease: the first report. *World J Gastroenterol*. 2017 May 21;23(19):3565–3568.
24. Siegmund B. Is intensity the solution for FMT in ulcerative colitis? *Lancet*. 2017 Mar 25;389(10075):1170–1172.
25. Paramsothy S, Kamm MA, Kaakoush NO, et al. Multidonor intensive faecal microbiota transplantation for active ulcerative colitis: a randomised placebo-controlled trial. *Lancet*. 2017 Mar 25;389(10075):1218–1228.
26. Rao K, Young VB, Malani PN. Capsules for fecal microbiota transplantation in recurrent *Clostridium difficile* infection: the new way forward or a tough pill to swallow? *JAMA*. 2017 Nov 28;318(20):1979–1980.
27. Kao D, Roach B, Silva M, et al. Effect of oral capsule- vs colonoscopy-delivered fecal microbiota transplantation on recurrent *Clostridium difficile* infection: a randomized clinical trial. *JAMA*. 2017 Nov 28;318(20):1985–1993.

28. Ott SJ, Waetzig GH, Rehman A, et al. Efficacy of sterile fecal filtrate transfer for treating patients with *Clostridium difficile* infection. *Gastroenterology.* 2017 Mar;152(4):799. e7–811.e7.

29. Van den Abbeele P, Verstraete W, El Aidy S, et al. Prebiotics, faecal transplants and microbial network units to stimulate biodiversity of the human gut microbiome. *Microb Biotechnol.* 2013 Jul;6(4):335–340.

30. Suez J, Zmora N, Zilberman-Schapira G, et al. Post-antibiotic gut mucosal microbiome reconstitution is impaired by probiotics and improved by autologous FMT. *Cell.* 2018 Sep 6;174(6):1406.e16–1423.e16.

31. Clemmensen C, Müller TD, Woods SC, et al. Gut-brain cross-talk in metabolic control. *Cell.* 2017 Feb 23;168(5):758–774.

32. Zeevi D, Korem T, Segal E. Talking about cross-talk: the immune system and the microbiome. Genome Biol. 2016 Mar 17;17:50.

33. Lee YS, Wollam J, Olefsky JM. An integrated view of immunometabolism. *Cell.* 2018 Jan 11;172(1–2):22–40.

34. Manfredo Vieira S, Hiltensperger M, Kumar V, et al. Translocation of a gut pathobiont drives autoimmunity in mice and humans. *Science.* 2018 Mar 9;359(6380):1156–1161.

35. Gianchecchi E, Fierabracci A. Recent advances on microbiota involvement in the pathogenesis of autoimmunity. Review. *Int J Mol Sci.* 2019 Jan 11;20(2); pii: E283. doi: 10.3390/ijms20020283.

36. Neuman H, Mor H, Bashi T, et al. Helminth-based product and the microbiome of mice with lupus. *mSystems.* 2019 Feb 19;4(1); pii: e00160-18, eCollection 2019 Jan–Feb. doi: 10.1128/mSystems.00160-18.

37. Schirmer M, Smeekens SP, Vlamakis H, et al. Linking the human gut microbiome to inflammatory cytokine production capacity. *Cell.* 2016 Dec 15;167(7):1897.

38. Levy M, Thaiss CA, Zeevi D, et al. Microbiota-modulated metabolites shape the intestinal microenvironment by regulating NLRP6 inflammasome signaling. *Cell.* 2015 Dec 3;163(6):1428–1443.

39. Geva-Zatorsky N, Sefik E, Kua L, et al. Mining the human gut microbiota for immuno-modulatory organisms. *Cell.* 2017 Feb 23;168(5):928.e11–943.e11.

40. Atarashi K, Tanoue T, Ando M, et al. Th17 cell induction by adhesion of microbes to intestinal epithelial cells. *Cell.* 2015 Oct 8;163(2):367–380.

41. Bystrom J, Taher TE, Muhyaddin MS, et al. Harnessing the therapeutic potential of Th17 cells. *Mediators Inflamm.* 2015;2015:205156.

42. Bischoff SC, Barbara G, Buurman W, et al. Intestinal permeability – a new target for disease prevention and therapy. *BMC Gastroenterol.* 2014 Nov 18;14:189.

43. Wyatt J, Vogelsang H, Hübl W, et al. Intestinal permeability and the prediction of relapse in Crohn's disease. *Lancet.* 1993 Jun 5;341(8858):1437–1439.

44. Damms-Machado A, Louis S, Schnitzer A, et al. Gut permeability is related to body weight, fatty liver disease, and insulin resistance in obese individuals undergoing weight reduction. *Am J Clin Nutr.* 2017 Jan;105(1):127–135.

45. Fasano A. Gut permeability, obesity, and metabolic disorders: who is the chicken and who is the egg? *Am J Clin Nutr.* 2017 Jan;105(1):3–4.

46. Jiang C, Wang X, Li X, et al. Dynamic human environmental exposome revealed by longitudinal personal monitoring. *Cell.* 2018 Sep 20;175(1):277.e31–291.e31.

47. Thaiss CA, Levy M, Korem T, et al. Microbiota diurnal rhythmicity programs host transcriptome oscillations. *Cell.* 2016 Dec 1;167(6):1495.e12–1510.e12.

48. Thaiss CA, Zeevi D, Levy M, et al. A day in the life of the meta-organism: diurnal rhythms of the intestinal microbiome and its host. *Gut Microbes.* 2015;6(2):137–142.

49. Liang X, Bushman FD, FitzGerald GA. Rhythmicity of the intestinal microbiota is regulated by gender and the host circadian clock. *Proc Natl Acad Sci U S A.* 2015 Aug 18;112(33):10479–10484.

50. Voigt RM, Forsyth CB, Green SJ, et al. Circadian disorganization alters intestinal microbiota. *PLoS One.* 2014 May 21;9(5):e97500.
51. Zmora N, Zeevi D, Korem T, et al. Taking it personally: personalized utilization of the human microbiome in health and disease. *Cell Host Microbe.* 2016 Jan 13;19(1):12–20.
52. Bäckhed F, Ding H, Wang T, et al. The gut microbiota as an environmental factor that regulates fat storage. *Proc Natl Acad Sci U S A.* 2004 Nov 2;101(44):15718–15723.
53. Org E, Blum Y, Kasela S, et al. Relationships between gut microbiota, plasma metabolites, and metabolic syndrome traits in the METSIM cohort. *Genome Biol.* 2017 Apr 13;18(1):70.
54. Wang Z, Bergeron N, Levison BS, et al. Impact of chronic dietary red meat, white meat, or non-meat protein on trimethylamine N-oxide metabolism and renal excretion in healthy men and women. *Eur Heart J.* 2019 Feb 14;40(7):583–594.
55. Yoshikata R, Myint KZ, Ohta H, et al. Inter-relationship between diet, lifestyle habits, gut microflora, and the equol-producer phenotype: baseline findings from a placebo-controlled intervention trial. *Menopause.* 2019 Mar;26(3):273–285.
56. Suez J, Elinav E. The path towards microbiome-based metabolite treatment. *Nat Microbiol.* 2017 May 25;2:17075.
57. Cani PD, Plovier H, Van Hul M, et al. Endocannabinoids – at the crossroads between the gut microbiota and host metabolism. *Nat Rev Endocrinol.* 2016 Mar;12(3):133–143.
58. Schroeder BO, Bäckhed F. Signals from the gut microbiota to distant organs in physiology and disease. *Nat Med.* 2016 Oct;22(10):1079–1089.
59. Mjösberg J, Rao A. Lung inflammation originating in the gut. *Science.* 2018 Jan 5;359(6371):36–37.
60. Christensen L, Roager HM, Astrup A, et al. Microbial enterotypes in personalized nutrition and obesity management. *Am J Clin Nutr.* 2018 Oct 1;108(4):645–651.
61. Komaroff AL. The microbiome and risk for obesity and diabetes. *JAMA.* 2017 Jan 24;317(4):355–356.
62. Gazzaniga FS, Kasper DL. Veggies and intact grains a day keep the pathogens away. *Cell.* 2016 Nov 17;167(5):1161–1162.
63. Desai MS, Seekatz AM, Koropatkin NM, et al. A dietary fiber-deprived gut microbiota degrades the colonic mucus barrier and enhances pathogen susceptibility. *Cell.* 2016 Nov 17;167(5):1339.e21–1353.e21.
64. Zhao L, Zhang F, Ding X, et al. Gut bacteria selectively promoted by dietary fibers alleviate type 2 diabetes. *Science.* 2018 Mar 9;359(6380):1151–1156.
65. Zmora N, Zilberman-Schapira G, Suez J, et al. Personalized gut mucosal colonization resistance to empiric probiotics is associated with unique host and microbiome features. *Cell.* 2018 Sep 6;174(6):1388.e21–1405.e21.
66. Zeevi D, Korem T, Zmora N, et al. Personalized nutrition by prediction of glycemic responses. *Cell.* 2015 Nov 19;163(5):1079–1094.
67. Mendes-Soares H, Raveh-Sadka T, Azulay S, et al. Assessment of a personalized approach to predicting postprandial glycemic responses to food among individuals without diabetes. *JAMA Netw Open.* 2019 Feb 1;2(2):e188102.
68. Korem T, Zeevi D, Zmora N, et al. Bread affects clinical parameters and induces gut microbiome-associated personal glycemic responses. *Cell Metab.* 2017 Jun 6;25(6):1243.e5–1253.e5.
69. Jobin C. Precision medicine using microbiota. *Science.* 2018 Jan 5;359(6371):32–34.
70. Routy B, Le Chatelier E, Derosa L, et al. Gut microbiome influences efficacy of PD-1-based immunotherapy against epithelial tumors. *Science.* 2018 Jan 5;359(6371):91–97.
71. Gopalakrishnan V, Spencer CN, Nezi L, et al. Gut microbiome modulates response to anti-PD-1 immunotherapy in melanoma patients. *Science.* 2018 Jan 5;359(6371):97–103.
72. Matson V, Fessler J, Bao R, et al. The commensal microbiome is associated with anti-PD-1 efficacy in metastatic melanoma patients. *Science.* 2018 Jan 5;359(6371):104–108.

73. Ramos A, Hemann MT. Drugs, bugs, and cancer: fusobacterium nucleatum promotes chemoresistance in colorectal cancer. *Cell.* 2017 Jul 27;170(3):411–413.

74. Jin C, Lagoudas GK, Zhao C, et al. Commensal microbiota promote lung cancer development via γδ t cells. *Cell.* 2019 Feb 21;176(5):998.e16–1013.e16.

75. Cani PD, de Vos WM. Next-generation beneficial microbes: the case of *Akkermansia muciniphila. Front Microbiol.* 2017 Sep 22;8:1765.

76. Anhê FF, Marette A. A microbial protein that alleviates metabolic syndrome. *Nat Med.* 2017 Jan 6;23(1):11–12.

77. Plovier H, Everard A, Druart C, et al. A purified membrane protein from *Akkermansia muciniphila* or the pasteurized bacterium improves metabolism in obese and diabetic mice. *Nat Med.* 2017 Jan;23(1):107–113.

78. Kolodziejczyk AA, Zheng D, Shibolet O, et al. The role of the microbiome in NAFLD and NASH. *EMBO Mol Med.* 2019 Feb;11(2); pii: e9302. doi: 10.15252/emmm.201809302.

79. Toribio-Mateas M. Harnessing the power of microbiome assessment tools as part of neuroprotective nutrition and lifestyle medicine interventions. Review. *Microorganisms.* 2018 Apr 25;6(2); pii: E35. doi: 10.3390/microorganisms6020035.

3 Immune Response to Microbial Toxins in Inflammatory and Neurodegenerative Disorders

Aristo Vojdani and Elroy Vojdani

CONTENTS

INTRODUCTION

Recent years have seen a rise in the incidence of many chronic diseases, including autoimmune and neurodegenerative disorders like Alzheimer's disease [Blaser 2017; Mednis 2017; van Oostrom et al. 2016; Meetoo 2008]. The National Institute on Aging lists Alzheimer's as the sixth leading cause of death in the United States, with recent estimates ranking it as high as third for the elderly population [NIH online]. Alzheimer's is a serious problem with no known cure and is now theorized by many to have an autoimmune origin catalyzed by environmental factors [Vojdani et al. 2018; Vojdani and Vojdani 2018a]. Pathogens like oral bacteria [Itzakhi et al. 2016; Pistollato et al. 2016]; Gram-negative bacteria like *E. coli, Salmonella* and their toxins; herpes type 1; herpes type 2; *H. pylori; Chlamydia; Cytomegalovirus;*

and *B. burgdorferi;* and other spirochetes are all reputed to play a role in autoimmune and neurodegenerative disorders, as summarized by Adams [2017]. According to Blaser [2017], the rise in inflammatory and autoimmune disorders could be associated with the disappearance of our ancestral microbiota, which includes the microorganisms in the oral cavity and the intestine. Blaser posits that the loss of our ancestral microbiota results in gut dysbiosis, the release of bacterial toxins such as lipopolysaccharides (LPS) and bacterial cytolethal distending toxins (BCdTs), and heightened immunological reactivity that manifests as disease immediately or later in life. Other studies have demonstrably associated infections and their resultant toxins with autoimmune and neurodegenerative disorders; for example, infection by microbial agents, namely *Campylobacter jejuni*, is linked to inflammatory bowel disease and Guillain-Barré syndrome [Souza 2018].

This chapter examines how the toxins released by oral pathogens, especially by our intestinal microbiota, may lead to inflammatory autoimmune and neurodegenerative disorders. Bacterial toxins including, among others, BCdTs and LPS send signals from the gut to distant organs like the brain, contributing to the breakdown of the gut lining and the blood–brain barrier (BBB). This may contribute not only to inflammatory bowel disease (IBD) and irritable bowel syndrome (IBS), but also to other autoimmune and neurodegenerative disorders like Alzheimer's [Schroeder and Bäckhed 2016]. In the case of inflammatory bowel disease, extra-intestinal manifestations occur in about one-third of individuals with the disease [Casella et al. 2014]. Indeed, neurological complications in inflammatory bowel disease are more frequent than commonly believed. Because of the neurologic and neuromuscular involvement, a serious number of these manifestations are potentially life-threatening and contribute to high levels of morbidity and permanent damage [Casella et al. 2014; Zois et al. 2010]. Furthermore, both ulcerative colitis and Crohn's disease have been shown to involve both the peripheral and central nervous systems [Zois et al. 2010]. Understanding the importance of the gut–brain–immune connection is vital to successfully combatting this silent epidemic; the crux of the matter lies in understanding the actual role our resident microbiota and the toxins they release play in the pathogenesis of gastrointestinal disorders and immune dysfunction, particularly neuroautoimmunities like Alzheimer's.

THE ROLE OF BACTERIAL TOXINS IN INFLAMMATORY AND AUTOIMMUNE DISORDERS

Bacterial toxins are a group of proteins, lipoproteins, and LPS that are produced by bacteria. Although they are an important component of the healthy immune system—as microbe-associated molecular patterns (MAMPs), they are recognized by pattern recognition receptors on epithelial and immune cells—overproduction of these toxins can damage the host at the site of a bacterial infection or at locations far from the source [Medzhitov 2007]. In this review, major emphasis will be placed on the BCdTs and LPS that are produced by enterobacters and other bacteria.

BCdT is a member of the family of toxins called cyclomodulins, which are produced by a group of Gram-negative bacteria. They play a role in the development of periodontitis, gastric ulcers, enteritis, irritable bowel syndrome (IBS), and small intestinal bacterial overgrowth (SIBO) by acting on and breaking down the tight junctions of intestinal epithelial cells [Pimentel et al. 2015a]. BCdT is a heterotrimeric complex of three subunits: CdtA, CdtB, and CdtC (Figure 3.1). Of these three subunits, CdtB is the active unit; the CdtA and CdtC subunits mediate the delivery of CdtB into the host epithelial cells, which may damage cytoskeletal proteins like vinculin, talin, and actinin. It enters a cell via receptor-mediated endocytosis and then travels deep into the cytosol, from where it subsequently enters the nucleus of the target cell [Haghjoo and Galan 2004]. Because CdtB also contains deoxyribonuclease enzymatic activity, it may cause damage to the DNA of a cell after penetrating the membrane and being transported into the nucleus.

Interestingly, CDTs are not unique to the gut microbiome; bacterial strains with CDT gene sequences and associated cytotoxic activity have frequently been found in individuals diagnosed with periodontal disease [Yamano et al. 2003]. When the gingival epithelium is damaged by bacterial toxins, bacteria and toxins collectively gain entry into the connective tissue, leading to activation of Th17 and other inflammatory cells. This invasion not only causes destruction of the tooth attachment apparatus, but may also make it possible for inflammatory cells and bacterial toxins to gain access to the blood [Geerts et al. 2002], the gastrointestinal tract [Edgar et al. 2004], and the brain [Dileepan et al. 2016]. New data increasingly indicates that changes in the oral microbiome may affect the underlying imbalances [Nikitakis et al. 2017] that drive the pathogenesis of systemic diseases like Alzheimer's [Ide et al. 2016; Itzhaki et al. 2016].

The systemic presence of CDTs and the immune reaction that produces antibodies against them are the best indicators that CDT-producing bacterial strains are present in the gingival epithelium or the gut mucosal tissue [Ando et al. 2010]. Circulating antibodies to CdtB from *E. coli, Salmonella, Shigella* and *Campylobacter jejuni* have been shown both in animal models and in humans with irritable bowel syndrome and small intestinal bacterial overgrowth, due to the fact that CDTs are also produced by the gut bacteria that are handled by the immune system [Pimentel et al. 2015b; Morales et al. 2013]. In both cases—locally aggressive periodontitis and patients with irritable bowel syndrome and small intestinal bacterial overgrowth—circulating antibodies to cytolethal distending toxin B correlated with the development and severity of the disease [Pimentel et al. 2015b; Morales et al. 2013; Ando et al. 2010]. Therefore, CDT and CDT antibodies in the blood may play a role in the early development of periodontal, gastrointestinal, and neurological diseases. The proposed mechanisms outlined above through which oral pathogens and their toxins

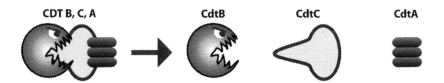

FIGURE 3.1   The cytolethal distending toxin (CDT is composed of 3 subunits: CdtB (the active unit), CdtC and CdtA.

contribute to the pathogenesis of autoimmune, neuroimmune, and neurodegenerative disorders are illustrated in Figure 3.2.

Lipopolysaccharides or endotoxins are structurally unique glycolipids produced by Gram-negative bacteria that can induce potent pathophysiological effects in humans. LPS is considered the prototypical pathogen-associated molecular pattern (PAMP), which is a molecule associated with groups of pathogens that can be recognized by

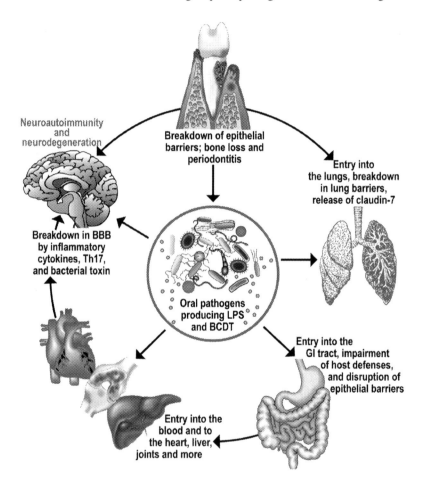

FIGURE 3.2 The role of oral pathogens and their toxins in the induction of autoimmune, neuroimmune, and neurodegenerative disorders beyond periodontitis. Oral pathogens damage the gingival epithelium, allowing their bacterial toxins (LPS and BCdT) to access not just the connecting tissue but also the bloodstream, allowing them entry into distal organs. In the lungs these toxins cause the breakdown of lung barriers and the release of claudin-7; a breakdown in the BBB leads to the activation of Th17 and other inflammatory cells; entry into the GI tract leads to the impairment of host defenses and the disruption of epithelial barriers. Thus, the penetration of bacterial toxins and their antibodies into the blood and their subsequent entry into the heart, liver, joints, brain and other organs may upset the immune balance and contribute to the pathogenesis of periodontal, gastrointestinal, neurological and autoimmune diseases.

receptors, monocytes, and macrophages. PAMPs can cause a rapid release of pro-inflammatory cytokines such as TNF-α, IL-1β, and IFN-γ. They can also activate complement, clotting, and fibrinolytic pathways [Raetz and Whitfield 2002].

Recent studies point to the role of abnormal microbiota, the release of particular LPS, and bacterial CDT as plausible mechanisms that could contribute to the pathogenesis of various autoimmune diseases [Vatanen et al. 2016]. A population-based microbiome study identified specific bacterial compounds, the absence or presence of which were associated with health status and disease [Vatanen et al. 2016]. The study followed the gut microbiome development of 222 infants in Northern Europe from birth until the age of three. Early-onset autoimmune diseases are common in Finland and Estonia, but less prevalent in Russia. One explanation for this disparity may have been found in the microbiome of the study participants. Researchers detected an abundance of *Bacteroides* species in the gut microbiomes of Finnish and Estonian children, while the Russian children showed a predominance of *E. coli*. It seems that *Bacteroides* LPS inhibits innate immune signaling and endotoxin tolerance, rendering immune response less effective. This study supports a model through which exposure to different subtypes of LPS produced by gut microbiota, particularly the LPS that is produced by the *Enterobacter* genus, can contribute to the development of intestinal inflammatory diseases and autoimmunities that affect sites distal to the gut such as lupus and arthritis [Kim et al. 2016; Rosser and Mauri 2016].

LPS may induce autoimmunities by making the gut more permeable and enhancing the production of proinflammatory cytokines. This idea is supported by a recent study involving macaques with compromised gastrointestinal integrity in association with increased microbial translocation and immune activation [Klatt et al. 2010]. This elegant study used pigtail macaques (PTMs) that had high levels of microbial translocation and LPS production, which correlated with significant damage to the structural barriers (occludin, zonulin, and claudin) of the gastrointestinal tract. The epithelial barriers of the gastrointestinal tract are composed of tight junctions of proteins that act as filters, preventing unwanted substances from entering circulation while allowing necessary nutrients to be absorbed [Turner 2009]. Researchers found that the diarrheic monkeys had increased LPS levels in the lamina propria (LP) section of the colon in comparison with the control monkeys. On average, LPS accounted for 13% of the lamina propria area in the infected PTM monkeys, while only 0.274% of the lamina propria was occupied by LPS in the control rhesus macaques (Figure 3.3). This finding strongly suggests that the mechanism underlying the increased microbial translocation involves structural damage to the gut epithelium in monkeys with diarrhea. The authors also demonstrated a significant positive correlation between damaged tight junction proteins and the level of LPS in the tissue and blood. Therefore, systemic LPS leads to both local and systemic effects, resulting in the progression of chronic inflammatory disorders. Fasano [2011] linked a compromised intestinal barrier to inflammation, autoimmunity, and even cancer.

Klatt et al.'s work focused on monkeys, so unfortunately their findings cannot be directly transferred to humans. However, a study by Magro et al. [2017] measured serum levels of LPS in Crohn's disease patients. This patient group similarly showed higher levels of LPS than healthy controls, and the level of LPS correlated

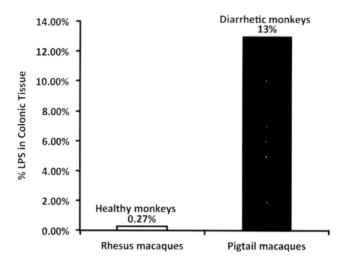

FIGURE 3.3 Correlation of tight junction breaches with LPS level. Uninfected control rhesus macaques □ showed only 0.27% LPS in their lamina propria, whereas pigtail macaques with diarrhea ■ showed 13% [Klatt et al. 2010].

with disease severity in the patient group. Maes et al. [2008] in turn connected LPS and the antibodies released against them to neurobehavioral disorders in their study, *The gut–brain barrier in major depression: Intestinal mucosal dysfunction with an increased translocation of LPS from gram negative enterobacteria (leaky gut) plays a role in the inflammatory pathophysiology of depression.* Their results suggested that the increased LPS translocation may mount an immune response, producing antibodies against LPS and thereby activating the inflammatory response system in some patients with major depression, inducing specific "sickness behavior" symptoms.

BACTERIAL TOXINS BREAKING THE GUT AND BLOOD–BRAIN BARRIERS

The gut has been called the gatekeeper to the brain, and the recent discovery of the gut–brain–immune axis has largely validated this contention. In fact, the link between the gut, the brain, and the immune system is now thought to be so important that Kipnis [2018] called the immune system, in connection with the brain, the body's "seventh sense" in a recent issue of *Scientific American*. However, this "seventh sense" is only as efficacious as the integrity of the barriers of both the gut and the blood–brain barrier. The structures of the intestinal barriers are composed of several layers. From the top of the cell to the bottom are the extracellular loop, tight junction (claudin, occludin, and zonulin), junctional adhesion molecule (JAM), adherens junction (E-cadherin, catenin, actin, α-actinin, talin, vinculin), desmosomes (actin, α-actinin, desmoplakin, plakophilin), and gap junctions. The tight junction, with its occludin and connected zonulin, is the most vulnerable of these structures to environmental assault. Unfortunately, this junction is also most responsible for the paracellular barrier function. One study using rats [Kimura et al. 1997] found that the interaction of LPS with the basolateral surface of intestinal epithelial cells disrupts occludin/zonulin function. As it turns out, the gates of the tight junction can be unlocked by both LPS and BCdTs.

In this regard, the CdtB subunit uses its DNase and other enzymatic properties to penetrate the epithelial cell membrane and reach the cell nucleus, where it can cause damage to the cells' DNA and to cytoskeletal proteins [Haghjoo and Galan 2004]. The presence of these bacterial cytotoxins and cytoskeletal proteins in the submucosa and in circulating blood can result in IgG, IgM, and IgA antibody production against these antigens. Furthermore, BCdTs can affect intestinal permeability through molecular mimicry of the vinculin–talin interaction. Talin and vinculin are two cytoskeletal proteins that are important bricks in the barrier wall, and their similarity to the bacterial toxin produced by a bacterium such as *Shigella* allows the toxin to bind to both vinculin and talin, producing a conformational change in these cytoskeletal proteins [Izard et al. 2006]. The resulting increased permeability of the intestinal epithelial barrier allows the passage of macromolecules such as bacterial toxins and dietary proteins into circulation. The uptake of immunogenic molecules such as bacterial cytotoxins, food antigens from lumen, and damaged cytoskeletal proteins results in immune response and antibody production against bacterial cytotoxins, tight junction proteins, cytoskeletal proteins, and possibly even food antigens. The excessive uptake of these antigens causes a breakdown in immunological tolerance or the suppression of immune responsiveness and can induce immunological activity both within the intestine and beyond—including in the nervous system—should these cross-reactive antibodies penetrate the blood–brain barrier (see Figure 3.4).

The Role of LPS in the Breakdown of the Blood–Brain Barrier and the Induction of Pathology in the CNS

The production of inflammatory cytokines like TNF-α is one of the gut's common inflammatory responses to LPS and other bacterial toxins. In this inflammatory environment, the enteric nervous system (ENS) responds to inflammatory mediators as well as to the LPS through TLR-4 complex engagement on the enteric neurons [Coquenlorge et al. 2014]. Systematically elevated levels of LPS, the production of inflammatory cytokines, and the activation of enteric neurons exert several undesirable effects on the blood–brain barrier, leading to increased permeability or outright disruption of endothelial cell tight junctions [Senturk et al. 2013]. Similar to its effect on mucosal intestinal epithelial cells [Jin et al. 2013], LPS downregulates the expression of tight junction proteins like occludins, resulting in increased permeability. LPS can also cause other structural and functional abnormalities in the blood–brain barrier: pathological alterations in blood-to-brain and brain-to-blood transporters; changes in blood–brain barrier protein, astrocytes, and in transcytolic and paracellular permeability; and the induction of cytokine release. All these LPS-related changes and abnormalities can have far-reaching consequences, including the breakdown of the blood–brain barrier and enhanced penetration of LPS, immune cells, and macromolecules into the brain and central nervous system [Jangula and Murphy 2013]. This results in an immune response via

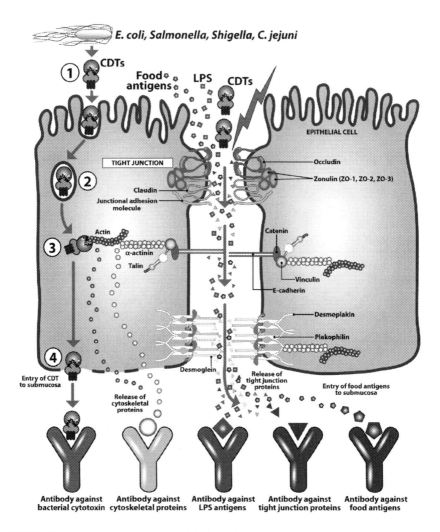

FIGURE 3.4 The mechanism by which bacteria or their toxins manage to penetrate the epithelial cells, resulting in immunological reactivity in the gut and beyond. CDT released by *E. coli* (1) undergoes endocytosis (2), attacks cytoskeletal proteins (3), and then enters the submucosa (4). CDT-assisted breakdown of the tight junctions results in the release of bacterial cytotoxins and cytoskeletal proteins, and the penetration of food antigens. Antibody production against these molecules can result in immunological activity within the gut and beyond, including the brain.

the production of antibodies against blood–brain barrier proteins (such as S100B, claudins), LPS, and other macromolecules. Furthermore, penetration of LPS into the brain provokes direct inflammatory responses in the hippocampus through increased TLR-4 expression and the upregulation of IL-1β and a range of MAPK kinases. Elevated levels of IL-1 β in this part of the brain have an inhibitory effect on long-term potentiation and synaptic activity, leading to cognitive dysfunction and eventual neurodegeneration [Chung et al. 2010].

CORRELATION OF INTESTINAL BACTERIAL LPS ANTIBODY WITH OCCLUDIN/ZONULIN, S100B AND AQUAPORIN 4

It has been established that a significant percentage of patients with inflammatory bowel disease suffer not only from enhanced intestinal permeability, but are also more prone to multiple autoimmunities [Citi 2018]. LPS from gut enterobacters have been shown to play a role in systemic inflammation, leading to the opening of the blood–brain barrier, the activation of astrocytes and microglia, and a potential contribution to neuroautoimmunity. In fact, the administration of as little as 1 μg/mL of LPS has been shown to generate a significant secretion of S100B, which easily becomes a target for autoimmunity [Guerra et al. 2011]. In a recent study presented by the corresponding author at the 11th International Congress of Autoimmunity [2018], 188 inflammatory bowel disease subjects and 196 healthy controls were tested for possible correlation between LPS, occludin/zonulin, aquaporin, and S100B antibodies [Lambert and Vojdani 2018]. Statistical analysis of the results showed that of the 188 inflammatory bowel disease subjects, 72%, 41%, and 33% tested positive for IgG, IgA, and IgM LPS antibodies, respectively, as opposed to 31%, 8%, and 6% for the controls, respectively. Of the 72% positive for IgG, 48% showed elevations for occludin + zonulin, 42% showed elevations for AQP4, and 34% showed elevations for S100B. If LPS antibodies were elevated, there was a significantly increased risk of having antibodies to barrier proteins occludin + zonulin, S100B, and AQP4. The risk ratio for IgG ranged from 1.2 to 1.7, for IgM from 2.3 to 2.7, and for IgA from 2.2 to 3.8, as shown in Table 3.1.

These results clearly demonstrate that excessive amounts of LPS not only affect the gut's structural proteins, but also disrupt the blood–brain barrier, which is the gateway to neuroinflammation, neuroautoimmunity, and neurodegeneration. In fact, the inflammatory effect of systemic LPS has been linked to multiple disorders ranging from the gut to the brain [Zhan et al. 2016; Klatt et al. 2010]. The increased levels of serum LPS antibodies in inflammatory bowel disease patients, therefore, may explain the increased prevalence of extra-intestinal autoimmune disorders that have been reported in patients with the condition [Wilson et al. 2016].

TABLE 3.1
Risk Analysis of Positive LPS IgG, IgM, and IgA with Positive Gut and BBB Protein Antibodies

	Occludin and Zonulin	Aquaporin	S100B
IgG	(1.2–2.0)	(1.3–2.2)	(0.9–1.6)
	1.5	1.7	1.2
	p = 0.001	p < 0.001	p = 0.1
IgM	(2.1–3.6)	(1.9–3.3)	(1.8–3.0)
	2.7	2.5	2.3
	p < 0.001	p < 0.0001	p < 0.0001
IgA	(1.6–2.9)	(3.0–4.9)	(2.5–4.1)
	2.2	3.8	3.2
	p < 0.0001	p < 0.0001	p = 0.0001

Inflammatory bowel disease and irritable bowel syndrome are thought to result from inappropriate activation of the mucosal immune system driven by intestinal bacterial toxins [Zois et al. 2010]. There is evidence to suggest that inflammatory bowel disease can manifest in the neurologic system, resulting in peripheral neuropathy and central nervous system disorders. This extra-intestinal manifestation of inflammatory bowel disease may occur in about one-third of patients living with the disease [Casella et al. 2014]. *Campylobacter jejuni* and its CDT are not only involved in exacerbations of inflammatory bowel disease and irritable bowel syndrome, but may also contribute to the development of autoimmune inflammatory demyelinating polyneuropathy [Masuda et al. 2002]. Furthermore, very recent research published in *JAMA Neurology* points toward an increased risk of Parkinson's disease in individuals who suffer from inflammatory bowel disease [Peter et al. 2018]. In comparison to unaffected controls, the incidence of Parkinson's was 28% higher among people with inflammatory bowel disease. Treatment with anti-TNF-α was associated with a reduction in the incidence of Parkinson's of 78%. Taken together, these studies indicate that the gut, immune system, and brain interact routinely, both in sickness and in health [Vojdani 2015].

Although the mechanisms that are involved in the pathogenesis of neurologic and neurodegenerative manifestations of inflammatory bowel disease and irritable bowel syndrome are not clear, they are likely related to the molecular mimicry between bacterial toxins and nervous system antigens [Vojdani and Vojdani 2018a, b].

ASSOCIATION OF GRAM-NEGATIVE BACTERIAL MOLECULES (LPS, BCDT) WITH ALZHEIMER'S DISEASE (AD)

It has been previously reported that infections such as *Streptococcus sanguinis, Streptococcus mutans, Borrelia burgdorferi, Chlamydia pneumoniae, Candida albicans*, EBV-EA, HSV-1, and HHV-6 are associated with sporadic, late-onset of Alzheimer's. The role that these pathogens play in the pathology of Alzheimer's was recently summarized in a review of the literature by Adams [2017] and a study by Readhead et al. [2018]. Pistollato et al. [2016] observed that the bacteria in the gut can release significant amounts of amyloids and LPS. Asti and Gioglio [2014] found that *in vitro* Aβ fibrillogenesis was potentiated by the *E. coli* endotoxin, showing the importance of infection events in the pathogenesis of Alzheimer's and implicating pathological factors in the underlying mechanisms of Aβ fibrillogenesis. Zhan et al. [2016] found that prominent Gram-negative bacteria like *E. coli* K99 and LPS were detected in brain parenchyma and vessels of Alzheimer's patients at much higher levels compared to healthy control brains ($p<0.01$). *E. coli* K99 was also localized in neuron-like cells in Alzheimer's, but not in the control brains. Furthermore, LPS co-localized with A$\beta_{1-40/42}$ in amyloid plaques around blood vessels in Alzheimer's brains. Based on these findings, another recent study led by the primary author [Vojdani et al. 2018] tested the immunoreactivity of AβP antibody with LPS and CDTs from *E. coli, S. typhosa, C. jejuni*, and *S. flexneri*, organisms that cause diarrheal illness in humans [Zhan et al. 2016]. These bacteria also produce BCdTs, which play a major role in the disruption of tight junction, cytoskeletal, and blood–brain barrier proteins. As mentioned earlier, these toxins share homology with junctional proteins like vinculin, talin, and enteric ganglia. Due to their structural similarity with junctional proteins, it is possible that they play a significant role in autoimmune reactivity in patients with irritable bowel syndrome [Smith and Bayles 2006].

The data presented in Figure 3.5 shows that the reaction of AβP antibody with E. coli, S. typhosa, C. jejuni antigens, and their pure LPS ranged from moderate to strong. Regarding the BCdT, immunoreactivity was strongest with C. jejuni BCdT, and strong with E. coli BCdT, as well as S. typhosa BCdT. Interestingly, the same dilution of antibody did not react with S. flexneri antigens nor its toxins. The study concluded that BCdTs, like LPS, may play an important role in the neuropathology of Alzheimer's and merit additional research [Vojdani et al. 2018].

The reaction of Aβ-42 antibody with bacterial LPS and BCdT may be related to the homology between peptide stretches of microbial origin and Aβ-42. We postulated that by crossing the gut and the blood–brain barrier, bacterial molecules may bind to Aβ protein, form small oligomers, encase pathogens and their molecules to finally form amyloid plaques, the tell-tale markers of Alzheimer's (Figure 3.6).

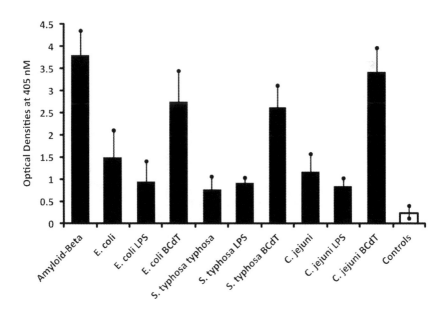

FIGURE 3.5 Degree of reactivity of rabbit monoclonal anti-β-amyloid peptide 1-42 with different bacterial antigens and toxins measured by ELISA. The mean ± 3SD of 12 determinations for each antigen is shown. Compared to the monoclonal antibody's reaction with amyloid-β, the reaction of this antibody with *Escherichia coli* LPS, *Salmonella typhosa*, *Salmonella* LPS, *Campylobacter jejuni*, and *C. jejuni LPS* is moderate (OD = 0.51–1.20), and with *E. coli*, *E. coli* BCdT, *Salmonella* BCdT, and *C. jejuni* BCdT is high (OD >1.20). Modified from Vojdani (2018a).

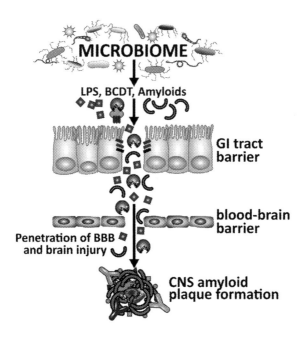

FIGURE 3.6   The role of microbial toxins in the induction of breaches in the gut and blood–brain barrier, and their binding to Aβ protein or peptides, forming amyloid plaque in the CNS.

CIRCULATING ANTIBODIES AGAINST BACTERIAL TOXINS MAY BECOME PATHOGENIC IN THE CONTEXT OF BBB BREAKDOWN

Antibodies against bacteria and other types of invaders have been found to be nearly ubiquitous in human sera and could induce pathology in the context of barrier breakdown [Levin et al. 2010]. These antibodies can circulate in the blood for years before the actual onset of autoimmune disorders [Ma et al. 2017]. The development of Alzheimer's may therefore depend on the specific inciting factors that lead to the breakdown of the barriers, including the blood–brain barrier. Nagele et al. [2011] pointed out that the normal function of a working blood–brain barrier is to restrict the entry of soluble molecules into the parenchyma of the brain, including immunoglobulins and blood-borne cells. In that study, they demonstrated that the binding of serum IgG to neurons in the cerebral cortex of Alzheimer's brains implicates cerebrovascular compromise in the pathogenesis of the disease. The widespread abundance of IgG-positive neurons detected in postmortem Alzheimer's brains implies that autoantibodies are able to consistently gain access to neurons in the brain through a compromised blood–brain barrier [Nagele et al. 2011]. In a previous study, Nagele et al. had already reported that the vast majority, if not all, of postmortem Alzheimer's brains show evidence of blood–brain barrier breakdown as evidenced by the presence of antibodies, complement, and soluble Aβ peptides such as $A\beta_{42}$ [Clifford et al. 2007]. Nagele states that it is reasonable then to speculate that healthy and non-demented individuals are free of these detectable materials because they possess an intact blood–brain barrier that prevented blood-borne brain-reactive autoantibodies from gaining access to the brain [Nagele et al. 2011]. Since many neurodegenerative diseases are accompanied by inflammation that could jeopardize the integrity of the blood–brain barrier [Weisman et al. 2006], this compromise may play a key role in the progression of many of these neurodegenerative diseases. The pre-requisite of enhanced blood–brain barrier permeability would explain why the presence of brain-reactive autoantibodies in the blood by itself may not result in central nervous system disease. However, in patients with breached blood–brain barriers, these same antibodies could have far-reaching effects that lead to neurodegenerative disorders such as Alzheimer's. Therefore, it becomes critical to identify the factors that can modulate the integrity and permeability of the blood–brain barrier toward permitting brain-reactive autoantibodies, macromolecules, and bacterial Aβ peptides to gain access to brain tissues [Nagele et al. 2011].

In another recent report [Vojdani and Vojdani 2018b], it was hypothesized that neuronal antibodies in the blood that cross-react with amyloid-beta peptide 1-42 (AβP-42) and other antigens—Aβ-proteins, tau protein, α-synuclein, and particularly beta nerve growth factor (β-NGF) and brain-derived neurotrophic factor (BDNF)—may play a pathogenic role in the onset and progression of Alzheimer's and other neurodegenerative disorders, if they penetrate the blood–brain barrier. Moreover, some of these antibodies may be generated in response to immunoreactivity against microbial transglutaminase (mTG) and/or enteric neuronal antigens that strongly react with proteins expressed in the central nervous system. Therefore, in individuals with compromised blood–brain barriers, these brain-reactive and cross-reactive autoantibodies may reach the interstitium of the brain, where they react with the key neural proteins or peptides (Figure 3.7), in much the same way that streptococcal antibodies—which are known to cross-react with ganglioside—have been shown to penetrate the blood–brain barrier and there interact with tissues of the basal ganglia [Gebhard et al. 2015]. The immunoreactivity of these cross-reactive autoantibodies with AβP-42, as shown in the authors' study [Vojdani and Vojdani 2018b], may contribute toward the deposition of AβP-42 and the formation of amyloid plaques that are the hallmark of Alzheimer's. Antigenic similarity or homology between the structures of LPS, BCdT, mTG, tissue antigens, and those of AβP-42 and other neuronal antigens could be the mechanism through which these brain-reactive auto-antibodies attack the brain's own cells.

This brings the focus back to the previously mentioned β-NGF and BDNF, two factors that are vital to neuronal regeneration [Rahmani et al. 2013]. β-NGF supports the survival and growth of neural cells, regulates cell growth, promotes differentiation of neurons, and aids in neuron migration [Yuan et al. 2013]. BDNF also plays a vital role in the growth, development, maintenance, and functioning of several neuronal systems [Halepoto et al. 2014]. This chapter proposes that due to the cross-reactivity of β-NGF and BDNF antibodies with AβP-42, these autoantibodies not only enhance the process of amyloidogenesis, but also may actually prevent the normal healing and replacement of these nerve cells. As one, all of the factors and processes outlined above can result in neurodegeneration and the neuropathology of Alzheimer's and other neurological disorders.

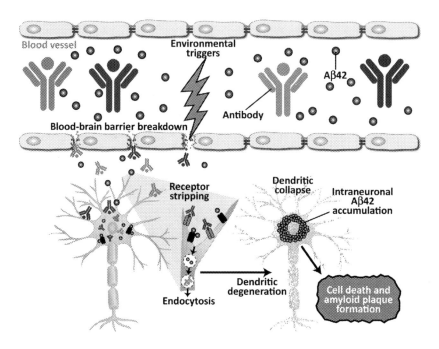

FIGURE 3.7 A mechanism for AD pathogenesis combining blood-barrier breakdown and the presence of neuron-binding autoantibodies in the serum. Modified from Nagele et al., *J Alzheimer's Dis*, 2011, 25:605–622. Breach of the BBB results in chronic extravasation of plasma components including autoantibodies and soluble Aβ42 peptide. Autoantibodies then bind to targets on neuronal surfaces. Neurons attempt receptor-mediated endocytosis to clear their surfaces of the bound autoantibodies; this results in internalization of the autoantibodies and Aβ42, as well as the stripping of key neuron surface membrane proteins, both of which jeopardize neuronal function. The internalized autoantibodies are readily degraded within lysosomes, but Aβ42 is non-degradable. The accumulated Aβ42 in neurons leads to dendritic collapse, synaptic loss, and eventual cell death. The resulting release of intraneruonal Aβ42 contributes to the formation of amyloid plaques.

Furthermore, Friedland [2015] proposes that the cross-reactivity between amyloids and brain tissue may be triggered by amyloid-containing bacteria in the nose and/or gut. Friedland's article states that in Parkinson's disease, the misfolding of α-synuclein may be caused by bacterial amyloids coming from the gut through the vagus and other nerves, or directly through the roof of the nose to the olfactory cortex. Friedland also talks about the desirability and potential of predicting the possibility of cross-seeding or cross-reactivity between two proteins through computer modeling and stresses the importance of assessing the role of microbiota on protein folding and inflammation.

Therefore, by identifying the triggers that induce the production of autoreactive antibodies, it could be possible to remove or limit these triggers and develop therapeutic protocols focused on recalibrating gut microbiota, restoring barrier integrity and ultimately alleviating the suffering of patients with inflammatory autoimmune and neurodegenerative disorders.

CONCLUSION

This chapter briefly discusses how oral pathogens, through their variety of resultant toxins, may make it possible for normally harmless but potentially autoreactive antibodies to gain access to the blood, the gastrointestinal tract, and the brain [Dileepan et al. 2016; Edgar et al. 2004; Geerts et al. 2002]. It also discusses how bacterial toxins such as LPS and BCdT are not only involved in inflammatory bowel disease, irritable bowel syndrome, and periodontitis, but also, due to their cross-reactivity with Aβ peptide and protein, may also play a crucial role in the induction of autoimmune and neurodegenerative disorders. In this chapter, evidence has been presented that ubiquitous brain-reactive or cross-reactive autoantibodies found in the blood may be harmless in otherwise healthy individuals, but can have catastrophic consequences should they cross the blood–brain barrier and cross-react with blood–brain barrier proteins, neuronal antigens, and Aβ-42 peptide. These ideas have significant potential for therapeutic application. Identification of the triggering bacteria or their components that react or cross-react with amyloid-β and neuronal antigens would allow the prescription of targeted therapeutic interventions to remove or diminish harmful bacteria or their metabolic byproducts. In addition, consideration should be made as it relates to prebiotics that enhance the growth of beneficial organisms, and designer probiotics that provide additional beneficial bacteria.

The development of strategies that will improve gut diversity and minimize the release of LPS, BCdT and other bacterial toxins by the gut microbiome may minimize immune reactivity with brain tissues such as amyloid-β peptide and brain growth factor. This approach may provide hope for preventing, or at least slowing, the progression of various neurodegenerative disorders like Alzheimer's, allowing many individuals to avoid years of suffering.

REFERENCES

Adams, J. U. 2017. Do microbes trigger Alzheimer's disease? *Scientist* 31(9):1–9.

Ando, E. S., L. A. De-Gennaro, M. Faveri, M. Feres, J. M. DiRienzo, and M. P. Mayer. 2010. Immune response to cytolethal distending toxin of *Aggregatibacter actinomycetemcomitans* in periodontitis patients. *J. Periodont. Res.* 45(4):471–80.

Asti, A., and L. Gioglio. 2014. Can a bacterial endotoxin be a key factor in the kinetics of amyloid fibril formation? *J. Alzheimers Dis.* 39(1):169–79. doi:10.3233/JAD-131394.

Blaser, M. J. 2017. The theory of disappearing microbiota and the epidemics of chronic diseases. *Nat. Rev. Immunol.* 17(8):461–63. doi: 10.1038/nri.2017.77.

Casella, G., G. E. Tontini, G. Bassotti, et al. 2014. Neurological disorders and inflammatory bowel diseases. *World J. Gastroenterol.* 20(27):8764–82. doi:10.3748/wjg.v20.i27.8764.

Chung, Y. C., S. R. Kim, and B. K. Jin. 2010. Paroxetine prevents loss of nigrostriatal dopaminergic neurons by inhibiting brain inflammation and oxidative stress in an experimental model of Parkinson's disease. *J. Immunol.* 185(2):1230–7. doi:10.4049/jimmunol.1000208.

Citi, S. 2018. Intestinal barriers protect against disease: Leaky cell-cell junctions contribute to inflammatory and autoimmune disease. *Science* 359(6380):1097–8. doi:10.1126/science.aat0835.

Clifford, P. M., S. Zarrabi, G. Siu, et al. 2007. Abeta peptides can enter the brain through a defective blood-brain barrier and bind selectively to neurons. *Brain Res.* 1142:223–36. doi:10.1016/j.brainres.2007.01.070.

Coquenlorge, S., E. Duchalais, J. Chevalier, F. Cossais, M. Rolli-Derkinderen, and M. Neunlist. 2014. Modulation of lipopolysaccharide-induced neuronal response by activation of the enteric nervous system. *J. Neuroinflamm.* 11:202. doi:10.1186/s12974-014-0202-7.

Dileepan, T., E. D. Smith, D. Knowland, et al. 2016. Group A *Streptococcus* intranasal infection promotes CNS infiltration by streptococcal-specific Th17 cells. *J. Clin. Invest.* 126(1):303–17. doi:10.1172/JCI80792.

Edgar, M., C. Dawes, and D. O'Mullane. 2004. *Saliva and Oral Health*, British Dental Association, 3rd Revised Edition, London.

Fasano, A. 2011. Leaky gut and autoimmune diseases. *Clin. Rev. Allergy Immunol.* 42(1):71–8. doi:10.1007/s12016-011-8291-x.

Friedland, R. P. 2015. Mechanisms of molecular mimicry involving the microbiota in neurodegeneration. *J. Alzheimers Dis.* 45(2):349–62. doi:10.3233/JAD-142481.

Gebhard, R., C. Huff, M. Osborne, L. Riegle, and M. Kelly-Worden. 2015. Streptococcal antibody probe crosses the blood brain barrier and interacts within the basal ganglia. *Open J. Pathol.* 5(2):42–9.

Geerts, S. O., M. Nys, P. de Mol, et al. 2002. Systemic release of endotoxins induced by gentle mastication: Association with periodontitis severity. *J. Periodontol.* 73:73–8.

Guerra, M. C., L. S. Tortorelli, F. Galland, et al. 2011. Lipopolysaccharide modulates astrocytic S100B secretion: A study in cerebrospinal fluid and astrocyte cultures from rats. *J. Neuroinflamm.* 8:128.

Haghjoo, E., and J. E. Galan. 2004. *Salmonella typhi* encodes a functional cytolethal distending toxin that is delivered into host cells by a bacterial-internalization pathway. *Proc. Natl Acad. Sci. U. S. A.* 101(13):4614–9.

Halepoto, D. M., S. Bashir, and L. Al-Ayadhi. 2014. Possible role of brain-derived neurotrophic factor (BDNF) in autism spectrum disorder: Current status. *J. Coll. Physicians Surg. Pak.* 24(4):274–8. doi:04.2014/JCPSP.274278.

Ide, M., M. Harris, A. Stevens, et al. 2016. Periodontitis and cognitive decline in Alzheimer's disease. *PLOS ONE* 11(3):e0151081.

Itzhaki, R. F., R. Lathe, B. J. Balin, et al. 2016. Microbes and Alzheimer's disease. *J. Alzheimers Dis.* 51(4):979–84. doi:10.3233/JAD-160152.

Izard, T., G. T. Van Nheiv, and P. R. J. Bois. 2006. *Shigella* applies molecular mimicry to subvert vinculin and invade host cells. *J. Cell Biol.* 175(3):465–75. doi:10.1083/jcb.200605091.

Jangula, A., and E. J. Murphy. 2013. Lipopolysaccharide-induced blood brain barrier permeability is enhanced by alpha-synuclein expression. *Neurosci. Lett.* 551:23–7. doi:10.1016/j.neulet.2013.06.058.

Jin, L., R. L. Nation, J. Li, and J. A. Nicolazzo. 2013. Species-dependent blood-brain barrier disruption of lipopolysaccharide: Amelioration by colistin in vitro and in vivo. *Antimicrob. Agents Chemother.* 57(9):4336–42. doi:10.1128/AAC.00765-13.

Kim, K. A., J. J. Jeong, S. Y. Yoo, and D. H. Kim. 2016. Gut microbiota lipopolysaccharide accelerates inflamm-aging in mice. *BMC Microbiol.* 16:9. doi:10.1186/s12866-016-0625-7.

Kimura, H., N. Sawada, H. Tobioka, et al. 1997. Bacterial lipopolysaccharide reduced intestinal barrier function and altered localization of 7H6 antigen in IEC-6 rat intestinal crypt cells. *J. Cell. Physiol.* 171(3):284–90. doi:10.1002/(SICI)1097-4652(199706)171:3<284::AID-JCP6>3.0.CO;2-K.

Kipnis, J. 2018. The seventh sense. *Sci. Am.* 319(2):28–35. doi:10.1038/scientificamerican0818-2.

Klatt, N. R., L. D. Harris, C. L. Vinton, et al. 2010. Compromised gastrointestinal integrity in pigtail macaques is associated with increased microbial translocation, immune activation, and IL-17 production in the absence of SIV infection. *Mucosal Immunol.* 3(4):387–98. doi:10.1038/mi.2010.14.

Lambert, J., and A. Vojdani. 2018. Correlation of intestinal bacterial lipopolysaccharide anti-bodies and blood-brain barrier antibodies in IBD subjects. 11th International Congress on Autoimmunity. Lisbon, Portugal, 16–20 May.

Levin, E. C., N. K. Acharya, M. Han, et al. 2010. Brain-reactive autoantibodies are nearly ubiquitous in human sera and may be linked to pathology in the context of blood-brain barrier breakdown. *Brain Res.* 1345:221–32. doi:10.1016/j.brainres.2010.05.038.

Ma, W.-T., C. Chang, M. E. Gershwin, and Z.-X. Lian. 2017. Development of autoantibodies precedes clinical manifestations of autoimmune diseases: A comprehensive review. *J. Autoimmun.* 83:95–112. doi:10.1016/j.jaut.2017.07.003.

Maes, M., M. Kubera, and J.-C. Leunis. 2008. The gut-brain barrier in major depression: Intestinal mucosal dysfunction with an increased translocation of LPS from gram neg-ative enterobacteria (leaky gut) plays a role in the inflammatory pathophysiology of depression. *Neuroendocrinol. Lett.* 29(1):117–24.

Magro, D. O., P. G. Kotze, C. A. R. Martinez, et al. 2017. Changes in serum levels of lipo-polysaccharides and CD26 in patients with Crohn's disease. *Intest. Res.* 15(3):352–7. doi:10.5217/ir.2017.15.3.352.

Masuda, H., U. Ishii, A. N. Nakayama, et al. 2002. Ulcerative colitis associated with Takayasu's disease in two patients who received proctocolectomy. *J. Gastroenterol.* 37(4):297–302.

Mednis, D. 2017. The growth of chronic conditions: Search for solutions to the problem. *Chronic Dis. Transl. Med.* 3(2):82–8. doi:10.1016/j.cdtm.2017.02.010.

Medzhitov, R. 2007. Recognition of microorganisms and activation of the immune response. *Nature* 449(7164):819–26. doi:10.1038/nature06246.

Meetoo, D. 2008. Chronic diseases: The silent global epidemic. *Br. J. Nurs.* 17(21):1320–5. doi:10.12968/bjon.2008.17.21.31731.

Morales, W., S. Weitsman, G. Kim, et al. 2013. Circulating antibodies to cytolethal distending toxin B correlate with the development of small intestinal bacterial overgrowth in a rat model of post-infectious IBS. *Gastroenterology* 144:S931–2.

Nagele, R. G., P. M. Clifford, G. Siu, et al. 2011. Brain-reactive autoantibodies prevalent in human sera increase intraneuronal amyloid-β (1–42) deposition. *J. Alzheimers Dis.* 25(4):605–22. doi:10.3233/JAD-2011-110098.

National Institute of Aging. Azheimer's disease fact sheet. https://www.nia.nih.gov/health/alzheimers-disease-fact-sheet.

Nikitakis, N. G., W. Papaioannou, L. I. Sakkas, and E. Kousvelari. 2017. The autoimmunity–oral microbiome connection. *Oral Dis.* 23(7):828–39. doi:10.1111/odi.12589. Epub 2016.

Ogrendik, M. 2014. Oral bacteria are responsible for the etiology of rheumatoid arthritis. *Open J. Rheumatol. Autoimmune Dis.* 4(3):162–9. doi:10.4236/ojra.2014.43023.

Peter, I., M. Dublinsky, S. Bressman, et al. 2018. Anti-tumor necrosis factor therapy and inci-dence of Parkinson's disease among patients with inflammatory bowel disease. *JAMA Neurol.* 75(8):939–46. doi:10.1001/jamaneurol.2018.0605.

Pimentel, M., W. Morales, V. Pokkunuri, et al. 2015b. Autoimmunity links vinculin to the pathophysiology of chronic functional bowel changes following Campylobacter jejuni infection in a rat model. *Dig. Dis. Sci.* 60(5):1195–205. doi:10.1007/s10620-014-3435-5.

Pimentel, M., W. Morales, A. Rezaie, et al. 2015a. Development and validation of a biomarker for diarrhea-predominant irritable bowel syndrome in human subjects. *PLOS ONE.* 10(5):e0126438. doi:10.1371/journal.pone.0126438.

Pistollato, F., S. Sumalla Cano, I. Elio, M. Masias Vergara, F. Giampieri, and M. Battino 2016. Role of gut microbiota and nutrients in amyloid formation and pathogenesis of Alzheimer disease. *Nutr. Rev.* 74(10):624–34.

Raetz, C. R., and C. Whitfield. 2002. Lipopolysaccharide endotoxins. *Annu. Rev. Biochem.* 71:635–700. doi:10.1146/annurev.biochem.71.110601.135414.

Rahmani, A., A. Shoae-Hassani, P. Keyhanvar, D. Kheradmand, and A. Darbandi-Azar 2013. Dehydroepiandrosterone stimulates nerve growth factor and brain derived neurotrophic factor in cortical neurons. *Adv. Pharmacol. Sci.* 2013:Article ID 506191. doi:10.1155/2013/506191.

Readhead, B., J.-V. Haure-Mirande, C. C. Funk, et al. 2018. Multiscale analysis of independent Alzheimer's cohorts finds disruption of molecular, genetic, and clinical networks by human herpesvirus. *Neuron* 99(1):1–19. doi:10.1016/j.neuron.2018.05.023.

Rosser, E. C., and C. Mauri. 2016. A clinical update on the significance of the gut microbiota in systemic autoimmunity. *J. Autoimmun.* 74:85–93. doi:10.1016/j.jaut.2016.06.009.

Schroeder, B. O., and F. Bäckhed. 2016. Signals from the gut microbiota to distant organs in physiology and disease. *Nat. Med.* 22(10):1079–89. doi:10.1038/nm.4185.

Senturk, E., F. Esen, P. Ergin Ozcan, et al. 2013. Effects of different doses and serotypes of LPS on blood-brain barrier permeability in Sprague-Dawley rats. *Crit. Care* 17(Suppl 2):P21. doi:10.1186/cc11959.

Smith, J. L., and D. O. Bayles. 2006. The contribution of cytolethal distending toxin to bacterial pathogenesis. *Crit. Rev. Microbiol.* 32(4):227–48. doi:10.1080/10408410601023557.

Souza, C. O., M. A. C. S. Vieira, F. M. A. Batista, et al. 2018. Serological markers of recent *Campylobacter jejuni* infection in patients with Guillain-Barré syndrome in the state of Piaui, Brazil, 2014–2016. *Am. J. Trop. Med. Hyg.* 98(2):586–8. doi:10.4269/ajtmh.17-0666.

Turner, J. R. 2009. Intestinal mucosal barrier function in health and disease. *Nat. Rev. Immunol.* 9(11):799–809. doi:10.1038/nri2653.

van Oostrom, S. H., R. Gijsen, I. Stirbu, et al. 2016. Time trends in prevalence of chronic diseases and multimorbidity not only due to aging: Data from general practices and health surveys. *PLOS ONE* 11(8):e0160264. doi:10.1371/journal.pone.0160264.

Vatanen, T., A. D. Kostic, E. d'Hennezel, et al. 2016. Variation in microbiome LPS immunogenicity contributes to autoimmunity in humans. *Cell* 165(4):842–53. doi:10.1016/j.cell.2016.04.007.

Vojdani, A. 2015. *Neuroimmunity and the Brain-Gut Connection.* Functional Neurology Series, Nova Science Publishers Inc., New York.

Vojdani, A. 2018. Antibodies against zonulin and other tight junction proteins in celiac disease. 11th International Congress on Autoimmunity. Lisbon, Portugal, 16–20 May.

Vojdani, A., and E. Vojdani. 2018a. Immunoreactivity of Anti-AβP-42 specific antibody with toxic chemicals and food antigens. *J. Alzheimers Dis. Parkinsonism* 8:3. doi:10.4172/2161-0460.1000441.

Vojdani, A., and E. Vojdani. 2018b. Amyloid-β 1–42 cross-reactive antibody prevalent in human sera may contribute to intraneuronal deposition of AβP-42. *Int. J. Alzheimers Dis.* 2018:Article ID 1672568, 12. doi:10.1155/2018/1672568.

Vojdani, A., E. Vojdani, E. Saidara, and D. Kharrazian. 2018. Reaction of amyloid-β peptide antibody witrh different infectious agents involved in Alzheimer's disease. *J. Alzheimers Dis.* 63(2):847–60. doi:10.3233/JAD-170961.

Weisman, D., E. Hakimian, and G. J. Ho. 2006. Interleukins, inflammation, and mechanisms of Alzheimer's disease. *Vitam. Horm.* 74:505–30. doi:10.1016/S0083-6729(06)74020-1.

Wilson, J. C., R. I. Furlano, S. S. Jick, and C. R. Meier. 2016. Inflammatory bowel disease and the risk of autoimmune diseases. *J. Crohns Colitis* 10:186–93. doi:10.1093/ecco-jcc/jjv193.

Yamano, R., M. Ohara, S. Nishikubo, et al. 2003. Prevalence of cytolethal distending toxin production in periodontopathogenic bacteria. *J. Clin. Microbiol.* 41(4):1391–8.

Yuan, J., G. Huang, Z. Xiao, L. Lin, and T. Han. 2013. Overexpression of β-NGF promotes differentiation of bone marrow mesenchymal stem cells into neurons through regulation of AKT and MAPK pathway. *Mol. Cell. Biochem.* 383(1–2):201–11. doi:10.1007/s11010-013-1768-6.

Zhan, X., B. Stamova, L.-W. Jin, C. DeCarrli, B. Phinney, and F. R. Sharp. 2016. Gram-negative bacterial molecules associate with Alzheimer disease pathology. *Neurology* 87(22):2324–32. doi:10.1212/WNL.0000000000003391.

Zois, C. D., K. H. Katsanos, M. Kosmidou, and E. V. Tsianos. 2010. Neurologic manifestations in inflammatory bowel diseases: Current knowledge and novel insights. *J. Crohns Colitis* 4(2):115–24. doi:10.1016/j.crohns.2009.10.005.

4 The Microbiome— Its Role in Neuroinflammation
The Autism Spectrum Disorder Paradigm

Maria R. Fiorentino and Alessio Fasano

CONTENTS

CROSS COMMUNICATION BETWEEN BRAIN AND GASTROINTESTINAL SYSTEM: THE GUT–BRAIN AXIS

The existence of a functional interaction between the brain and the digestive system has been long-accepted. Historically, scientific interest has been primarily focused on motility and secretion. It is well established that the brain uses the pathways of endocrine, paracrine, and neurocrine signaling to communicate with the gastrointestinal (GI) tract to regulate its primary functions: digestion and the absorption of nutrients. These pathways involve hormonal secretion (i.e., gastrin, secretin, cholecystokinin), the engagement of the autonomic nervous system—which is divided into parasympathetic innervation supplied primarily by the vagus nerve and sympathetic innervation—and the enteric nervous system, whose elements are grouped into networks embedded in the wall of the intestine. These neural networks work together to integrate sensory signals into the brain for the control and/or modulation of GI motility and secretion. Famous are Pavlov's experiments of behavioral conditioning in dogs, in which visive or auditory cues, such as the presentation of food or the sound of a bell associated with the later food presentation, induced the activation of the digestive system through salivation [1], demonstrating the functional connection between the brain and gut secretory processes. It is only relatively recently that scientists have started to really appreciate the fact that the gut can communicate with and affect brain function, suggesting the existence of a bidirectional communication pathway between the gut and the brain.

Over the past decade, research into the gut-brain axis has grown exponentially; we have learned that as the brain communicates with the gut, thereby altering gut functions. So too does the gut communicate with the brain influencing brain functions, largely because of the influence of gut bacteria. However, this notion is not new at all. The reported association between mental health and gut issues dates back to Hippocrates (460–377 BC), who tied together liver diseases and behavioral disturbances. He might have observed "hepatic encephalopathy (HE)," a neuropsychiatric syndrome caused by acute or chronic hepatic insufficiency and whose current first-line treatment includes antibiotics, dietary supplements, and/or ammonia reducers aimed at removing toxic substances from the gut. At the beginning of the 1900s, scientists believed that waste accumulation in the colon was linked to anxiety, depression, and psychosis and although this theory was eventually dismissed it showed that there existed a sense that the gut was influencing brain function, even at that time.

Nowadays, scientists have a better sense of the participants in and mechanisms of this bidirectional communication. A prime example of the current understanding of gut–brain connection comes from an elegant study from Hsiao's group [2] on the effect of dietary interventions on refractory epilepsy (RE), a condition in which disabling seizures continue despite medically appropriate treatment. Dietary interventions for the treatment of seizures, including fasting and starvation, date back to the 5th century B.C. [3]. In the early 1900s, clinicians proposed that the anti-seizure effect of starvation was due to ketone bodies in the blood and the ketogenic diet (KD) was developed and deployed as a treatment for epilepsy in the 1920s and 1930s until it was replaced by pharmacological therapies [4]. Nevertheless, numerous reports in the literature point to a beneficial effect of this diet in reducing seizures [5–11] and over the last decade, the ketogenic diet has gained popularity as an alternative treatment for this subset of patients. Hsiao's group described how the ketogenic diet, by modifying the gut microbiota, confers protection against seizures in mice models of epilepsy. The authors showed that the ketogenic diet increases the abundance of groups of beneficial bacteria, like *Akkermansia muciniphila* and *Parabacteroides*, and that gut microbiota is necessary for the anti-epileptic effect since germ-free (GF) and/or antibiotic-treated specific pathogen-free (SPF) mice placed on the ketogenic diet show no protection to seizures. They also suggested that ketogenic diet-induced protection might be associated with increased levels of GABA in the brain, indicating a potential mechanism through which gut microbiota affect brain function [12].

The coexistence of gastrointestinal and neurological manifestations of neuroinflammation has been described in animal models and human diseases, including celiac disease (CD), multiple sclerosis (MS), Parkinson's (PD), amyotrophic lateral sclerosis (ALS), and autism spectrum disorders (ASD). One recent study, conducted on a small cohort of patients, demonstrated that gastrointestinal symptoms typical of ALS, including delayed gastric emptying and slower colonic transit, [13, 14] precede neurological manifestations and are correlated with reduced gut microbiota diversity [15, 16]. In PD, gastrointestinal symptoms, particularly constipation, represent one of the earliest signs of the disease, appearing as early as 15 years before the onset of motor symptoms [17, 18]. Furthermore, some of the clinical presentations of celiac disease include behavioral alterations, anxiety, depression, sleep disturbances, cognitive impairment, psychosis, and attention-deficit disorder [19]. Gastrointestinal symptoms including dysphagia and bladder and bowel dysfunction have been reported in MS patients [20–22] and the gastrointestinal manifestations in the ASD population described in the literature as well, ranging from constipation to gastroesophageal reflux to gastritis to intestinal inflammation to flatulence to abdominal pain or discomfort and diarrhea [23, 24]. Finally, increased serum levels of LPS have been reported in both ALS and Alzheimer's disease-affected patients, and are associated with monocyte activation [25], suggesting defects in the gut epithelial barrier.

Although neurological diseases have generally been considered and investigated exclusively within the central nervous system (CNS), research is beginning to uncover the influence of the gut in the onset and/or progression of brain disorders. In particular, the composition of the gut microbiota seems to have an impact on several pathologies affecting the brain [14, 26–33]. In humans, strong evidence of a gut microbiota–brain interaction can be found in the observation of the remarkable symptomatic improvement in patients affected by hepatic encephalopathy upon administration of antibiotics [34]. Further compelling evidence of the influence of the gut microbiota in brain development, function, and behavior came from studies with germ-free, and antibiotic-treated SPF animal models. Although, it is well established that animal gut physiology and microbiota composition are remarkably different from humans and that the use of animal models (i.e., mice) poses limitations to the applicability to human diseases, animal models can be easily subjected to manipulations and are still extremely valuable to the process of understanding the mechanisms of disease.

Germ-free mice in particular have been a tremendously useful tool for studying the influence of the gut microbiota on the development and functioning of the central nervous system. It has been reported that germ-free mice have defects in both the intestine and the brain and they exhibit an enlarged cecum, smaller and fewer Peyer's patches, reduced intestinal surface area and villi number [35–39], lower levels of serotonin, and reduced gut epithelial cell turnover [40–42]. The brains of germ-free and antibiotic-treated SPF mice show altered hippocampal neurogenesis that leads to compromised spatial and object recognition [43–46] and exhibit altered microglial function, an impaired blood–brain barrier, and alterations in cortical myelination [47–50]; this in turn leads to abnormalities in sociability, repetitive and stereotyped behavior, anxiety and an exaggerated hypothalamus-pituitary-adrenal axis (HPA) response to stress [51–54]. Most of the behavioral changes observed in germ-free mice are normalized, at least partially and in an age-dependent manner, by microbial colonization that also has beneficial effects on gut health [51, 52, 55–58], supporting the critical role of the microbiota in brain function and behavior. An elegant study by Mazmanian's group in a mouse model of Parkinson's Disease overexpressing α-synuclein showed that "gut microbiota is required for motor deficits, microglia activation, and α-synuclein pathology." The authors showed that administration of microbiota metabolites induced neuroinflammation and motor deficits and that fecal transplant from Parkinson's Disease patients into germ-free α-synuclein-overexpressing mice increases physical impairment, suggesting gut microbiota dysbiosis as a risk factor for Parkinson's Disease [59].

Historically, it has been well documented that stress affects gastrointestinal function—specifically motility, secretions, and blood flow signals—through HPA axis activation, and that, once integrated by the brain, these signals translate into visceral manifestations like nausea, pain, satiety [60, 61]. However, a number of studies have reported the effect of physical and psychological stress on the gut microbiota composition in animal models [52, 62–69], further evidencing the notion that the interaction of gut bacteria with the brain is bidirectional and can involve multiple lines of communications. Several pathways have been suggested to be involved in the gut-brain axis, including the enteric nervous system (ENS), the vagus nerve, the immune system, and the metabolic processes of gut bacteria. We know that microbiota can directly affect the immune system and therefore the activation of immune cells and subsequent cytokine release may be a pathway for transmitting microbial signals to the brain [70].

Microorganisms can also communicate with the brain via neurotransmitters and neuromodulators like serotonin, dopamine, bacterial metabolites like short-chain fatty acids (SCFAs) [40, 71], or by inducing the secretion of a variety of gut peptides, including leptin and neuropeptide Y by enteroendocrine cells located in the gut epithelium. Several of these peptides are known to affect anxiety levels and behavior via the host nervous system [44, 72, 73]. SCFAs are produced by gut bacterial fermentation of dietary fibers in the large intestine and it has been shown that SCFAs can improve neurodevelopment and cognition in animal models of neurodegenerative disorders [74]. However, experiments involving the injection of propionate, a specific type of SCFA, into the brain of rats induces ASD-like behaviors and chemical alterations in the brain typical of neuroinflammation [75]. Indeed, SCFAs can regulate the maturation and function of microglia, the brain resident immune cells, thereby affecting brain function [47, 76]. Furthermore, gut SCFA-producing bacteria increase the expression of brain endothelial tight-junction proteins contributing to the overall strengthening of the BBB [77] and have been shown to alter host gene expression in the brain, supporting their role in influencing brain function [74].

Finally, the gut directly communicates with the brain through the vagus nerve [78] and there is strong evidence from animal studies to suggest that gut bacteria can activate the vagus nerve, affecting brain function and behavior. It has been shown that the positive behavioral effects observed in mice after probiotic administration were reverted following vagotomy [79, 80]. Nohr *et al.* have described the SCFA receptor GPR41/FFAR3 in vagal ganglia, suggesting a communication pathway between the microbiota and the central nervous system [81]. In humans, a study by Svensson *et al.*, reported on a Danish cohort of patients who underwent vagotomy between 1977 and 1995 and found that patients who had been subjected to full truncal vagotomy had a lower risk of developing Parkinson's Disease compared to patients who had only undergone partial vagotomy and the general population, suggesting a pivotal role played by the vagal pathway in the pathogenesis of Parkinson's [82]. It has also been suggested that intestinal pathologies may induce Parkinson's and that microbiota plays a fundamental role in the onset of the condition [83]. Dysbiosis of the gut microbial composition has been reported in Parkinson's [84–87] as well as in other diseases characterized by neuroinflammation affecting the central nervous system, such as ALS [16], MS [88–90], AD [91–93], ASD [29, 94–98] and schizophrenia [99].

COMBINED GUT AND BLOOD–BRAIN BARRIERS DEFECTS

Several species of commensals have the ability to strengthen or weaken gut barrier function [100–107], thereby altering intestinal permeability. Intestinal dysbiosis and inflammation are associated with a dysfunctional epithelial barrier, and increased intestinal permeability may contribute to the onset of neuroinflammation and the progression to neurological disease [108, 109]. An increased antigen trafficking through an impaired gut barrier connected with a shifted microbiota composition allows harmful substances from the intestinal lumen into the bloodstream [103, 110, 111], activation of immune cells leading to systemic inflammation that can in turn can affect blood–brain barrier integrity and function and promote neuroinflammation and disease [112–114].

Defects in gut barrier function, often associated with defects in blood–brain barrier integrity, have been reported in many inflammatory neurological diseases. Severance *et al.* and Melkersson *et al.* suggested the role of an impaired gut and blood–brain barrier in schizophrenia, respectively [115, 116]. In ALS patients, high levels of LPS have been detected in the serum, consistent with increased gut permeability [14, 117] and both the blood–brain barrier and the blood–spinal-cord–barrier (BSCB) exhibited reduced expression of intercellular junctional proteins, a sign of reduced barrier integrity [118–120]. The blood–brain barrier defects correlated with infiltration of macrophages and mast cells into the brain and spinal cord and exacerbated brain inflammation [118, 121]. Likewise, disruption of the blood–brain barrier has been reported in Parkinson's Disease [14, 122], MS [123, 124], Alzheimer's Disease [125, 126], and in autism spectrum disorders [127].

ASD AS A PROTOTYPICAL EXAMPLE OF GUT–BRAIN AXIS DYSFUNCTION

Autism spectrum disorders are complex neurodevelopmental conditions characterized by deficits in communication, social interaction, and cognition, the etiology of which is not known. Therapeutic approaches are extremely limited due to our limited understanding of the mechanisms leading to the condition. The prevalence of autism spectrum disorders has increased dramatically over time, to a current rate of 1:59, and affect boys at an even higher rate [128]. Genetics are thought to account for about 10–20% of autism spectrum disorders cases [129]. Identical twins share about an 80% chance of having autism [130–132], confirming a strong genetic hereditability for autism spectrum disorders, and scientists have identified roughly 65 genes related to the risk of developing autism spectrum disorders [133]. A study on 1,000 families with autism spectrum disorder-affected children linked regions from two chromosomes to pathogenesis of the condition with 90% certainty. One of the two is chromosome 16 and the study points to the importance of this chromosome, in particular the 16p11.2 region, in autism spectrum disorders. This region has been frequently associated with these disorders as most of the alterations are in this region, and all but one of those is in a male [134]. Scientists have identified a segment of 25 genes on chromosome 16, encompassing genes expressed in the brain to genes involved in immunity, that was deleted or duplicated in about 1% of autism spectrum disorder subjects [135]. However, while the genetic makeup of an individual plays an important role, the timeline of the autism spectrum disorders "epidemic" suggests that genes alone cannot account for this phenomenon. The interplay between host genetics, immune response, intestinal microbiota composition and function, and exposure to environmental factors seems to synergistically play a critical role in the onset of autism spectrum disorders. Environmental stimuli that have been associated with increased autism spectrum disorder risk include toxic exposure, antibiotic use or maternal infection during pregnancy, inflammatory conditions, and exposure to chemicals [136–141]. Among the many co-morbidities associated with autism spectrum disorders, immune and gastrointestinal dysfunctions are particularly interesting because of their reported prevalence and association with symptom severity [142–146]. Kohane *et al.* reported increased prevalence of intestinal bowel disease (IBD) and other gastrointestinal symptoms in a population of over 14,000 autism spectrum disorder subjects [147].

Despite numerous research efforts, there is no clearly defined explanation of how environmental triggers can lead to the development and progression of these neurobehavioral conditions. However, gut bacteria may be involved, as a number of studies report dysbiosis of the gut microbiota in autism spectrum disorders [29, 32, 33, 98, 148–151]. One general hypothesis, based on the interconnectivity of the gut-brain axis, suggests that inappropriate antigen trafficking through an impaired intestinal barrier, followed by the passage of bacterial/dietary antigens or activated immune complexes through a permissive blood–brain barrier, are part of the chain of events leading to neuroinflammation and disease. Increased intestinal permeability has been reported in autism spectrum disorders [152, 153] and is associated with altered expression of TJ components in the intestine [127] and hypothesized to have damaging effects not only locally but also systemically, with potential intestinal bacteria and/or dietary antigens translocation and consequent immune activation.

In recent years, we and others have indicated that children with an autism spectrum disorder diagnosis have brain pathology suggestive of ongoing neuroinflammation in different regions of the brain [127, 154–158], suggesting that the blood–brain barrier is breached in autism spectrum disorders pathogenesis [127, 159–161]. Zonulin, the precursor of haptoglobin 2 (pre-HP2) [162], is the only human protein known to date that can reversibly regulate gut epithelial and endothelial permeability by modulating intercellular TJ [162–165] both in the gut and the blood–brain barrier. Interestingly, the zonulin gene maps on chromosome 16, and genes related to autoimmune diseases, neoplastic conditions, and diseases affecting the brain—such as multiple sclerosis, schizophrenia, and autism spectrum disorders—have been mapped on chromosome 16 [166], strongly indicating alterations on chromosome 16 as a risk factor for disease development. Esnafoglu *et al.* used serum zonulin as a biomarker of gut permeability in subjects with autism spectrum disorders and showed that zonulin was elevated in patients with autism spectrum disorders compared to typically developed children [167].

Recently, increased serum zonulin has also been reported in association with hyperactivity and social dysfunctions in children with attention deficit hyperactivity disorder (ADHD) [168]. Zonulin increases the permeability of the blood–brain barrier *in vitro* [169] and has been shown to be involved in brain tumors, specifically gliomas [170, 171]. Skardelly *et al.* showed increased expression of zonulin in gliomas, which correlated with the degree of malignancy and degradation of the blood–brain barrier [171]. *In vitro* studies on a glioma cell line showed high zonulin expression compared to non-glioma control [170]. Furthermore, zonulin has been shown to induce transmigration of neuronal progenitor cells across the blood–brain barrier [170], which plays a critical role as one line of defense against circulating substances and immune cells that could negatively affect brain function. Dysfunctions of the blood–brain barrier have been associated with numerous neurological disorders, such as epilepsy, multiple sclerosis, and Parkinson's and Alzheimer's Disease [14, 122–126, 172–174], in which microbiota alterations have also been described [29, 84–99]. We reported a dysfunctional gut–brain axis associated with neuroinflammation in autism spectrum disorders, and our data pointed to barrier defects in both the blood–brain barrier and the intestine in *postmortem* brain samples and duodenal biopsies from autism spectrum disorders and typically developed subjects. This supports the notion that there is a differential regulation of the pathways associated with a gut–brain axis dysfunction involving the intestinal barrier, BBB integrity/function, and neuroinflammation in autism spectrum disorders, possibly leading to behavioral abnormalities [127].

Intestinal permeability is frequently associated with alterations in the immune response [175], and the involvement of the immune system in autism spectrum disorders has been well documented [176, 177]. Numerous studies have reported immune dysregulation, neuroinflammation, autoimmunity, and allergies in autism spectrum disorders [154, 155, 157, 177–183]. Furthermore, increased proinflammatory cytokines have been measured in serum, brain tissue, and cerebral spinal fluid in children afflicted with autism spectrum disorders [155, 184–186]. Maternal infection during pregnancy is one of the risk factors for autism spectrum disorders that has gained the most attention as a major candidate for the onset of immune system alterations in the offspring. Prenatal exposure to viral infections increases the risk of autism spectrum disorders and it has been postulated that the prenatal viral infection is the leading non-genetic cause of the condition [137, 187, 188]. Elevated levels of inflammatory cytokines in maternal blood, placenta, and amniotic fluid have been associated with increased risk of autism spectrum disorders [189–194]. Over 50 articles have reported that maternal inflammation may contribute to the neurochemical and behavioral changes that accompany mental retardation, schizophrenia, and/or autism spectrum disorders. Furthermore, the damaging effects of maternal inflammation on the fetal brain have been reported [195, 196] and are likely the result of pro-inflammatory molecules that could easily transfer between the mother and the fetus [197, 198].

The MIA (Maternal-Immune-Activation) mouse model exhibits core behavioral alterations of autism spectrum disorders in the offspring [199, 200] as well as gut microbial alterations similar to those reported in autism spectrum disorders. They also exhibit increased intestinal permeability that is corrected upon administration of *Bacteroides fragilis* [201], a commensal shown to exert neuroinflammatory and gastrointestinal disease protective effects in mouse models of multiple sclerosis [202] and colitis [203], respectively. Mazmanian's group shows that *B. fragilis* treatment in the MIA mouse model has a positive effect on behavioral alterations typical of autism spectrum disorders, suggesting "microbiome-mediated therapies as a safe and effective treatment for ASD" [201]. Furthermore, Smith *et al.* reported that the effects of MIA on the fetal brain are mediated mainly by the proinflammatory interleukin(IL)-6 [204]. Altered cytokine profiles have been reported in autism spectrum disorders subjects [183, 186] associated with more severe behavioral abnormalities [205].

In a collaborative study with Ashwood's group, we have shown that children with autism spectrum disorders *and* gastrointestinal symptoms (ASD[GI]) have an immune and gut microbial signature distinct from children with autism spectrum disorders without gastrointestinal (ASD[NoGI]) disturbances and typical developed subjects. The ASD[GI] group exhibited differences in gut microbiota composition compared to TD[GI] children and had the ability to produce elevated levels of mucosal-relevant cytokines compared to the ASD[NoGI] cohort. Furthermore, the ASD[GI] group scored higher for irritability and agitation, social withdrawal and lethargy, and hyperactivity compared to children in the ASD[NoGI] group, suggesting a possible relationship between the microbiome, the immune system and behavioral outcome in autism spectrum disorders [97]. We also observed a significant difference in the *HP2* gene representation between ASD[GI] children and TD[GI] children, suggesting that the presence of the *HP2* gene (either in heterozygosis or homozygosis) may lead to a predisposition toward increased intestinal permeability. Increased blood levels of LPS, a byproduct of the cell walls of gram-negative bacteria, has been found in some autism spectrum disorders children, a finding that was associated with increased IL-6 production [206]. Increased gastrointestinal permeability in autism spectrum disorders may be another mechanism through which microbiota and the immune system interact in some children. It is interesting to note that the zonulin promoter is under IL-6 control [207] and, therefore, the increased IL-6 in ASD[GI] children may lead to the overexpression of the zonulin (*HP2*) gene in patients who have at least one copy [97]. Elevated levels of IL-6 are known to modify neuronal function and have been associated with increased behavioral impairment in autism spectrum disorders [145].

A small, open-label study in children with autism spectrum disorders showed that treatment with oral vancomycin, a non-absorbable antibiotic that only acts in the gut, temporarily improved both gastrointestinal and behavioral symptoms, suggesting the importance of gut microbiota in the development and progression of the disease [208]. Numerous manipulations of the gut microbiota have been proposed as effective intervention strategies to treat autism spectrum disorders. Among these, the use of probiotics has been considered the most promising and feasible long-term intervention. A study from Pärtty *et al.*, in which infants receiving *Lactobacillus rhamnosus* GG (LGG) or placebo for six months following birth were followed and screened for microbiota and psycho-behavioral diagnoses 2 and 13 years later, showed that about 17% of placebo-treated children had attention deficits or Asperger's syndrome, compared to LGG treated group in which none of the participants received either diagnosis [209]. In this same vein, important insights can be gleaned from our recent exploratory open-label study involving microbiota transfer from typically developed children without gastrointestinal disorders to children with autism spectrum disorders and gastrointestinal problems [210]. This study showed that fecal material transfer shifted gut microbiota of children with autism spectrum disorders toward that of typically developed children, remarkably improving both gastrointestinal and autism spectrum disorder-related behavioral symptoms, providing supporting evidence to the involvement of microbiota in the pathogenesis of these conditions.

CONCLUSION

We are on the verge of transformational science in many fields of human biology. One of the most promising and challenging new frontiers of discovery is the leveraging of the human microbiome to potentially mitigate inflammatory processes pathogenetically linked to a variety of human diseases. One of the most fascinating aspects of the symbiotic relationship between individuals and their microbiome is related to brain functions affecting behavior and performance. An appreciation of the idea that the gut–brain axis facilitates a bidirectional discussion opened new paradigms of science supported by a variety of animal studies and human observations, ultimately suggesting that microbiome composition and, most importantly, function can influence brain performance and state of health. These observations open unprecedented therapeutic opportunities for mitigating a variety of the neurological and behavioral diseases for which we currently only have limited interventions. The major challenge we face in exploiting these opportunities is moving existing microbiome studies from observation to causation in order to mechanistically link microbiome function, metabolic profiles, and clinical outcomes. If we can achieve this goal, we may well identify potential therapeutic targets that can be exploited to manipulate microbiome composition using prebiotic, probiotic or symbiotic interventions specifically formulated to re-establish the physiological gut-brain axis cross-talk.

REFERENCES

1. Pavlov, I. P. *Conditioned Reflexes: An Investigation of the Physiological Activity of the Cerebral Cortex.* 1927. Oxford: Oxford University Press.
2. Olson, C.A., et al., The gut microbiota mediates the anti-seizure effects of the ketogenic diet. *Cell*, 2018. **173**(7): p. 1728–41.e13.
3. Prasad, A.N., C.F. Stafstrom, and G.L. Holmes, Alternative epilepsy therapies: The ketogenic diet, immunoglobulins, and steroids. *Epilepsia*, 1996. **37**(Suppl 1): p. S81–95.
4. Swink, T.D., E.P. Vining, and J.M. Freeman, The ketogenic diet: 1997. *Adv Pediatr*, 1997. **44**: p. 297–329.
5. Liu, Y.M., and H.S. Wang, Medium-chain triglyceride ketogenic diet, an effective treatment for drug-resistant epilepsy and a comparison with other ketogenic diets. *Biomed J*, 2013. **36**(1): p. 9–15.
6. Neal, E.G., and J.H. Cross, Efficacy of dietary treatments for epilepsy. *J Hum Nutr Diet*, 2010. **23**(2): p. 113–9.
7. Schwartz, R.H., et al., Ketogenic diets in the treatment of epilepsy: Short-term clinical effects. *Dev Med Child Neurol*, 1989. **31**(2): p. 145–51.
8. Martin-McGill, K.J., et al., Ketogenic diets for drug-resistant epilepsy. *Cochrane Database Syst Rev*, 2018. **11**: p. CD001903.
9. Lambrechts, D.A., et al., The MCT-ketogenic diet as a treatment option in refractory childhood epilepsy: A prospective study with 2-year follow-up. *Epilepsy Behav*, 2015. **51**: p. 261–6.

10. Wijnen, B.F.M., et al., Long-term clinical outcomes and economic evaluation of the ketogenic diet *versus* care as usual in children and adolescents with intractable epilepsy. *Epilepsy Res*, 2017. **132**: p. 91–9.

11. Martin, K., et al., Ketogenic diet and other dietary treatments for epilepsy. *Cochrane Database Syst Rev*, 2016. **2**: p. CD001903.

12. Olson, C.A., et al., The gut microbiota mediates the anti-seizure effects of the ketogenic diet. *Cell*, 2018. **174**(2): p. 497.

13. Toepfer, M., et al., Gastrointestinal dysfunction in amyotrophic lateral sclerosis. *Amyotroph Lateral Scler Other Motor Neuron Disord*, 1999. **1**(1): p. 15–9.

14. Fang, X., Potential role of gut microbiota and tissue barriers in Parkinson's disease and amyotrophic lateral sclerosis. *Int J Neurosci*, 2016. **126**(9): p. 771–6.

15. Fang, X., et al., Evaluation of the microbial diversity in amyotrophic lateral sclerosis using high-throughput sequencing. *Front Microbiol*, 2016. **7**: p. 1479.

16. Rowin, J., et al., Gut inflammation and dysbiosis in human motor neuron disease. *Physiol Rep*, 2017. **5**(18).

17. Fasano, A., et al., Gastrointestinal dysfunction in Parkinson's disease. *Lancet Neurol*, 2015. **14**(6): p. 625–39.

18. Mertsalmi, T.H., et al., More than constipation – Bowel symptoms in Parkinson's disease and their connection to gut microbiota. *Eur J Neurol*, 2017. **24**(11): p. 1375–83.

19. Zingone, F., et al., Psychological morbidity of celiac disease: A review of the literature. *United European Gastroenterol J*, 2015. **3**(2): p. 136–45.

20. Kurtzke, J.F., Rating neurologic impairment in multiple sclerosis: An expanded disability status scale (EDSS). *Neurology*, 1983. **33**(11): p. 1444–52.

21. Bergamaschi, R., et al., The DYMUS questionnaire for the assessment of dysphagia in multiple sclerosis. *J Neurol Sci*, 2008. **269**(1–2): p. 49–53.

22. Nusrat, S., et al., Anorectal dysfunction in multiple sclerosis: A systematic review. *ISRN Neurol*, 2012. **2012**: p. 376023.

23. Buie, T., et al., Recommendations for evaluation and treatment of common gastrointestinal problems in children with ASDs. *Pediatrics*, 2010. **125**(Suppl 1): p. S19–29.

24. Molloy, C.A., and P. Manning-Courtney, Prevalence of chronic gastrointestinal symptoms in children with autism and autistic spectrum disorders. *Autism*, 2003. **7**(2): p. 165–71.

25. Zhang, R., et al., Circulating endotoxin and systemic immune activation in sporadic amyotrophic lateral sclerosis (sALS). *J Neuroimmunol*, 2009. **206**(1–2): p. 121–4.

26. Dinan, T.G., and J.F. Cryan, The impact of gut microbiota on brain and behaviour: Implications for psychiatry. *Curr Opin Clin Nutr Metab Care*, 2015. **18**(6): p. 552–8.

27. Desbonnet, L., et al., Gut microbiota depletion from early adolescence in mice: Implications for brain and behaviour. *Brain Behav Immun*, 2015. **48**: p. 165–73.

28. Li, L., et al., Gut microbes in correlation with mood: Case study in a closed experimental human life support system. *Neurogastroenterol Motil*, 2016. **28**(8): p. 1233–40.

29. Kang, D.W., et al., Reduced incidence of *Prevotella* and other fermenters in intestinal microflora of autistic children. *PLOS ONE*, 2013. **8**(7): p. e68322.

30. Hill, J.M., et al., The gastrointestinal tract microbiome and potential link to Alzheimer's disease. *Front Neurol*, 2014. **5**: p. 43.

31. Williams, B.L., et al., Application of novel PCR-based methods for detection, quantitation, and phylogenetic characterization of *Sutterella species* in intestinal biopsy samples from children with autism and gastrointestinal disturbances. *MBio*, 2012. **3**(1).

32. Finegold, S.M., J. Downes, and P.H. Summanen, Microbiology of regressive autism. *Anaerobe*, 2012. **18**(2): p. 260–2.

33. Parracho, H.M., et al., Differences between the gut microflora of children with autistic spectrum disorders and that of healthy children. *J Med Microbiol*, 2005. **54**(Pt 10): p. 987–91.

34. Morgan, M.Y., The treatment of chronic hepatic encephalopathy. *Hepatogastroenterology*, 1991. **38**(5): p. 377–87.

35. Shanahan, F., The host-microbe interface within the gut. *Best Pract Res Clin Gastroenterol*, 2002. **16**(6): p. 915–31.

36. Gordon, H.A., and E. Bruckner-Kardoss, Effect of normal microbial flora on intestinal surface area. *Am J Physiol*, 1961. **201**: p. 175–8.

37. Gordon, H.A., and E. Bruckner-Kardoss, Effect of the normal microbial flora on various tissue elements of the small intestine. *Acta Anat (Basel)*, 1961. **44**: p. 210–25.

38. Wostmann, B., and E. Bruckner-Kardoss, Development of cecal distention in germ-free baby rats. *Am J Physiol*, 1959. **197**: p. 1345–6.

39. Abrams, G.D., H. Bauer, and H. Sprinz, Influence of the normal flora on mucosal morphology and cellular renewal in the ileum. A comparison of germ-free and conventional mice. *Lab Invest*, 1963. **12**: p. 355–64.

40. Yano, J.M., et al., Indigenous bacteria from the gut microbiota regulate host serotonin biosynthesis. *Cell*, 2015. **161**(2): p. 264–76.

41. Reigstad, C.S., et al., Gut microbes promote colonic serotonin production through an effect of short-chain fatty acids on enterochromaffin cells. *FASEB J*, 2015. **29**(4): p. 1395–403.

42. Rakoff-Nahoum, S., et al., Recognition of commensal microflora by toll-like receptors is required for intestinal homeostasis. *Cell*, 2004. **118**(2): p. 229–41.

43. Mohle, L., et al., Ly6C(hi) monocytes provide a link between antibiotic-induced changes in gut microbiota and adult hippocampal neurogenesis. *Cell Rep*, 2016. **15**(9): p. 1945–56.

44. Frohlich, E.E., et al., Cognitive impairment by antibiotic-induced gut dysbiosis: Analysis of gut microbiota-brain communication. *Brain Behav Immun*, 2016. **56**: p. 140–55.

45. O'Leary, O.F., and J.F. Cryan, A ventral view on antidepressant action: Roles for adult hippocampal neurogenesis along the dorsoventral axis. *Trends Pharmacol Sci*, 2014. **35**(12): p. 675–87.

46. Moser, M.B., et al., Spatial learning with a minislab in the dorsal hippocampus. *Proc Natl Acad Sci U S A*, 1995. **92**(21): p. 9697–701.

47. Erny, D., et al., Host microbiota constantly control maturation and function of microglia in the CNS. *Nat Neurosci*, 2015. **18**(7): p. 965–77.

48. Braniste, V., et al., The gut microbiota influences blood-brain barrier permeability in mice. *Sci Transl Med*, 2014. **6**(263): p. 263ra158.

49. Hoban, A.E., et al., Regulation of prefrontal cortex myelination by the microbiota. *Transl Psychiatry*, 2016. **6**: p. e774.

50. Lu, J., et al., Microbiota influence the development of the brain and behaviors in C57BL/6J mice. *PLOS ONE*, 2018. **13**(8): p. e0201829.

51. Desbonnet, L., et al., Microbiota is essential for social development in the mouse. *Mol Psychiatry*, 2014. **19**(2): p. 146–8.

52. Sudo, N., et al., Postnatal microbial colonization programs the hypothalamic-pituitary-adrenal system for stress response in mice. *J Physiol*, 2004. **558**(Pt 1): p. 263–75.

53. Clarke, G., et al., The microbiome-gut-brain axis during early life regulates the hippocampal serotonergic system in a sex-dependent manner. *Mol Psychiatry*, 2013. **18**(6): p. 666–73.

54. Neufeld, K.M., et al., Reduced anxiety-like behavior and central neurochemical change in germ-free mice. *Neurogastroenterol Motil*, 2011. **23**(3): p. 255–64.e119.

55. Bercik, P., et al., The intestinal microbiota affect central levels of brain-derived neurotropic factor and behavior in mice. *Gastroenterology*, 2011. **141**(2): p. 599–609, 609.e1–3.

56. Luk, B., et al., Postnatal colonization with human "infant-type" *Bifidobacterium species* alters behavior of adult gnotobiotic mice. *PLOS ONE*, 2018. **13**(5): p. e0196510.

57. Chang, B., et al., The protective effect of VSL#3 on intestinal permeability in a rat model of alcoholic intestinal injury. *BMC Gastroenterol*, 2013. **13**: p. 151.
58. Uronis, J.M., et al., Gut microbial diversity is reduced by the probiotic *VSL#3* and correlates with decreased TNBS-induced colitis. *Inflamm Bowel Dis*, 2011. **17**(1): p. 289–97.
59. Sampson, T.R., et al., Gut microbiota regulate motor deficits and neuroinflammation in a model of Parkinson's disease. *Cell*, 2016. **167**(6): p. 1469–80.e12.
60. Drossman, D.A., Presidential address: Gastrointestinal illness and the biopsychosocial model. *Psychosom Med*, 1998. **60**(3): p. 258–67.
61. Bhatia, V., and R.K. Tandon, Stress and the gastrointestinal tract. *J Gastroenterol Hepatol*, 2005. **20**(3): p. 332–9.
62. Takajo, T., et al., Depression promotes the onset of irritable bowel syndrome through unique dysbiosis in rats. *Gut Liver*, 2019.
63. De Palma, G., et al., Microbiota and host determinants of behavioural phenotype in maternally separated mice. *Nat Commun*, 2015. **6**: p. 7735.
64. Watanabe, Y., et al., Chronic psychological stress disrupted the composition of the murine colonic microbiota and accelerated a murine model of inflammatory bowel disease. *PLOS ONE*, 2016. **11**(3): p. e0150559.
65. Moya-Perez, A., et al., *Bifidobacterium* CECT 7765 modulates early stress-induced immune, neuroendocrine and behavioral alterations in mice. *Brain Behav Immun*, 2017. **65**: p. 43–56.
66. Dodiya, H.B., et al., Chronic stress-induced gut dysfunction exacerbates Parkinson's disease phenotype and pathology in a rotenone-induced mouse model of Parkinson's disease. *Neurobiol Dis*, 2018.
67. Galley, J.D., et al., The structures of the colonic mucosa-associated and luminal microbial communities are distinct and differentially affected by a prolonged murine stressor. *Gut Microbes*, 2014. **5**(6): p. 748–60.
68. Bailey, M.T., et al., Exposure to a social stressor alters the structure of the intestinal microbiota: Implications for stressor-induced immunomodulation. *Brain Behav Immun*, 2011. **25**(3): p. 397–407.
69. Bailey, M.T., and C.L. Coe, Maternal separation disrupts the integrity of the intestinal microflora in infant rhesus monkeys. *Dev Psychobiol*, 1999. **35**(2): p. 146–55.
70. Forsythe, P., and J. Bienenstock, Immunomodulation by commensal and probiotic bacteria. *Immunol Invest*, 2010. **39**(4–5): p. 429–48.
71. Bhattacharjee, S., and W.J. Lukiw, Alzheimer's disease and the microbiome. *Front Cell Neurosci*, 2013. **7**: p. 153.
72. Borre, Y.E., et al., The impact of microbiota on brain and behavior: Mechanisms & therapeutic potential. *Adv Exp Med Biol*, 2014. **817**: p. 373–403.
73. Reichmann, F., et al., Environmental enrichment induces behavioural disturbances in neuropeptide Y knockout mice. *Sci Rep*, 2016. **6**: p. 28182.
74. Stilling, R.M., T.G. Dinan, and J.F. Cryan, Microbial genes, brain & behaviour – Epigenetic regulation of the gut-brain axis. *Genes Brain Behav*, 2014. **13**(1): p. 69–86.
75. Macfabe, D.F., Short-chain fatty acid fermentation products of the gut microbiome: Implications in autism spectrum disorders. *Microb Ecol Health Dis*, 2012. **23**.
76. Castillo-Ruiz, A., et al., The microbiota influences cell death and microglial colonization in the perinatal mouse brain. *Brain Behav Immun*, 2018. **67**: p. 218–29.
77. Al-Asmakh, M., and L. Hedin, Microbiota and the control of blood-tissue barriers. *Tissue Barriers*, 2015. **3**(3): p. e1039691.
78. Forsythe, P., J. Bienenstock, and W.A. Kunze, Vagal pathways for microbiome-brain-gut axis communication. *Adv Exp Med Biol*, 2014. **817**: p. 115–33.
79. Bravo, J.A., et al., Ingestion of *Lactobacillus strain* regulates emotional behavior and central GABA receptor expression in a mouse via the vagus nerve. *Proc Natl Acad Sci U S A*, 2011. **108**(38): p. 16050–5.

80. Bercik, P., et al., The anxiolytic effect of *Bifidobacterium longum* NCC3001 involves vagal pathways for gut-brain communication. *Neurogastroenterol Motil*, 2011. **23**(12): p. 1132–9.

81. Nohr, M.K., et al., Expression of the short chain fatty acid receptor GPR41/FFAR3 in autonomic and somatic sensory ganglia. *Neuroscience*, 2015. **290**: p. 126–37.

82. Svensson, E., et al., Vagotomy and subsequent risk of Parkinson's disease. *Ann Neurol*, 2015. **78**(4): p. 522–9.

83. Holmqvist, S., et al., Direct evidence of Parkinson pathology spread from the gastrointestinal tract to the brain in rats. *Acta Neuropathol*, 2014. **128**(6): p. 805–20.

84. Cassani, E., et al., Increased urinary indoxyl sulfate (indican): New insights into gut dysbiosis in Parkinson's disease. *Parkinsonism Relat Disord*, 2015. **21**(4): p. 389–93.

85. Keshavarzian, A., et al., Colonic bacterial composition in Parkinson's disease. *Mov Disord*, 2015. **30**(10): p. 1351–60.

86. Scheperjans, F., et al., Gut microbiota are related to Parkinson's disease and clinical phenotype. *Mov Disord*, 2015. **30**(3): p. 350–8.

87. Unger, M.M., et al., Short chain fatty acids and gut microbiota differ between patients with Parkinson's disease and age-matched controls. *Parkinsonism Relat Disord*, 2016. **32**: p. 66–72.

88. Miyake, S., et al., Dysbiosis in the gut microbiota of patients with multiple sclerosis, with a striking depletion of species belonging to *Clostridia* XIVa and IV clusters. *PLOS ONE*, 2015. **10**(9): p. e0137429.

89. Chen, J., et al., Multiple sclerosis patients have a distinct gut microbiota compared to healthy controls. *Sci Rep*, 2016. **6**: p. 28484.

90. Jangi, S., et al., Alterations of the human gut microbiome in multiple sclerosis. *Nat Commun*, 2016. **7**: p. 12015.

91. Vogt, N.M., et al., Gut microbiome alterations in Alzheimer's disease. *Sci Rep*, 2017. **7**(1): p. 13537.

92. Cattaneo, A., et al., Association of brain amyloidosis with pro-inflammatory gut bacterial taxa and peripheral inflammation markers in cognitively impaired elderly. *Neurobiol Aging*, 2017. **49**: p. 60–8.

93. Zhuang, Z.Q., et al., Gut microbiota is altered in patients with Alzheimer's disease. *J Alzheimers Dis*, 2018. **63**(4): p. 1337–46.

94. Wang, L., et al., Increased abundance of *Sutterella spp.* and *Ruminococcus torques* in feces of children with autism spectrum disorder. *Mol Autism*, 2013. **4**(1): p. 42.

95. Tomova, A., et al., Gastrointestinal microbiota in children with autism in Slovakia. *Physiol Behav*, 2015. **138**: p. 179–87.

96. Luna, R.A., et al., Distinct microbiome-neuroimmune signatures correlate with functional abdominal pain in children with autism spectrum disorder. *Cell Mol Gastroenterol Hepatol*, 2017. **3**(2): p. 218–30.

97. Rose, D.R., et al., Differential immune responses and microbiota profiles in children with autism spectrum disorders and co-morbid gastrointestinal symptoms. *Brain Behav Immun*, 2018. **70**: p. 354–68.

98. Kang, D.W., et al., Differences in fecal microbial metabolites and microbiota of children with autism spectrum disorders. *Anaerobe*, 2018. **49**: p. 121–31.

99. Lv, F., et al., The role of microbiota in the pathogenesis of schizophrenia and major depressive disorder and the possibility of targeting microbiota as a treatment option. *Oncotarget*, 2017. **8**(59): p. 100899–907.

100. Jakobsson, H.E., et al., The composition of the gut microbiota shapes the colon mucus barrier. *EMBO Rep*, 2015. **16**(2): p. 164–77.

101. Alvarez, C.S., et al., Outer membrane vesicles and soluble factors released by probiotic *Escherichia coli* Nissle 1917 and commensal ECOR63 enhance barrier function by regulating expression of tight junction proteins in intestinal epithelial cells. *Front Microbiol*, 2016. **7**: p. 1981.

102. Everard, A., et al., Cross-talk between *Akkermansia muciniphila* and intestinal epithelium controls diet-induced obesity. *Proc Natl Acad Sci U S A*, 2013. **110**(22): p. 9066–71.

103. Bischoff, S.C., et al., Intestinal permeability–A new target for disease prevention and therapy. *BMC Gastroenterol*, 2014. **14**: p. 189.

104. Deng, H., et al., *Bacteroides fragilis* prevents *Clostridium difficile* infection in a mouse model by restoring gut barrier and microbiome regulation. *Front Microbiol*, 2018. **9**: p. 2976.

105. Chiaro, T.R., et al., A member of the gut mycobiota modulates host purine metabolism exacerbating colitis in mice. *Sci Transl Med*, 2017. **9**(380).

106. Martin, R., et al., *Bifidobacterium animalis ssp.* lactis CNCM-I2494 restores gut barrier permeability in chronically low-grade inflamed mice. *Front Microbiol*, 2016. **7**: p. 608.

107. Karczewski, J., et al., Regulation of human epithelial tight junction proteins by *Lactobacillus plantarum in vivo* and protective effects on the epithelial barrier. *Am J Physiol Gastrointest Liver Physiol*, 2010. **298**(6): p. G851–9.

108. Marizzoni, M., et al., Microbiota and neurodegenerative diseases. *Curr Opin Neurol*, 2017. **30**(6): p. 630–8.

109. Sochocka, M., et al., The gut microbiome alterations and inflammation-driven pathogenesis of Alzheimer's disease–A critical review. *Mol Neurobiol*, 2019. **56**(3): p. 1841–51.

110. Potgieter, M., et al., The dormant blood microbiome in chronic, inflammatory diseases. *FEMS Microbiol Rev*, 2015. **39**(4): p. 567–91.

111. Konig, J., et al., Human intestinal barrier function in health and disease. *Clin Transl Gastroenterol*, 2016. **7**(10): p. e196.

112. Wardill, H.R., et al., Cytokine-mediated blood brain barrier disruption as a conduit for cancer/chemotherapy-associated neurotoxicity and cognitive dysfunction. *Int J Cancer*, 2016. **139**(12): p. 2635–45.

113. Elahy, M., et al., Blood-brain barrier dysfunction developed during normal aging is associated with inflammation and loss of tight junctions but not with leukocyte recruitment. *Immun Ageing*, 2015. **12**: p. 2.

114. Wang, J., et al., Connection between systemic inflammation and neuroinflammation underlies neuroprotective mechanism of several phytochemicals in neurodegenerative diseases. *Oxid Med Cell Longev*, 2018. **2018**: p. 1972714.

115. Severance, E.G., et al., Discordant patterns of bacterial translocation markers and implications for innate immune imbalances in schizophrenia. *Schizophr Res*, 2013. **148**(1–3): p. 130–7.

116. Melkersson, K., and S. Bensing, Signs of impaired blood-brain barrier function and lower IgG synthesis within the central nervous system in patients with schizophrenia or related psychosis, compared to that in controls. *Neuro Endocrinol Lett*, 2018. **39**(1): p. 33–42.

117. Wu, S., et al., Leaky intestine and impaired microbiome in an amyotrophic lateral sclerosis mouse model. *Physiol Rep*, 2015. **3**(4).

118. Bataveljic, D., et al., Novel molecular biomarkers at the blood-brain barrier in ALS. *BioMed Res Int*, 2014. **2014**: p. 907545.

119. Henkel, J.S., et al., Decreased mRNA expression of tight junction proteins in lumbar spinal cords of patients with ALS. *Neurology*, 2009. **72**(18): p. 1614–6.

120. Garbuzova-Davis, S., et al., Impaired blood-brain/spinal cord barrier in ALS patients. *Brain Res*, 2012. **1469**: p. 114–28.

121. Graves, M.C., et al., Inflammation in amyotrophic lateral sclerosis spinal cord and brain is mediated by activated macrophages, mast cells and T cells. *Amyotroph Lateral Scler Other Motor Neuron Disord*, 2004. **5**(4): p. 213–9.

122. Gray, M.T., and J.M. Woulfe, Striatal blood-brain barrier permeability in Parkinson's disease. *J Cereb Blood Flow Metab*, 2015. **35**(5): p. 747–50.
123. Soon, D., et al., Quantification of subtle blood-brain barrier disruption in non-enhancing lesions in multiple sclerosis: A study of disease and lesion subtypes. *Mult Scler*, 2007. **13**(7): p. 884–94.
124. Minagar, A., and J.S. Alexander, Blood-brain barrier disruption in multiple sclerosis. *Mult Scler*, 2003. **9**(6): p. 540–9.
125. Wada, H., Blood-brain barrier permeability of the demented elderly as studied by cerebrospinal fluid-serum albumin ratio. *Intern Med*, 1998. **37**(6): p. 509–13.
126. Bell, R.D., and B.V. Zlokovic, Neurovascular mechanisms and blood-brain barrier disorder in Alzheimer's disease. *Acta Neuropathol*, 2009. **118**(1): p. 103–13.
127. Fiorentino, M., et al., Blood-brain barrier and intestinal epithelial barrier alterations in autism spectrum disorders. *Mol Autism*, 2016. **7**: p. 49.
128. Baio, J., et al., Prevalence of autism spectrum disorder among children aged 8 years – autism and developmental disabilities monitoring network, 11 sites, United States, 2014. *MMWR Surveill Summ*, 2018. **67**(6): p. 1–23.
129. Abrahams, B.S., and D.H. Geschwind, Advances in autism genetics: On the threshold of a new neurobiology. *Nat Rev Genet*, 2008. **9**(5): p. 341–55.
130. Muhle, R., S.V. Trentacoste, and I. Rapin, The genetics of autism. *Pediatrics*, 2004. **113**(5): p. e472–86.
131. Rosenberg, R.E., et al., Trends in autism spectrum disorder diagnoses: 1994–2007. *J Autism Dev Disord*, 2009. **39**(8): p. 1099–111.
132. Ronald, A., and R.A. Hoekstra, Autism spectrum disorders and autistic traits: A decade of new twin studies. *Am J Med Genet B Neuropsychiatr Genet*, 2011. **156B**(3): p. 255–74.
133. Sanders, S.J., et al., Insights into autism spectrum disorder genomic architecture and biology from 71 risk loci. *Neuron*, 2015. **87**(6): p. 1215–33.
134. Sebat, J., et al., Strong association of de novo copy number mutations with autism. *Science*, 2007. **316**(5823): p. 445–9.
135. Weiss, L.A., et al., Association between microdeletion and microduplication at 16p11.2 and autism. *N Engl J Med*, 2008. **358**(7): p. 667–75.
136. Raz, R., et al., Autism spectrum disorder and particulate matter air pollution before, during, and after pregnancy: A nested case-control analysis within the Nurses' Health Study II cohort. *Environ Health Perspect*, 2015. **123**(3): p. 264–70.
137. Atladottir, H.O., et al., Autism after infection, febrile episodes, and antibiotic use during pregnancy: An exploratory study. *Pediatrics*, 2012. **130**(6): p. e1447–54.
138. Shelton, J.F., et al., Neurodevelopmental disorders and prenatal residential proximity to agricultural pesticides: The CHARGE study. *Environ Health Perspect*, 2014. **122**(10): p. 1103–9.
139. Arndt, T.L., C.J. Stodgell, and P.M. Rodier, The teratology of autism. *Int J Dev Neurosci*, 2005. **23**(2–3): p. 189–99.
140. Chess, S., Autism in children with congenital rubella. *J Autism Child Schizophr*, 1971. **1**(1): p. 33–47.
141. Roberts, E.M., et al., Maternal residence near agricultural pesticide applications and autism spectrum disorders among children in the California Central Valley. *Environ Health Perspect*, 2007. **115**(10): p. 1482–9.
142. Hsiao, E.Y., Gastrointestinal issues in autism spectrum disorder. *Harv Rev Psychiatry*, 2014. **22**(2): p. 104–11.
143. White, J.F., Intestinal pathophysiology in autism. *Exp Biol Med (Maywood)*, 2003. **228**(6): p. 639–49.
144. Buie, T., et al., Evaluation, diagnosis, and treatment of gastrointestinal disorders in individuals with ASDs: A consensus report. *Pediatrics*, 2010. **125**(Suppl 1): p. S1–18.

145. Onore, C., M. Careaga, and P. Ashwood, The role of immune dysfunction in the patho-physiology of autism. *Brain Behav Immun*, 2012. **26**(3): p. 383–92.
146. Mead, J., and P. Ashwood, Evidence supporting an altered immune response in ASD. *Immunol Lett*, 2015. **163**(1): p. 49–55.
147. Kohane, I.S., et al., The co-morbidity burden of children and young adults with autism spectrum disorders. *PLOS ONE*, 2012. **7**(4): p. e33224.
148. Adams, J.B., et al., Gastrointestinal flora and gastrointestinal status in children with autism–Comparisons to typical children and correlation with autism severity. *BMC Gastroenterol*, 2011. **11**: p. 22.
149. Gondalia, S.V., et al., Molecular characterisation of gastrointestinal microbiota of chil-dren with autism (with and without gastrointestinal dysfunction) and their neurotypical siblings. *Autism Res*, 2012. **5**(6): p. 419–27.
150. Williams, B.L., et al., Impaired carbohydrate digestion and transport and mucosal dys-biosis in the intestines of children with autism and gastrointestinal disturbances. *PLOS ONE*, 2011. **6**(9): p. e24585.
151. Iovene, M.R., et al., Intestinal dysbiosis and yeast isolation in stool of subjects with autism spectrum disorders. *Mycopathologia*, 2017. **182**(3–4): p. 349–63.
152. de Magistris, L., et al., Alterations of the intestinal barrier in patients with autism spec-trum disorders and in their first-degree relatives. *J Pediatr Gastroenterol Nutr*, 2010. **51**(4): p. 418–24.
153. D'Eufemia, P., et al., Abnormal intestinal permeability in children with autism. *Acta Paediatr*, 1996. **85**(9): p. 1076–9.
154. Pardo, C.A., D.L. Vargas, and A.W. Zimmerman, Immunity, neuroglia and neuroin-flammation in autism. *Int Rev Psychiatry*, 2005. **17**(6): p. 485–95.
155. Vargas, D.L., et al., Neuroglial activation and neuroinflammation in the brain of patients with autism. *Ann Neurol*, 2005. **57**(1): p. 67–81.
156. Zimmerman, A.W., et al., Cerebrospinal fluid and serum markers of inflammation in autism. *Pediatr Neurol*, 2005. **33**(3): p. 195–201.
157. Chez, M.G., et al., Elevation of tumor necrosis factor-alpha in cerebrospinal fluid of autistic children. *Pediatr Neurol*, 2007. **36**(6): p. 361–5.
158. Morgan, J.T., et al., Microglial activation and increased microglial density observed in the dorsolateral prefrontal cortex in autism. *Biol Psychiatry*, 2010. **68**(4): p. 368–76.
159. Singer, H.S., et al., Antibodies against fetal brain in sera of mothers with autistic chil-dren. *J Neuroimmunol*, 2008. **194**(1–2): p. 165–72.
160. Zimmerman, A.W., et al., Maternal antibrain antibodies in autism. *Brain Behav Immun*, 2007. **21**(3): p. 351–7.
161. Braunschweig, D., and J. Van de Water, Maternal autoantibodies in autism. *Arch Neurol*, 2012. **69**(6): p. 693–9.
162. Tripathi, A., et al., Identification of human zonulin, a physiological modulator of tight junctions, as prehaptoglobin-2. *Proc Natl Acad Sci U S A*, 2009. **106**(39): p. 16799–804.
163. Sturgeon, C., and A. Fasano, Zonulin, a regulator of epithelial and endothelial barrier functions, and its involvement in chronic inflammatory diseases. *Tissue Barriers*, 2016. **4**(4): p. e1251384.
164. Ciccia, F., et al., Dysbiosis and zonulin upregulation alter gut epithelial and vascu-lar barriers in patients with ankylosing spondylitis. *Ann Rheum Dis*, 2017. **76**(6): p. 1123–32.
165. Fasano, A., Regulation of intercellular tight junctions by zonula occludens toxin and its eukaryotic analogue zonulin. *Ann N Y Acad Sci*, 2000. **915**: p. 214–22.
166. Fasano, A., Zonulin and its regulation of intestinal barrier function: The biological door to inflammation, autoimmunity, and cancer. *Physiol Rev*, 2011. **91**(1): p. 151–75.
167. Esnafoglu, E., et al., Increased serum zonulin levels as an intestinal permeability marker in autistic subjects. *J Pediatr*, 2017. **188**: p. 240–4.

168. Ozyurt, G., et al., Increased zonulin is associated with hyperactivity and social dysfunctions in children with attention deficit hyperactivity disorder. *Compr Psychiatry*, 2018. **87**: p. 138–42.

169. Rahman, M.T., et al., IFN-gamma, IL-17A, or zonulin rapidly increase the permeability of the blood-brain and small intestinal epithelial barriers: Relevance for neuro-inflammatory diseases. *Biochem Biophys Res Commun*, 2018. **507**(1–4): p. 274–9.

170. Diaz-Coranguez, M., et al., Transmigration of neural stem cells across the blood brain barrier induced by glioma cells. *PLOS ONE*, 2013. **8**(4): p. e60655.

171. Skardelly, M., et al., Expression of zonulin, c-kit, and glial fibrillary acidic protein in human gliomas. *Transl Oncol*, 2009. **2**(3): p. 117–20.

172. Moor, A.C., et al., The blood-brain barrier and multiple sclerosis. *Biochem Pharmacol*, 1994. **47**(10): p. 1717–24.

173. Weissberg, I., et al., Blood-brain barrier dysfunction in epileptogenesis of the temporal lobe. *Epilepsy Res Treat*, 2011. **2011**: p. 143908.

174. Heinemann, U., D. Kaufer, and A. Friedman, Blood-brain barrier dysfunction, TGFbeta signaling, and astrocyte dysfunction in epilepsy. *Glia*, 2012. **60**(8): p. 1251–7.

175. Turner, J.R., Intestinal mucosal barrier function in health and disease. *Nat Rev Immunol*, 2009. **9**(11): p. 799–809.

176. Patterson, P.H., Immune involvement in schizophrenia and autism: Etiology, pathology and animal models. *Behav Brain Res*, 2009. **204**(2): p. 313–21.

177. Atladottir, H.O., et al., Association of family history of autoimmune diseases and autism spectrum disorders. *Pediatrics*, 2009. **124**(2): p. 687–94.

178. Croen, L.A., et al., Maternal autoimmune diseases, asthma and allergies, and childhood autism spectrum disorders: A case-control study. *Arch Pediatr Adolesc Med*, 2005. **159**(2): p. 151–7.

179. Garbett, K.A., et al., Effects of maternal immune activation on gene expression patterns in the fetal brain. *Transl Psychiatry*, 2012. **2**: p. e98.

180. Noriega, D.B., and H.F. Savelkoul, Immune dysregulation in autism spectrum disorder. *Eur J Pediatr*, 2014. **173**(1): p. 33–43.

181. Estes, M.L., and A.K. McAllister, Immune mediators in the brain and peripheral tissues in autism spectrum disorder. *Nat Rev Neurosci*, 2015. **16**(8): p. 469–86.

182. Kern, J.K., et al., Relevance of neuroinflammation and encephalitis in autism. *Front Cell Neurosci*, 2015. **9**: p. 519.

183. Wang, T.T., et al., [Research advances in immunological dysfunction in children with autism spectrum disorders]. *Zhongguo Dang Dai Er Ke Za Zhi*, 2014. **16**(12): p. 1289–93.

184. Li, X., et al., Elevated immune response in the brain of autistic patients. *J Neuroimmunol*, 2009. **207**(1–2): p. 111–6.

185. Xu, N., X. Li, and Y. Zhong, Inflammatory cytokines: Potential biomarkers of immunologic dysfunction in autism spectrum disorders. *Mediators Inflamm*, 2015. **2015**: p. 531518.

186. Ashwood, P., et al., Associations of impaired behaviors with elevated plasma chemokines in autism spectrum disorders. *J Neuroimmunol*, 2011. **232**(1–2): p. 196–9.

187. Moy, S.S., and J.J. Nadler, Advances in behavioral genetics: Mouse models of autism. *Mol Psychiatry*, 2008. **13**(1): p. 4–26.

188. Ciaranello, A.L., and R.D. Ciaranello, The neurobiology of infantile autism. *Annu Rev Neurosci*, 1995. **18**: p. 101–28.

189. Abdallah, M.W., et al., Neonatal levels of cytokines and risk of autism spectrum disorders: An exploratory register-based historic birth cohort study utilizing the Danish Newborn Screening biobank. *J Neuroimmunol*, 2012. **252**(1–2): p. 75–82.

190. Jones, K.L., et al., Autism with intellectual disability is associated with increased levels of maternal cytokines and chemokines during gestation. *Mol Psychiatry*, 2017. **22**(2): p. 273–9.

191. Bronson, S.L., and T.L. Bale, Prenatal stress-induced increases in placental inflammation and offspring hyperactivity are male-specific and ameliorated by maternal antiinflammatory treatment. *Endocrinology*, 2014. **155**(7): p. 2635–46.

192. Ponzio, N.M., et al., Cytokine levels during pregnancy influence immunological profiles and neurobehavioral patterns of the offspring. *Ann N Y Acad Sci*, 2007. **1107**: p. 118–28.

193. Buehler, M.R., A proposed mechanism for autism: An aberrant neuroimmune response manifested as a psychiatric disorder. *Med Hypotheses*, 2011. **76**(6): p. 863–70.

194. Goines, P.E., et al., Increased midgestational IFN-gamma, IL-4 and IL-5 in women bearing a child with autism: A case-control study. *Mol Autism*, 2011. **2**: p. 13.

195. Wang, X., et al., Lipopolysaccharide-induced inflammation and perinatal brain injury. *Semin Fetal Neonatal Med*, 2006. **11**(5): p. 343–53.

196. Huleihel, M., H. Golan, and M. Hallak, Intrauterine infection/inflammation during pregnancy and offspring brain damages: Possible mechanisms involved. *Reprod Biol Endocrinol*, 2004. **2**: p. 17.

197. Wang, X., et al., Effects of intrauterine inflammation on the developing mouse brain. *Brain Res*, 2007. **1144**: p. 180–5.

198. Inder, T.E., et al., Defining the nature of the cerebral abnormalities in the premature infant: A qualitative magnetic resonance imaging study. *J Pediatr*, 2003. **143**(2): p. 171–9.

199. Shi, L., et al., Activation of the maternal immune system alters cerebellar development in the offspring. *Brain Behav Immun*, 2009. **23**(1): p. 116–23.

200. Malkova, N.V., et al., Maternal immune activation yields offspring displaying mouse versions of the three core symptoms of autism. *Brain Behav Immun*, 2012. **26**(4): p. 607–16.

201. Hsiao, E.Y., et al., Microbiota modulate behavioral and physiological abnormalities associated with neurodevelopmental disorders. *Cell*, 2013. **155**(7): p. 1451–63.

202. Ochoa-Reparaz, J., et al., Central nervous system demyelinating disease protection by the human commensal *Bacteroides fragilis* depends on polysaccharide A expression. *J Immunol*, 2010. **185**(7): p. 4101–8.

203. Mazmanian, S.K., J.L. Round, and D.L. Kasper, A microbial symbiosis factor prevents intestinal inflammatory disease. *Nature*, 2008. **453**(7195): p. 620–5.

204. Smith, S.E., et al., Maternal immune activation alters fetal brain development through interleukin-6. *J Neurosci*, 2007. **27**(40): p. 10695–702.

205. Ashwood, P., et al., Elevated plasma cytokines in autism spectrum disorders provide evidence of immune dysfunction and are associated with impaired behavioral outcome. *Brain Behav Immun*, 2011. **25**(1): p. 40–5.

206. Emanuele, E., et al., Low-grade endotoxemia in patients with severe autism. *Neurosci Lett*, 2010. **471**(3): p. 162–5.

207. Oliviero, S., and R. Cortese, The human haptoglobin gene promoter: Interleukin-6-responsive elements interact with a DNA-binding protein induced by interleukin-6. *EMBO J*, 1989. **8**(4): p. 1145–51.

208. Sandler, R.H., et al., Short-term benefit from oral vancomycin treatment of regressive-onset autism. *J Child Neurol*, 2000. **15**(7): p. 429–35.

209. Partty, A., et al., Probiotic *Lactobacillus rhamnosus* GG therapy and microbiological programming in infantile colic: A randomized, controlled trial. *Pediatr Res*, 2015. **78**(4): p. 470–5.

210. Kang, D.W., et al., Microbiota transfer therapy alters gut ecosystem and improves gastrointestinal and autism symptoms: An open-label study. *Microbiome*, 2017. **5**(1): p. 10.

5 Nutrition and the Microbiome — Implications for Autism Spectrum Disorder

Kirsten Berding and Sharon Donovan

CONTENTS

INTRODUCTION

Autism spectrum disorder (ASD) is a neurodevelopmental disorder characterized by the presence of repetitive or restrictive behaviors and deficits in social and communication skills.[1] There has been a pervasive increase over the last decade in the number of children being diagnosed with ASD. In 2010, 1-in-68 children were diagnosed with ASD, while new estimates completed in 2014 reported that 1-in-59 children received an ASD diagnosis.[2] Although the underlying causes of this increase in the prevalence of ASD are unknown, genetic heritability, exposure to environmental risk factors, gene–environment interactions, improved clinical testing and diagnostic methods, and broader diagnostic criteria are all thought to have contributed, apart or in some combination, to the rise of ASD prevalence.[3]

Furthermore, emerging evidence points to a potential new environmental risk factor, the gastrointestinal (GI) microbiota.[4] The last decade has brought about an increasing emphasis on the importance of the bidirectional communication in the microbiota-gut-brain axis.[5] In ASD, evidence of this gut-brain communication can be found in many studies reporting the commonality of GI abnormalities in the ASD population, as well as differences in the fecal microbiota composition and microbial metabolites of children with ASD in comparison to unaffected controls.[6–8] Furthermore, the known association of specific bacterial taxa and the severity of ASD symptoms further suggests the potential role of the GI microbiota in influencing ASD pathophysiology.[6,9]

A number of environmental factors can shape the composition and function of the GI microbiota, including diet. More than half of microbial changes are attributable to diet[10] and diet-induced changes in the GI microbiota composition have been linked to the risk of developing certain diseases.[11] In the ASD population, diet has the potential to play an even more critical role in modulating the microbiome due to the high prevalence of challenging feeding behaviors and the common use of dietary interventions (i.e., Gluten-free/Casein-free diet) to manage symptoms of ASD.[12,13] One recent study found that dietary patterns and nutrient intake predicted a unique microbial profile that could be linked to some GI symptoms in children with ASD,[6] demonstrating the existence of a triangular relationship between diet, GI microbiota, and symptoms of ASD. This chapter seeks to summarize the current understanding of the role of the GI microbiota and microbial metabolites in ASD and will explore the role of dietary interventions in moderating the interaction between the GI microbiota and symptoms of ASD.

ASD AND MICROBIOTA

In 1997, Bolte first hypothesized that *Clostridium tetani* might be involved in ASD symptomology.[14] Since then, a number of studies have shown that the fecal microbiota of children with ASD differs from unaffected, age-matched controls at both the bacterial phylum and genus levels. Specifically, observations of children with ASD have shown a higher abundance of Bacteroidetes, Proteobacteria, Clostridia, *Prevotella, Coprococcuss, Enterococcus, Lactobacillus, Streptococcus, Lactococcus, Staphylococcus, Ruminococcus* and *Bifidobacterium*, and a lower abundance of Firmicutes and Actinobacteria, and *Sutterella* and *Desulfovibrio*.[15–19] However, no succinct explanation of this dysbiosis has since emerged.

Microbiome research in ASD has offered a particular focus on the class Clostridia and the genus *Clostridium*, due to the fact that *Clostridium* was one of the first and most consistent microbes shown to be elevated in children with ASD.[20,21] One hypothesis for the involvement of Clostridial species in ASD pathophysiology and symptom development posits that immunosuppressed, at-risk children are infected with Clostridial spores from their immediate environment, which, in turn, produce enterotoxins and neurotoxins and provide a potential mechanism through which *Clostridium* contributes to the development of ASD symptoms.[20] An observed increase in the abundance of Clostridiales in children who developed GI symptoms around the same time as their ASD diagnosis supports this infection hypothesis.[22] A higher abundance of Clostridia was associated with increased severity of ASD symptoms, further evidencing the link between *Clostridium* and ASD.[23]

Clostridium does not represent the only link between the GI microbiota and ASD pathophysiology. Reduced overall bacterial richness; a higher abundance of *Desulfovibrio, Faecalibacterium*, and Peptostreptococcaceae; and a lower Bacteroidetes/Firmicutes ratio have all also been associated with ASD symptom severity.[6,16,24–26] Due to the common co-occurrence of GI symptoms in children with ASD, deciphering whether ASD symptoms and microbial dysbiosis are directly related to one another or are potentially mediated through GI symptoms is often difficult. This dynamic can be seen in various studies reporting a decrease of beneficial bacteria only in children with ASD and co-morbid GI symptoms.[23,24]

In addition to the previously discussed differences in fecal bacterial composition in children, yeast and fungi are also suspected of being involved in the gut-to-brain communication pathways in ASD. Differences in the β-diversity of the GI mycobiota, evidenced by overall higher yeast abundance with a higher presence of *Candida* spp., have been described in children with ASD versus unaffected controls.[23–27] Furthermore, some yeast, such as *Candida krusei* or *Candida glabrate*, were present in the stool samples of children with ASD, but not in those from control children.[27] One mechanism through which yeast and fungi could impact ASD symptom development is the link between higher levels of *Candida* and decreased absorption of carbohydrates and minerals and increased absorption of toxins.[28]

Because human studies only allow us to draw conclusions about associations between the microbiota and ASD behaviors, animal models are an invaluable tool to further investigate the role of the GI microbiota in ASD symptomology. For example, germ-free (GF) mice exhibit significant social impairments, a core symptom of ASD,[29] and the GI microbiota composition present in mouse models of ASD is often different from commensal mice.[30] A dysbiotic microbiota similar to that observed in human studies of ASD with IBD was observed in a poly I:C and valproic acid (VPA) mouse model of ASD, mimicking widely used environmental risk factors for ASD development.[31] Lastly, GI barrier defects and alterations in microbiota composition observed in the maternal immune activation (MIA) mouse model of ASD were shown to be correctable via oral administration of *Bacteroides fragilis*, suggesting that the GI microbiota could contribute to the development of symptoms associated with ASD.[32]

ASD AND MICROBIAL METABOLITES

In addition to microbial dysbiosis, significant differences have been reported in the concentrations of bacterial metabolites, such as short-chain fatty acids (SCFA) and serotonin, in the blood, urine, and feces of individuals with ASD. This variance suggests that bacterial metabolites could play a role in microbiota-to-brain communication in the development and progression of ASD.[7,33,34]

SCFAs like acetate, propionate, and butyrate are the end-products of microbial fermentation in the colon and have the potential to confer health benefits to their host, including weight control, balancing lipid profiles, and improving colon health.[35] SCFAs are rapidly absorbed in the large intestine and can be detected in the blood.[36] Once in the blood, SCFAs can cross the blood–brain barrier (BBB) via monocarboxylic acid transporters or through passive diffusion, where they can impact nervous system physiology and cause developmental delay or seizures.[37,38] Likewise, SCFAs could also interact with G protein-coupled membrane receptors (GPR), such as GPR-41, -43, or -109, triggering the activation of gene expression of pathways implicated in ASD, including neurotransmitter systems (e.g., serotonergic/cholinergic system), neuronal cell adhesion molecules, inflammation, oxidative stress, lipid metabolism, and mitochondrial function.[39] In animal studies, propionate has been shown to cause brain events similar to those observed in individuals with ASD, and intraventricular administration of propionate provoked ASD-like behaviors in animals, including repetitive interests and impaired social interactions.[39–41]

Serotonin, or 5-hydroxytryptamine (5-HT), modulates neurodevelopment and could play a critical role in governing social function and repetitive behaviors.[42] Elevated levels of whole blood and platelet 5-HT are consistently observed in a subset of children with ASD, making it the first known biomarker identified in ASD.[34,42] Genetic, GI, or immune changes have all been proposed as contributing factors to the hyperserotonemia observed in children with ASD.[43–45] It has been proposed that a dysfunctional serotonergic system can contribute to ASD symptomology, including decreased binding to platelet and brain 5-HT receptors, worsening of symptoms with tryptophan depletion, and alleviation of symptoms with selective serotonin inhibitors and genetic abnormalities.[43] Because most serotonin is produced in the GI tract, and some bacterial strains that are known to influence 5-HT metabolism (e.g., Clostridial spp., *Lactobacillus*) are more prevalent in the stool of affected children, it could also be suggested that the GI microbiota plays a role in serotonin metabolism in ASD.

Other bacterial metabolites of amino acids, carbohydrates, and bile acids metabolism were altered in children with ASD, including taurocholenate sulfate, 3-(3-hydroxyphenyl)-3-hydroxypropionic acid (HPHPA), and 5-aminovalerate.[46,47] Evidence for a potential role in ASD has been presented for HPHPA, a metabolic by-product of the genus *Clostridium*, a microbe often implicated in ASD. It has been suggested that HPHPA could induce ASD symptoms by depleting catecholamine concentrations in the brain.[47] Moreover, a specific bacterial metabolite (4-ethylphenylsulphate; 4EPS) caused ASD-related behaviors in an animal model of ASD.[32]

GASTROINTESTINAL SYMPTOMS AND ASD

GI distress, including diarrhea, constipation or abdominal pain, and functional abnormalities like reduced enzyme expression are prevalent among individuals with ASD and could contribute to behavioral problems and symptom severity.[8,9,22,48–50] Estimates show that individuals with ASD experience GI symptoms four times as often as individuals without ASD[8] and frequency estimates for GI distress range from 15% to 90% among individuals with ASD.[50–52] However, pinning down the exact prevalence of GI disorders in the ASD population is challenging due to social communication difficulties, interpretation discrepancies in GI problems, and differences in sample characteristics and methodological approaches.

Anecdotal reports by parents claim that GI problems and behavioral symptoms manifest in parallel; one study reported that in 67% of cases the onset of GI symptoms occurred before or at the time of ASD diagnosis.[22] The underlying connection between GI distress and ASD symptoms is not well understood, but it is hypothesized to include intestinal inflammation, mitochondrial dysfunction, or microbial dysbiosis. Mitochondrial dysfunction (e.g., dysfunction of mitochondrial enzymes or carriers) is prevalent in the ASD population and many mitochondrial diseases are associated with GI disorders.[53] Intestinal inflammation could also be triggered by an accumulation of undigested carbohydrates, due to reduced carbohydrate digestive capacity.[22] Inflammatory mucosal pathology, increased T-cell activation, cytokines, immunoglobulins, and histological changes were all found in intestinal biopsies in a subset of children with ASD suffering from co-morbid GI symptoms.[54] Furthermore, concentrations of pro-inflammatory cytokines, tumor necrosis factor-alpha (TNFα), interferon-gamma (IFNγ), and interleukins-4 (IL-4) and -5 (IL-5), in intestinal mucosal biopsies and blood were similar to those observed in neurotypical children with Crohn's Disease,[54] suggesting both local and systemic immune activation.

Lastly, studies that consistently report a link between GI distress and microbial dysbiosis could be suggestive of the idea that the microbiota is involved in the relationship between GI and ASD symptoms. For example, constipation is associated with higher levels of *Escherichia/Shigella* and Clostridium Cluster XVIII, and *Clostridium perfringens* and its toxin-producing genes were found in higher abundances in children with ASD and co-morbid GI symptoms.[26,55] One study reporting parallel onset of ASD and GI symptoms also suggested that the timing of the onset of GI symptoms relative to the onset of ASD symptoms could be associated with an increased abundance of the order Clostridiales, namely the families *Lachnospiraceae* and *Ruminococcacaea*.[22] Furthermore, a unique mucosa-associated microbiome in children with ASD and GI disorders, characterized by an increased abundance of Clostridiales and reduced abundance of the genera *Dorea*, *Blautia*, and *Sutterella*, was correlated with peripheral cytokine and tryptophan levels, suggesting a potential relationship between GI symptoms, microbiota composition and peripheral immune and metabolic markers.[56]

NUTRITIONAL CHALLENGES IN CHILDREN WITH ASD

Approximately 90% of children with ASD experience some type of feeding-related symptomology, like picky eating, food selectivity (based on color, shape, texture, or temperature) and restrictive eating; some children consume as little as five different foods.[12,57–59] Children with ASD often require specialized utensils, specific presentation of their food, or seating at a specific place at the table.[58–60] The most common reason children with ASD are referred to a registered dietitian is to alleviate concerns about food selectivity and dietary adequacy.[61] These eating difficulties in children with ASD are often attributed to the co-occurrence of GI symptoms, food allergies, metabolic abnormalities, and sensory sensitivities or behaviors, such as repetitive, ritualistic or externalizing behaviors.[60] Some research suggests that the magnitude of food selectivity and feeding problems could be associated with the severity of ASD symptoms and temper tantrums,[62–64] while other studies found that the severity of ASD symptoms might be related to the type and duration of refusal behavior, but not directly to food selectivity.[60,65] Furthermore, some eating problems resolve over time, as older children with ASD tend to have fewer eating problems than younger children with ASD, possibly due to the success of behavioral therapies.[66]

Feeding problems in children with ASD can influence the amount and types of foods children consume. Children with ASD strongly prefer starches, snack, and processed foods, while often rejecting fruits, vegetables, and protein-rich foods when compared to unaffected children.[67–69] Lower macro- and micronutrient consumption in children with ASD compared to unaffected children have also been reported; some studies have reported lower intakes of some vitamins (e.g., folate, vitamin B12, vitamin D, vitamin E), minerals (e.g., calcium, magnesium, iron), and omega-3 fatty acids (DHA, EPA) in children with ASD compared to unaffected controls.[6,67,69–74] However, the results are not conclusive and nutrient intakes above, below, or at the same level as neurotypical children have been documented in children with ASD.[69–72] In addition, these eating behaviors can also lead to an increased risk of being underweight, overweight, or obese, and of developing obesity-related complications like hypertension and diabetes.[67,71,75–77]

Due to the dearth of effective medical treatments, parents often seek alternative treatment options for their children after a diagnosis of ASD, often including dietary interventions. The most common dietary interventions include the Gluten-free/Casein-free diet, low FODMAP (Fermentable Oligo-, Di-, Mono-saccharides, And Polyols) diet, elimination diets, Ketogenic diet, a specific carbohydrate diet (e.g., lactose- or sucrose-free), or the use of nutrition and fatty acid supplements.[4,13,76] Specialty diets used in the ASD population, along with the nutrients at risk for deficient or excessive intake, are summarized in Table 5.1. Some animal and human studies have provided evidence for the efficacy of dietary interventions to alleviate some symptoms of ASD, but other studies demonstrated no changes in behavioral outcomes or even reported insufficient or excessive nutrient intake in response to interventions.[78–80] Nevertheless, dietary interventions are often adopted by parents of children with ASD; it has been estimated that one-third of children with ASD have been treated with some type of dietary intervention after ASD diagnosis.[13,81]

INFLUENCE OF DIET ON MICROBIOTA COMPOSITION

Diet is one of the most influential environmental factors in shaping microbiota composition and function, with protein, fat, carbohydrates/fiber/prebiotics, and bioactive components all influencing the microbiota.[82] Although microbiota composition has been linked to long-term dietary patterns,[83] acute changes in dietary intake, like switching to solely plant or animal-based foods, modifies microbiota composition and gene expression within 24 hours, but the changes revert once subjects return to their habitual diet.[84] Furthermore, the early postnatal period is a critically important time for establishing the microbiota. Nutrition in early life regulates the development of the GI microbiota, and distinct differences have been observed between breast- and formula-fed infants, due in part to the oligosaccharides (human milk oligosaccharides [HMO]) in human milk.[85] However, how diet shapes microbiota composition after the first year of life, particularly in longitudinal studies, has been less well studied.[86]

A recent study of 903 children between 3 and 46 months of age showed that the developing GI microbiota undergoes three distinct phases of composition: the developmental phase between months 3 and 14, a transitional phase from months 15 to 30, and a stable phase from months 31 to 46. Breastfeeding, either exclusively or alongside formula feeding, was the most significant factor influencing the microbiota structure. Breastfeeding was associated with higher levels of *Bifidobacterium* spp., and the cessation of breast milk resulted in faster maturation of the GI microbiota, as marked by the phylum Firmicutes.[86] It is commonly stated in the literature

TABLE 5.1

Potential Nutritional Implications of Diets Used to Manage Symptoms of Autism Spectrum Disorder

Diet	Description of the Diet	Nutrients at Risk for Inadequate or Excessive Intake	
		Inadequate	Excessive
Gluten-free/ Casein-free	Avoidance of foods containing gluten (wheat, rye, barley, oats) or casein (all dairy products; foods with added milk, casein)	Calcium, vitamin D, phosphorus, fiber, some B vitamins (riboflavin, niacin, B_{12}), iron, zinc, folate, protein	Depending on food consumed to compensate for elimination of gluten- and casein-containing foods
Low FODMAP	Avoidance of foods high in FODMAPS (carbohydrates and sugar alcohols)	Fiber, calcium, antioxidants (e.g., flavonoids, carotenoids), vitamin C, vitamin D, B-vitamins	Not usually reported; depending on foods consumed with low FODMAP content
Ketogenic	High fat, low carbohydrate, moderate protein diet. The macronutrient ratio for ketogenic diets varies, but can range from 60–90% of calories from fat, 4–10% carbohydrates and 6–30% protein	Carbohydrates, fiber, calcium, magnesium, potassium, vitamin D, folate, vitamin C	Fat, potentially saturated fatty acids, depending on which high-fat foods are consumed
Specific carbohydrate reduction or avoidance	Avoidance of many carbohydrate-containing foods (grains, simple carbohydrates, lactose, and processed foods. Diet is composed of monosaccharides, solid protein, fats, vegetables with high amylose:amylopectin ratio, fruits, and nuts	Calcium vitamin D, fiber, folate, potassium, vitamin A, vitamin C (if fruits are avoided)	Depending on individual diet
Vitamin, mineral or fatty acid supplements	Supplementation with vitamins, minerals or fatty acids in capsules, powders. Drinks or bars	Depending on type and dose of supplement	

Abbreviations: FODMAP – Fermentable oligo-, di-, mono-saccharides and polyols that the microbiota becomes relatively stable and resembles that of adults by three years of age.[86,87] However, other studies show that the GI microbiota has a more prolonged development, lasting well into adolescence.[88,89] For example, the fecal microbiota of pre-adolescent children between the ages of 7 and 12 was enriched in *Bifidobacterium* spp., *Faecalibacterium* spp., and members of the *Lachnospiraceae*, while adults harbored greater abundances of *Bacteroides* spp.[88]

Recently, our laboratory investigated the relationships between dietary patterns and the fecal microbiota composition and microbial metabolites in healthy four-to-eight-year-old children[90] and two-to-seven-year-old children with ASD[6] at three time points over a six-month period. In both cases, we identified two dietary patterns using Principal component and Factor analysis that were associated with distinct microbiome compositions and concentration of volatile fatty acids (VFAs). In children with ASD, higher intake of vegetables, legumes, nuts and seeds, fruit, starchy vegetables, grains, juice, and dairy was associated with lower abundance of *Enterobacteriaceae*, *Lactococcus*, *Roseburia*, *Leuconostoc*, and *Ruminococcus*, plus lower total GI severity and constipation scores. On the other hand, a diet comprised of less healthful foods, such as fried foods, "kids' meals," condiments, snacks, starchy foods, and protein foods, was linked to higher abundance of *Barnesiellaceae* and *Alistipes* and lower abundance of *Streptophyta*.[6] Higher levels of VFAs (propionate, isobutyrate, valerate, and isovalerate) were also observed in children consuming a diet filled with less-healthy foods. In children without ASD, temporal stability of the microbiota over a six-month period was also associated with baseline dietary patterns.[90] Although diet-induced microbial profiles were not associated with social deficits scores in children with ASD, these studies suggest that habitual diet in early life is linked to the establishment of the microbiota and that some dietary patterns maybe be associated with a more stable microbial profile than others. Future studies with larger cohorts are warranted to decipher whether diet can moderate the relationship between microbiota and symptoms in diseases associated with microbial dysbiosis.

INTERVENTIONS TARGETING THE MICROBIOTA IN ASD TO MANAGE SYMPTOMS

The emerging evidence suggesting that microbial dysbiosis influences symptom development in children with ASD, coupled with the association of specific microbes with the severity of ASD symptoms, has positioned dietary interventions aimed at manipulating the GI microbiota as a promising therapeutic avenue to ameliorate some symptoms of ASD. The term "microbiome nutrition" was recently proposed as a way to express the fundamental role of diet in microbiota-targeted interventions, due to the GI microbiota's role as a key mediator in the diet–brain health connection.[91,92] Dietary interventions aimed at modulating the GI microbiota and improving health outcomes have shown that diet-induced changes in microbiota composition and function were associated with altered host metabolic or GI health.[93] Data from animal models and human studies suggest that diet-induced changes in the GI microbiota could contribute to behavioral changes and affect brain activity.[94,95] Furthermore, a healthy long-term dietary pattern might be more beneficial in promoting a microbial profile that could protect against diseases, and, conversely, consuming a diet high in processed foods is associated with decreased microbial diversity and an increased risk for mental disorders.[11,91]

In individuals with ASD, dietary interventions have shown some promise in managing symptoms. Although the underlying mechanisms are largely unknown, changes in the microbiota composition could be the link between dietary interventions and reduction in ASD symptom severity. In murine models of ASD, a ketogenic diet reversed the microbial profile associated with ASD[96] and improved ASD-like behaviors.[97] Importantly, one recent animal study demonstrated that a ketogenic diet did not protect against seizures in the absence of microbiota, demonstrating that the GI microbiota is required to bring about the anti-seizure effect of the dietary intervention.[97] Although these studies indicate that the microbiota could be an important link between dietary interventions and improvements in ASD symptoms, future intervention studies like randomized controlled trials or cross-over studies are necessary to elucidate the interplay between diet, the microbiota, and symptoms of ASD.

In addition to dietary interventions, pre- and probiotics are efficacious in modifying the microbiota and influencing behavior and cognitive function. Probiotics are a common adjuvant therapy in the ASD population, with approximately 20% of physicians recommending probiotics for the treatment of ASD symptoms.[98,99] Several research groups using human studies and animal models have explored the role of probiotics in alleviating symptoms of ASD, showing some improvement in symptoms and modulation of microbial and metabolite imbalances after probiotic treatment.[9,31,100–102] Furthermore, in an *in vitro* model using fecal inoculum of children with ASD, the prebiotic B-GOS increased potentially beneficial bacteria (e.g., *Bifidobacterium*) and decreased ASD-associated microbes (e.g., *Sutterella, Ruminococcus*).[103] However, it is difficult for clinicians to provide definitive recommendations on the amount and kind of probiotic to use in treating ASD due to the significant differences in the dose and intervention length between studies.

Lastly, there is a new approach to manipulating the GI microbiota and managing ASD symptoms: fecal microbial transfer (FMT) (see Chapter 11). FMT has been consistently shown to be successful in treating *Clostridium difficile* infections in elderly patients; however, only one study has examined the effectiveness of FMT in ASD treatment. An eight-week, open-label study investigating the tolerability and efficacy of FMT in children with ASD showed improvements in GI symptoms, the parents' perceived behavior of their children, overall severity of symptoms, social impairments, and other ASD-associated behaviors like irritability, lethargy, stereotypy, hyperactivity, and inappropriate speech.[104]

POTENTIAL ROLE OF NUTRITION IN THE MICROBIOTA-TO-BRAIN COMMUNICATION IN ASD

An interrelationship between dietary intake, neurodevelopment, and cognitive function has been observed in healthy children and ensuring adequate nutrition has been suggested as an important aspect in the treatment and etiology of some psychiatric disorders.[105,106] Therefore, the interaction between diet and behavior could be due to altered metabolism of dietary components and changes in metabolic products, as well as direct interaction of the GI microbiota with enteric neurons.[107,108] Mice receiving microbiota transfers from high fat-fed mice showed increased anxiety-like behaviors compared to mice receiving microbiota from chow-fed mice,[109] suggesting that diet-induced changes in the GI microbiota could lead to neurological and behavioral changes. Similarly, inoculation of GI microbiota from undernourished children to GF mice precipitated changes in host metabolism and the immune system, offering additional evidence that diet-induced microbiota composition affects host systems and processes.[110]

There is limited evidence for the role of nutrition in moderating the microbiota-to-brain signaling in ASD. However, several important findings regarding ASD physiology support the development of hypotheses on the potential link between diet, microbiota, and ASD symptomology. First, dietary interventions and prebiotic supplementation, two factors known to shape the GI microbial profile, alleviated some ASD symptoms and normalized microbiota composition and systemic bacterial metabolites in the maternal immune activation model of ASD and a human population.[96,111] Second, SCFAs, which are altered in stool samples of children with ASD and can elicit ASD-like behaviors in animal models, are a major by-product of bacterial carbohydrate fermentation.[7,41] Likewise, fiber (e.g., inulin, pectin) present in fruits and vegetables, which are usually consumed in low amount by children with ASD, decreased propionate production *in vitro*.[112] Therefore, substrate availability could drive microbial activity in ASD. Lastly, it has been hypothesized that the serotonergic system is dysfunctional in ASD and the capability of the GI microbiota to produce serotonin and regulate the metabolism of tryptophan could suggest a role of the microbiota in influencing the serotonergic system.[42] Alterations in tryptophan metabolism related to microbiota composition were associated with social behavioral deficits observed in a mouse model of ASD.[113]

In murine models, diet-induced changes in GI microbiota composition were associated with behavioral changes observed in the animals.[114–116] Interestingly, feeding a high-fat or high-sucrose diet to mice resulted in higher percentages of Clostridiales and Bacteroidales, two bacterial orders that were observed at higher levels in children with ASD, compared to mice fed a normal chow diet. These mice also displayed poorer cognitive flexibility compared to controls.[116] In contrast, evidence for the role of nutrition in the microbiota-brain communication in ASD in humans is limited. In a six-month pilot study, vitamin A intervention in children with ASD resulted in changes in the microbiota composition and ASD-related biochemical markers (e.g., CD38), but ASD behavioral symptoms did not improve after the intervention.[117] Furthermore, an observational study conducted in our laboratory reported that dietary patterns are associated with microbiota composition in children with ASD. Although an association between diet-induced microbial profiles and ASD symptoms was not observed, children with ASD who consumed fewer foods from the "healthy dietary pattern" reported higher prevalence of GI symptoms.[6] Because of the strong positive correlation between GI and ASD symptoms, these results suggest that nutrition might be an important moderator of the microbiota-gut-brain axis in ASD.

CONCLUSIONS AND FUTURE DIRECTIONS

Significant advances have been made in the past decade towards uncovering the role of the GI microbiota in the gut-to-brain communication. We summarized the current evidence for the involvement of the GI microbiota in ASD, potential underlying mechanisms, and the role of nutrition in the ASD population and the microbiota-to-brain communication. Although multiple studies report an aberrant microbiota composition in the ASD population, no clear trend has emerged describing which microbes could consistently elicit ASD symptoms.

Therefore, large population studies are required to provide sufficient evidence to define an "ASD microbiome." These studies should also seek to collect information on dietary intake and other environmental factors, like medication use, to delineate whether or not the microbial differences observed in children with ASD are due to environmental factors or are inherent to ASD itself. Furthermore, large-scale human studies could also lead to the identification of a microbial profile that can serve as a biomarker for individuals at increased risk of developing ASD. By identifying an easily manipulated biomarker, early intervention strategies, such as diet or probiotics, could be used to reduce the severity of ASD symptoms. Furthermore, the use of GF and gnotobiotic animal models will be of fundamental importance to depict underlying mechanisms of the microbiota-to-brain communication in ASD and provide new information on the potential causality of the microbiota-gut-brain axis in ASD.

Due to our rapidly expanding understanding of the critical role of the microbiota in ASD symptomology, studies aimed at harnessing the microbiota as a treatment option have emerged, including the use of probiotics, prebiotics, or FMT. Studies using dietary intervention strategies like the ketogenic diet have shown improvement in some ASD behaviors. Because diet is a key determinant of the GI microbiota composition, it could be hypothesized that the diet-mediated improvements can be mediated through the microbiota after dietary intervention. In animal models, diet-induced changes in the microbiota composition led to behavioral changes, supporting the idea that diet could be used as a future therapeutic avenue for psychiatric disorders. Some studies have started to shed light on the complex relationship between diet and microbiota in ASD symptomology, but the evidence for this interaction is in its infancy. Future clinical research using well-designed randomized controlled trials or cross-over design studies could be very helpful in delineating the potential of diet to manage some of the symptoms of ASD through manipulation of the GI microbiota. These multidisciplinary studies should collect fecal samples for microbiota sequencing, use validated questionnaires to quantify ASD symptom severity, and collect other biological samples in order to assess potential mechanisms like bacterial metabolites and immune markers. Whether diet therapy can be used to alleviate symptoms of ASD alone or in conjunction with other therapies remains to be determined. However, dietary interventions are readily available, low cost, and non-invasive treatment strategies that could provide exciting new options for individuals with ASD.

REFERENCES

1. American Psychiatric Association. *Diagnostic and Statistical Manual of Mental Disorders.* 5th ed. Arlington, VA: American Psychiatric Publishing, 2013.
2. Center for Disease Control. Autism spectrum disorder. Data and statistics: Prevalence. 2014. Retrieved from: http://www.cdc.gov/ncbddd/autism/data.html. Accessed: September 14, 2016.

3. Hallmayer J, Cleveland S, Torres A, Philips J, Cohen B, Torigoe T, Miller J, Fedele A, Collins J, Smith K, Lotspeich L, Croen LA, Ozonoff S, Lajonchere C, Grether JK, Risch N. Genetic heritability and shared environmental factors among twin pairs with autism. *Arch Gen Psychiatry.* 2011; 68(11): 1095–1102.

4. Berding K, Donovan SM. Microbiome and nutrition in autism spectrum disorder: Current knowledge and research needs. *Nutr Rev.* 2016; 74(12): 723–736.

5. Martin CR, Osadchiy V, Kalani A, Mayer EA. The brain-gut-microbiome axis. *Cell Mol Gastroenterol Hepatol.* 2018; 6(2): 133–148.

6. Berding K, Donovan SM. Diet can impact microbiota composition in children with autism spectrum disorder. *Front Neurosci.* 2018; 12: 515. doi: 10.3389/fnins.2018.00515.

7. Wang L, Christophersen CT, Sorich MJ, Gerber JP, Angley MT, Conlon MA. Elevated fecal short chain fatty acid and ammonia concentrations in children with autism spectrum disorder. *Dig Dis Sci.* 2012; 57(8): 2096–2102.

8. McElhanon BO, McCracken C, Karpen S, Sharp WG. Gastrointestinal symptoms in autism spectrum disorder: A meta-analysis. *Pediatrics.* 2014; 133(5): 872–883.

9. Tomova A, Husarova V, Lakatosova S, Bakos J, Vlkova B, Babinska K, Ostatnikova D. Gastrointestinal microbiota in children with autism in Slovakia. *Physiol Behav.* 2015; 138: 179–187.

10. Zhang C, Zhang M, Wang S, Han R, Cao Y, Hua W, Mao Y, Zhang X, Pang X, Wei C, Zhao G, Chen Y, Zhao L. Interactions between gut microbiota, host genetics and diet relevant to development of metabolic syndromes in mice. *ISME J.* 2010; 4(2): 232–241.

11. Albenberg LG, Wu GD. Diet and the intestinal microbiome: Associations, functions, and implications for health and disease. *Gastroenterology.* 2014; 146(6): 1564–1572.

12. Ledford JR, Gast DL. Feeding problems in children with autism spectrum disorders a review. *Focus Autism Other Dev Disabl.* 2006; 21(3): 153–166.

13. Stewart PA, Hyman SL, Schmidt BL, Macklin EA, Reynolds A, Johnson CR, James SJ, Manning-Courtney P. Dietary supplementation in children with autism spectrum disorders: Common, insufficient, and excessive. *J Acad Nutr Diet.* 2015; 115(8): 1237–1248.

14. Bolte ER. Autism and *Clostridium tetani. Med Hypotheses.* 1998; 51(2): 133–134.

15. Finegold SM, Dowd SE, Gontcharova V, Liu C, Henley KE, Wolcott RD, Youn E, Summanen PH, Granpeesheh D, Dixon D, Liu M, Molitoris DR, Green JA 3rd. Pyrosequencing study of fecal microflora of autistic and control children. *Anaerobe.* 2010; 16(4): 444–453.

16. Kang DW, Park JG, Ilhan ZE, Wallstrom G, LaBaer J, Adams JB, Krajmalnik-Brown R. Reduced incidence of *Prevotella* and other fermenters in intestinal microflora of autistic children. *PLOS ONE.* 2013; 8(7): e68322. doi: 10.1371/journal.pone.0068322.

17. De Angelis M, Piccolo M, Vannini L, Siragusa S, De Giacomo A, Serrazzanetti DI, Cristofori F, Guerzoni ME, Gobetti M, Francavilla R. Fecal microbiota and metabolome of children with autism and pervasive developmental disorder not otherwise specified. *PLOS ONE.* 2013; 8(10): e76993.

18. Wang L, Christophersen CT, Sorich MJ, Gerber JP, Angley MT, Conlon MA. Low relative abundances of the mucolytic bacterium *Akkermansia muciniphila* and *Bifidobacterium* spp. in feces of children with autism. *Appl Environ Microbiol.* 2011; 77(18): 6718–6721.

19. Parracho HM, Bingham MO, Gibson GR, McCartney AL. Differences between the gut microflora of children with autistic spectrum disorders and that of healthy children. *J Med Microbiol.* 2005; 54(10): 987–991.

20. Finegold SM. Therapy and epidemiology of autism–clostridial spores as key elements. *Med Hypotheses.* 2008; 70(3): 508–511.

21. Sandler RH, Finegold SM, Bolte ER, Buchanan CP, Maxwell AP, Väisänen ML, Nelson MN, Wexler HM. Short-term benefit from oral vancomycin treatment of regressive-onset autism. *J Child Neurol.* 2000; 15(7): 429–435.

22. Williams BL, Hornig M, Buie T, Bauman ML, Cho Paik M, Wick I, Bennett A, Jabado O, Hirschberg DL, Lipkin WI. Impaired carbohydrate digestion and transport and mucosal dysbioisis in the intestines of children with autism and gastrointestinal disturbances. *PLOS ONE.* 2011; 6(9): e24585. doi: 10.1371/journal.pone.0024585.
23. Iovene MR, Bombace F, Maresca R, Sapone A, Iardino P, Picardi A, Marotta R, Schiraldi C, Siniscalco D, Serra N, de Magistris L, Bravaccio C. Intestinal dysbiosis and yeast isolation in stool of subjects with autism spectrum disorders. *Mycopathologia.* 2017; 182(3–4): 349–363.
24. Gondalia SV, Palombo EA, Knowles SR, Cox SB, Meyer D, Austin DW. Molecular characterisation of gastrointestinal microbiota of children with autism (with and without gastrointestinal dysfunction) and their neurotypical siblings. *Autism Res.* 2012; 5(6): 419–427.
25. Son JS, Zheng LJ, Rowehl LM, Tian X, Zhang Y, Zhu W, Litcher-Kelly L, Gadow KD, Gathungu G, Robertson CE, Ir D, Frank DN, Li E. Comparison of fecal microbiota in children with autism spectrum disorders and neurotypical siblings in the simons simplex collection. *PLOS ONE.* 2015; 10(10): e0137725. doi: 10.1371/journal.pone.0137725.
26. Strati F, Cavalieri D, Albanese D, De Felice C, Donati C, Hayek J, Jousson O, Leoncini S, Renzi D, Calabrò A, De Filippo C. New evidences on the altered gut microbiota in autism spectrum disorders. *Microbiome.* 2017; 5(1). doi: 10.1186/s40168-017-0242-1: 24.
27. Kantarcioglu AS, Kiraz N, Aydin A. Microbiota–gut–brain axis: Yeast species isolated from stool samples of children with suspected or diagnosed autism spectrum disorders and in vitro susceptibility against nystatin and fluconazole. *Mycopathologia.* 2016; 181(1–2): 1–7. doi: 10.1007/s11046-015-9949-3.
28. Burrus CJ. A biochemical rationale for the interaction between gastrointestinal yeast and autism. *Med Hypotheses.* 2012; 79(6): 784–785.
29. Desbonnet L, Clarke G, Shanahan F, Dinan TG, Cryan JF. Microbiota is essential for social development in the mouse. *Mol Psychiatry.* 2014; 19(2): 146–148.
30. de Theije CG, Wopereis H, Ramadan M, van Eijndthoven T, Lambert J, Knol J, Garssen J, Kraneveld AD, Oozeer R. Altered gut microbiota and activity in a murine model of autism spectrum disorders. *Brain Behav Immun.* 2014; 37: 197–206.
31. Lim JS, Lim MY, Choi Y, Ko G. Modeling environmental risk factors of autism in mice induces IBD-related gut microbial dysbiosis and hyperserotonemia. *Mol Brain.* 2017; 10(1): 14. doi: 10.1186/s13041-017-0292-0.
32. Hsiao EY, McBride SW, Hsien S, Sharon G, Hyde ER, McCue T, Codelli JA, Chow J, Reisman SE, Pretrosino JF, Patterson PH, Mazmanian SK. Microbiota modulate behavioral and physiological abnormalities associated with neurodevelopmental disorders. *Cell.* 2013; 155(7): 1451–1463.
33. Zhao R, Chu L, Wang Y, Song Y, Liu P, Li C, Huang J, Kang X. Application of packed-fiber solid-phase extraction coupled with GC–MS for the determination of short-chain fatty acids in children's urine. *Clin Chim Acta.* 2017; 468: 120–125.
34. Gabriele S, Sacco R, Persico AM. Blood serotonin levels in autism spectrum disorder: A systematic review and meta-analysis. *Eur Neuropsychopharmacol.* 2014; 24(6): 919–929.
35. Byrne CS, Chambers ES, Morrison DJ, Frost G. The role of short chain fatty acids in appetite regulation and energy homeostasis. *Int J Obes.* 2015; 39(9): 1331–1338.
36. Tsukahara T, Matsukawa N, Tomonaga S, Inoue R, Ushida K, Ochiai K. High-sensitivity detection of short-chain fatty acids in porcine ileal, cecal, portal and abdominal blood by gas chromatography-mass spectrometry. *Anim Sci J.* 2014; 85(4): 494–498.
37. Deroover L, Boets E, Tie Y, Vandermeulen G, Verbeke K. Quantification of plasma or serum short-chain fatty acids: Choosing the correct blood tube. *J Nutr Health Food Sci.* 2017; 5(6): 1–6.

38. Feliz B, Witt DR, Harris BT. Propionic acidemia: A neuropathology case report and review of prior cases. *Arch Pathol Lab Med.* 2003; 127(8): e325–e328.
39. Nankova BB, Agarwal R, MacFabe DF, La Gamma EE. Enteric bacterial metabolites propionic and butyric acid modulate gene expression, including CREB-dependent cate-cholaminergic neurotransmission, in PC12 cells-possible relevance to autism spectrum disorders. *PLOS ONE.* 2014; 9(8): e103740. doi: 10.1371/journal.pone.0103740.
40. Thomas RH, Meeking MM, Mepham JR, Tichenoff L, Possmayer F, Liu S, MacFabe DF. The enteric bacterial metabolite propionic acid alters brain and plasma phospho-lipid molecular species: Further development of a rodent model of autism spectrum disorders. *J Neuroinflammation.* 2012; 9: 1–18.
41. MacFabe DF, Cain NE, Boon F, Ossenkopp KP, Cain DP. Effects of the enteric bac-terial metabolic product propionic acid on object-directed behavior, social behavior, cognition, and neuroinflammation in adolescent rats: Relevance to autism spectrum disorder. *Behav Brain Res.* 2011; 217(1): 47–54.
42. Muller CL, Anacker AMJ, Veenstra-VanderWeele J. The serotonin system in autism spectrum disorder: From biomarker to animal models. *Neuroscience.* 2016; 321: 24–41.
43. Schain RJ, Freedman DX. Studies on 5-hydroxyindole metabolism in autistic and other mentally retarded children. *J Pediatr.* 1961; 58: 315–320.
44. Anderson GM, Freedman DX, Cohen DJ, Volkmar FR, Hoder EL, McPhedran P, Minderaa RB, Hansen CR, Young JG. Whole blood serotonin in autistic and normal subjects. *J Child Psychol Psychiatry.* 1987; 28(6): 885–900.
45. Hanley HG, Stahl SM, Freedman DX. Hyperserotonemia and amine metabolites in autistic and retarded children. *Arch Gen Psychiatry.* 1977; 34(5): 521–531.
46. Ming X, Stein TP, Barnes V, Rhodes N, Guo L. Metabolic perturbance in autism spec-trum disorders: A metabolomics study. *J Proteome Res.* 2012; 11(12): 5856–5862.
47. Keşli R, Gökçen C, Buluğ U, Terzi Y. Investigation of the relation between anaerobic bacteria genus clostridium and late-onset autism etiology in children. *J Immunoassay Immunochem.* 2014; 35(1): 101–109.
48. Adams JB, Johansen LJ, Powell LD, Quig D, Rubin RA. Gastrointestinal flora and gastrointestinal status in children with autism–Comparisons to typical chil-dren and correlation with autism severity. *BMC Gastroenterol.* 2011; 11: 22. doi: 10.1186/1471-230X-11-22.
49. Buie T, Campbell DB, Fuchs GJ, Furuta GT, Levy J, Vandewater J, Whitaker AH, Atkins D, Bauman ML, Beaudet AL, Carr EG, Gershon MD, Hyman SL, Jirapinyo P, Jyonouchi H, Kooros K, Kushak R, Levitt P, Levy SE, Lewis JD, Murray KF, Natowicz MR, Sabra A, Wershil BK, Weston SC, Zeltzer L, Winter H. Evaluation, diagnosis, and treatment of gastrointestinal disorders in individuals with ASDs: A consensus report. *Pediatrics.* 2010; 125(Suppl 1): S1–S18.
50. Horvath K, Perman JA. Autism and gastrointestinal symptoms. *Curr Gastroenterol Rep.* 2002; 4(3): 251–258. doi: 10.1007/s11894-002-0071-6.
51. Fombonne E, Chakrabarti S. No evidence for a new variant of measles-mumps-rubella-induced autism. *Pediatrics.* 2001; 108(4): e58. doi: 10.1542/peds.108.4.e58.
52. de Theije CG, Wu J, da Silva SL, Kamphuis PJ, Garssen J, Korte SM, Kraneveld AD. Pathways underlying the gut-to-brain connection in autism spectrum disorders as future targets for disease management. *Eur J Pharmacol.* 2011; 668(Suppl 1): S70–S80.
53. Rossignol DA, Bradstreet JJ. Evidence of mitochondrial dysfunction in autism and implications for treatment. *Am J Biochem Biotechnol.* 2008; 4(2): 208–217.
54. Ashwood P, Wakefield AJ. Immune activation of peripheral blood and mucosal CD3+ lymphocyte cytokine profiles in children with autism and gastrointestinal symptoms. *J Neuroimmunol.* 2006; 173(1): 126–134.

55. Finegold SM, Summanen PH, Downes J, Corbett K, Komoriya T. Detection of *Clostridium perfringens* toxin genes in the gut microbiota of autistic children. *Anaerobe*. 2017; 45: 133–137.
56. Luna RA, Oezguen N, Balderas M, Venkatachalam A, Runge JK, Versalovic J, Veenstra-VanderWeele J, Anderson GM, Savidge T, Williams KC. Distinct microbiome-neuroimmune signatures correlate with functional abdominal pain in children with autism spectrum disorder. *Cell Mol Gastroenterol Hepatol*. 2017; 3(2): 218–230.
57. Nadon G, Feldman DE, Dunn W, Gisel E. Mealtime problems in children with autism spectrum disorder and their typically developing siblings: A comparison study. *Autism*. 2011; 15(1): 98–113.
58. Cermak SA, Curtin C, Bandini LG. Food selectivity and sensory sensitivity in children with autism spectrum disorders. *J Am Diet Assoc*. 2010; 110(2): 238–246.
59. Schreck KA, Williams K, Smith AF. A comparison of eating behaviors between children with and without autism. *J Autism Dev Disord*. 2004; 34(4): 433–438.
60. Johnson CR, Turner K, Stewart PA, Schmidt B, Shui A, Macklin E, Reynolds A, James J, Johnson SL, Courtney PM, Hyman SL. Relationships between feeding problems, behavioral characteristics and nutritional quality in children with ASD. *J Autism Dev Disord*. 2014; 44(9): 2175–2184.
61. Bowers L. An audit of referrals of children with autistic spectrum disorder to the dietetic service. *J Hum Nutr Diet*. 2002; 15(2): 141–144.
62. Crasta JE, Benjamin TE, Suresh APC, Alwinesh MT, Kanniappan G, Padankatti SM, Russell PS, Nair MK. Feeding problems among children with autism in a clinical population in India. *Indian J Pediatr*. 2014; 81(2): 169–172.
63. Postorino V, Sanges V, Giovagnoli G, Fatta LM, De Peppo L, Armando M, Vicari S, Mazzone L. Clinical differences in children with autism spectrum disorder with and without food selectivity. *Appetite*. 2015; 92: 126–132.
64. Dominick KC, Davis NO, Lainhart J, Tager-Flusberg H, Folstein S. Atypical behaviors in children with autism and children with a history of language impairment. *Res Dev Disabil*. 2007; 28(2): 145–162.
65. Aponte CA, Romanczyk RG. Assessment of feeding problems in children with autism spectrum disorder. *Res Autism Spec Disord*. 2016; 21: 61–72.
66. Laud RB, Girolami PA, Boscoe JH, Gulotta CS. Treatment outcomes for severe feeding problems in children with autism spectrum disorder. *Behav Modif*. 2009; 33(5): 520–536.
67. Bicer AH, Alsaffar AA. Body mass index, dietary intake and feeding problems of Turkish children with autism spectrum disorder (ASD). *Res Dev Disabil*. 2013; 34(11): 3978–3987.
68. Al-Farsi YM, Al-Sharbati MM, Waly MI, Al-Farsi OA, Al Shafaee MA, Deth RC. Malnutrition among preschool-aged autistic children in Oman. *Res Autism Spectr Disord*. 2011; 5(4): 1549–1552.
69. Malhi P, Venkatesh L, Bharti B, Singhi P. Feeding problems and nutrient intake in children with and without autism: A comparative study. *Indian J Pediatr*. 2017; 84(4): 283–288.
70. Liu X, Liu J, Xiong X, Yang T, Hou N, Liang X, Chen J, Cheng Q, Li T. Correlation between nutrition and symptoms: Nutritional survey of children with autism spectrum disorder in Chongqing, China. *Nutrients*. 2016; 8(5): E294. doi: 10.3390/nu8050294.
71. Zimmer MH, Hart LC, Manning-Courtney P, Murray DS, Bing NM, Summer S. Food variety as a predictor of nutritional status among children with autism. *J Autism Dev Disord*. 2012; 42(4): 549–556.
72. Emond A, Emmett P, Steer C, Golding J. Feeding symptoms, dietary patterns, and growth in young children with autism spectrum disorders. *Pediatrics*. 2010; 126(2): e337–e342.

73. Ranjan S, Nasser JA. Nutritional status of individuals with autism spectrum disorders: Do we know enough? *Adv Nutr.* 2015; 6(4): 397–407.

74. Esparham AE, Smith T, Belmont JM, Haden M, Wagner LE, Evans RG, Drisko JA. Nutritional and metabolic biomarkers in autism spectrum disorders: An exploratory study. *Integr Med (Encinitas).* 2015; 14(2): 40–53.

75. Curtin C, Anderson SE, Must A, Bandini L. The prevalence of obesity in children with autism: A secondary data analysis using nationally representative data from the National Survey of Children's Health. *BMC Pediatr.* 2010; 10: 11. doi: 10.1186/1471-2431-10-11.

76. Berry RC, Novak P, Withrow N, Schmidt B, Rarback S, Feucht S, Criado KK, Sharp WG. Nutrition management of gastrointestinal symptoms in children with autism spectrum disorder: Guideline from an expert panel. *J Acad Nutr Diet.* 2015; 115(12): 1919–1927.

77. Shmaya Y, Eilat-Adar S, Leitner Y, Reif S, Gabis L. Nutritional deficiencies and over-weight prevalence among children with autism spectrum disorder. *Res Dev Disabil.* 2015; 38: 1–6.

78. Millward C, Ferriter M, Calver S, Connell-Jones G. Gluten-and casein-free diets for autistic spectrum disorder. *Cochrane Database Syst Rev.* 2008; (2): CD003498. doi: 10.1002/14651858.CD003498.pub3.

79. Mousain-Bosc M, Roche M, Polge A, Pradal-Prat D, Rapin J, Bali JP. Improvement of neurobehavioral disorders in children supplemented with magnesium-vitamin B6. II. Pervasive developmental disorder-autism. *Magnes Res.* 2006; 19(1): 53–62.

80. Srinivasan P. A review of dietary interventions in autism. *Ann Clin Psychiatry.* 2009; 21(4): 237–247.

81. Levy SE, Mandell DS, Merhar S, Ittenbach RF, Pinto-Martin JA. Use of complementary and alternative medicine among children recently diagnosed with autistic spectrum disorder. *J Dev Behav Pediatr.* 2003; 24(6): 418–423.

82. Singh RK, Chang HW, Yan D, Lee KM, Ucmak D, Wong K, Abrouk M, Farahnik B, Nakamura M, Zhu TH, Bhutani T, Liao W. Influence of diet on the gut microbiome and implications for human health. *J Transl Med.* 2017; 15(1): 73.

83. Wu GD, Chen J, Hoffmann C, Bittinger K, Chen YY, Keilbaugh SA, Bewtra M, Knights D, Walters WA, Knight R, Sinha R, Gilroy E, Gupta K, Baldassano R, Nessel L, Li H, Bushman FD, Lewis JD. Linking long-term dietary patterns with gut microbial enterotypes. *Science.* 2011; 334(6052): 105–108.

84. David LA, Maurice CF, Carmody RN, Gootenberg DB, Button JE, Wolfe BE, Ling AV, Devlin AS, Varma Y, Fischbach MA, Biddinger SB, Dutton RJ, Turnbaugh PJ. Diet rapidly and reproducibly alters the human gut microbiome. *Nature.* 2014; 505(7484): 559–563.

85. Davis EC, Wang M, Donovan SM. The role of early life nutrition in the establishment of gastrointestinal microbial composition and function. *Gut Microbes.* 2017; 8(2): 143–171.

86. Stewart CJ, Ajami NJ, O'Brien JL, Hutchinson DS, Smith DP, Wong MC, Ross MC, Lloyd RE, Doddapaneni H, Metcalf GA, Muzny D, Gibbs RA, Vatanen T, Huttenhower C, Xavier RJ, Rewers M, Hagopian W, Toppari J, Ziegler AG, She JX, Akolkar B, Lernmark A, Hyoty H, Vehik K, Krischer JP, Petrosino JF. Temporal development of the gut microbiome in early childhood from the TEDDY study. *Nature.* 2018; 562(7728): 583–588.

87. Yatsunenko T, Rey FE, Manary MJ, Trehan I, Dominguez-Bello MG, Contreras M, Magris M, Hidalgo G, Baldassano RN, Anokhin AP, Heath AC, Warner B, Reeder J, Kuczynski J, Caporaso JG, Lozupone CA, Lauber C, Clemente JC, Knights D, Knight R, Gordon JI. Human gut microbiome viewed across age and geography. *Nature.* 2012; 486(7402): 222–227.

88. Hollister EB, Riehle K, Luna RA, Weidler EM, Rubio-Gonzales M, Mistretta TA, Raza S, Doddapaneni HV, Metcalf GA, Muzny DM, Gibbs RA, Petrosino JF, Shulman RJ, Versalovic J. Structure and function of the healthy pre-adolescent pediatric gut microbiome. *Microbiome.* 2015; 3: 36.

89. Agans R, Rigsbee L, Kenche H, Michail S, Khamis HJ, Paliy O. Distal gut microbiota of adolescent children is different from that of adults. *FEMS Microbiol Ecol.* 2011; 77(2): 404–412.

90. Berding K, Holscher HD, Arthur AE, Donovan SM. Fecal microbiome composition and stability in 4- to 8-year old children is associated with dietary patterns and nutrient intakes. *J Nutr Biochem.* 2018; 56: 165–174.

91. Dawson SL, Dash SR, Jacka FN. Chapter Fifteen–The importance of diet and gut health to the treatment and prevention of mental disorders. *Int Rev Neurobiol.* 2016; 131: 325–346.

92. Lam YY, Zhang C, Zhao L. Causality in dietary interventions-building a case for gut microbiota. *Genome Med.* 2018; 10(1): 62.

93. Zhao L, Zhang F, Ding X, Wu G, Lam YY, Wang X, Fu H, Xue X, Lu C, Ma J, Yu L, Xu C, Ren Z, Xu Y, Xu S, Shen H, Zhu X, Shi Y, Shen Q, Dong W, Liu R, Ling Y, Zeng Y, Wang X, Zhang Q, Wang J, Wang L, Wu Y, Zeng B, Wei H, Zhang M, Peng Y, Zhang C. Gut bacteria selectively promoted by dietary fibers alleviate type 2 diabetes. *Science.* 2018; 359(6380): 1151–1156.

94. Ohland CL, Kish L, Bell H, Thiesen A, Hotte N, Pankiv E, Madsen KL. Effects of Lactobacillus helveticus on murine behavior are dependent on diet and genotype and correlate with alterations in the gut microbiome. *Psychoneuroendocrinology.* 2013; 38(9): 1738–1747.

95. Newell C, Bomhof MR, Reimer RA, Hittel DS, Rho JM, Shearer J. Ketogenic diet modifies the gut microbiota in a murine model of autism spectrum disorder. *Mol Autism.* 2016; 7(1): 37.

96. Ruskin DN, Murphy MI, Slade SL, Masino SA. Ketogenic diet improves behaviors in a maternal immune activation model of autism spectrum disorder. *PLOS ONE.* 2017; 12(2): e0171643. doi: 10.1186/s13229-016-0099-3.

97. Olson CA, Vuong HE, Yang JM, Liang QY, Nusbaum DJ, Hsiao EY. The gut microbiota mediates the anti-seizure effects of the ketogenic diet. *Cell.* 2018; 173(7): 1728–1741.

98. Critchfield JW, van Hemert S, Ash M, Mulder L, Ashwood P. The potential role of probiotics in the management of childhood autism spectrum disorders. *Gastroenterol Res Pract.* 2011; 2011: 161358. doi: 10.1155/2011/161358.

99. Golnik AE, Ireland M. Complementary alternative medicine for children with autism: A physician survey. *J Autism Dev Disord.* 2009; 39(7): 996–1005.

100. Kałużna-Czaplińska J, Błaszczyk S. The level of arabinitol in autistic children after probiotic therapy. *Nutrition.* 2012; 28(2): 124–126.

101. West R, Roberts E, Sichel LS, Sichel J. Improvements in gastrointestinal symptoms among children with autism spectrum disorder receiving the Delpro® probiotic and immunomodulatory formulation. *J Probiotics Health.* 2013; 1: 2. doi: 10.4172/2329-8901.1000102.

102. Russo AJ. Decreased plasma myeloperoxidase associated with probiotic therapy in autistic children. *Clin Med Insights Pediatr.* 2015; 9: 13–17.

103. Grimaldi R, Cela D, Swann JR, Vulevic J, Gibson GR, Tzortzis G, Costabile A. In vitro fermentation of B-GOS: Impact on faecal bacterial populations and metabolic activity in autistic and non-autistic children. *FEMS Microbiol Ecol.* 2017; 93(2). pii: fiw233. doi.org/10.1093/femsec/fiw233.

104. Kang DW, Adams JB, Gregory AC, Borody T, Chittick L, Fasano A, Khoruts A, Geis E, Maldonado J, McDonough-Means S, Pollard EL, Roux S, Sadowsky MJ, Lipson KS, Sullivan MB, Caporaso JG, Krajmalnik-Brown R. Microbiota transfer therapy alters gut ecosystem and improves gastrointestinal and autism symptoms: An open-label study. *Microbiome.* 2017; 5(1): 10. doi: 10.1186/s40168-016-0225-7.

105. Khan NA, Raine LB, Drollette ES, Scudder MR, Hillman CH. The relation of saturated fats and dietary cholesterol to childhood cognitive flexibility. *Appetite.* 2015; 93: 51–56.

106. Khan NA, Raine LB, Drollette ES, Scudder MR, Kramer AF, Hillman CH. Dietary fiber is positively associated with cognitive control among prepubertal children. *J Nutr.* 2015; 145(1): 143–149.

107. Hanstock TL, Clayton EH, Li KM, Mallet PE. Anxiety and aggression associated with the fermentation of carbohydrates in the hindgut of rats. *Physiol Behav.* 2004; 82(2–3): 357–368.

108. Furness JB, Kunze WA, Clerc N. Nutrient tasting and signaling mechanisms in the gut. II. The intestine as a sensory organ: Neural, endocrine, and immune responses. *Am J Physiol.* 1999; 277(5): G922–G928.

109. Bruce-Keller AJ, Salbaum JM, Luo M, Blanchard E 4th, Taylor CM, Welsh DA, Berthoud HR. Obese-type gut microbiota induce neurobehavioral changes in the absence of obesity. *Biol Psychiatry.* 2015; 77(7): 607–615.

110. Kau AL, Planer JD, Liu J, Rao S, Yatsunenko T, Trehan I, Manary MJ, Liu TC, Stappenbeck TS, Maleta KM, Ashorn P, Dewey KG, Houpt ER, Hsieh CS, Gordon JI. Functional characterization of IgA-targeted bacterial taxa from undernourished Malawian children that produce diet-dependent enteropathy. *Sci Transl Med.* 2015; 7(276): 276ra24. doi: 10.1126/scitranslmed.aaa4877.

111. Grimaldi R, Gibson GR, Vulevic J, Giallourou N, Castro-Mejía JL, Hansen LH, Gibson EL, Nielsen DS, Costabile A. A prebiotic intervention study in children with autism spectrum disorders (ASDs). *Microbiome.* 2018; 6(1): 133. doi: 10.1186/s40168-018-0523-3.

112. Yang J, Marınez I, Walter J, Keshavarzian A, Rose DJ. In vitro characterization of the impact of selected dietary fibers on fecal microbiota composition and short chain fatty acid production. *Anaerobe.* 2013; 23: 74–81.

113. Golubeva AV, Joyce SA, Moloney G, Burokas A, Sherwin E, Arboleya S, Flynn I, Khochanskiy D, Moya-Pérez A, Peterson V, Rea K, Murphy K, Makarova O, Buravkov S, Hyland NP, Stanton C, Clarke G, Gahan CGM, Dinan TG, Cryan JF. Microbiota-related changes in bile acid & tryptophan metabolism are associated with gastrointestinal dysfunction in a mouse model of autism. *EBioMedicine.* 2017; 24: 166–178.

114. Li W, Dowd SE, Scurlock B, Acosta-Martinez V, Lyte M. Memory and learning behavior in mice is temporally associated with diet-induced alterations in gut bacteria. *Physiol Behav.* 2009; 96(4–5): 557–567.

115. Pyndt Jørgensen B, Hansen JT, Krych L, Larsen C, Klein AB, Nielsen DS, Josefsen K, Hansen AK, Sørensen DB. A possible link between food and mood: Dietary impact on gut microbiota and behavior in BALB/c mice. *PLOS ONE.* 2014; 9(8): e103398. doi: 10.1371/journal.pone.0103398.

116. Magnusson KR, Hauck L, Jeffrey BM, Elias V, Humphrey A, Nath R, Perrone A, Bermudez LE. Relationships between diet-related changes in the gut microbiome and cognitive flexibility. *Neuroscience.* 2015; 300: 128–140.

117. Liu J, Liu X, Xiong XQ, Yang T, Cui T, Hou NL, Lai X, Liu S, Guo M, Liang XH, Cheng Q, Chen J, Li TY. Effect of vitamin A supplementation on gut microbiota in children with autism spectrum disorders-a pilot study. *BMC Microbiol.* 2017; 17(1): 204. doi: 10.1186/s12866-017-1096-1.

6 Alzheimer's Disease, the Microbiome, and 21st Century Medicine

Dale Bredesen

CONTENTS

It has become increasingly clear over the last few decades that humans are not the discrete, individual organisms we imagined ourselves to be. Rather, we are much more akin to the colonial man-o-war, that ethereal creature that sometimes stings us as we swim or surf in the ocean. The man-o-war consists of several specialized organisms that cooperate to perform the predatory and digestive functions necessary for its survival. Similarly, our thoughts, moods, sense of self-preservation, and our disease processes are all the result of a complex collaboration between more than 1,000 different organisms, both prokaryotes and eukaryotes. This perspective of humans as collectives rather than individuals gives new, non-singular definitions to the terms "I" and "me."

Unfortunately, this beautifully orchestrated, complex collaboration breaks down frequently, especially as we age. This disintegration in turn causes some of the most common illnesses that plague us today, including Alzheimer's disease, depression, inflammatory bowel disease, and type 2 diabetes. However, deepening our understanding of this collaborative system offers a glimmer of hope, as the system holds the promise of more effective preventive and therapeutic strategies for these very same diseases.

In what is almost surely a reductive approach, we define the microbiome as the assemblage of non-Homo sapiens organisms that make up the human organismal system. In doing so, however, we also must recognize nonetheless that neither part could function effectively without the other. More than 1,000 species that comprise the human gut microbiome include anaerobic and aerobic bacteria, fungi, protozoa, archaea, viruses, and bacteriophages. Anaerobic bacteria, such as those from the phyla Firmicutes, Actinobacteria, and Bacteroidetes dominate the overall microbial composition. As described in detail below, these species contribute to illness in numerous ways. In addition to these species, there are of course important contributions from the mitochondria, a major member of the "intracytoplasmic microbiome."

Alzheimer's disease is now a global pandemic, and recent studies suggest that it is the third leading cause of death in the United States (James et al., 2014). However, our conception of Alzheimer's disease is evolving rapidly: the amyloid-β that is vilified as the "cause" of Alzheimer's has been shown to, in fact, be an anti-microbial, a component of the innate immune system (Kumar et al., 2016); additional subtypes of Alzheimer's disease have been identified (Bredesen, 2015); and monotherapeutics have failed repeatedly in clinical trials, while therapeutic programs have been shown to be effective for both prevention (Ngandu et al., 2015) and reversal (Bredesen, 2014; Bredesen et al., 2016) of the cognitive decline associated with Alzheimer's.

As noted above, as we have come to better understand Alzheimer's disease, multiple subtypes of the condition have been identified. Since the subtypes were identified using metabolic profiling, further increases in data set size-through characterization of the microbiome of each patient, whole-genome sequencing, expanded toxicological profiles, and extensive PCR studies for occult pathogens—is likely to provide additional dissection of subtypes and/or additional subtypes. Type 1 (inflammatory) Alzheimer's is characterized by increased C-reactive protein, interleukin-6, and tumor necrosis factor-alpha, as well as other markers of systemic inflammation. As shown by Fiala and his colleagues, the M1/M2 ratio from peripheral blood mononuclear cells is increased, reflecting the pro-inflammatory state (Famenini et al., 2017). This inflammation may occur due to specific pathogens, such as *Porphyromonas gingivalis* or *Fusobacterium nucleatum* from the oral microbiome; alternatively, the inflammation may be sterile, for example from the ingestion of trans fats (in contrast, ingestion of omega-3 fats, along with lipoic acid, slows cognitive decline (Shinto et al., 2014)). Patients with type 1 Alzheimer's disease often carry the epsilon-4 allele of apolipoprotein E (ApoE4+), may have other inflammation-associated conditions such as arthritis or cardiovascular disease, often experience their first symptoms in their seventh decade, and typically present with an amnestic syndrome. Mechanistically, the activation of NF-κB induces up-regulation of the β-secretase and γ-secretase complex, thus shifting the cleavage pattern of the amyloid precursor protein, APP, toward the amyloidogenic pathway. The microbiome may contribute to type 1 Alzheimer's in numerous ways, such as the leaking of LPS or bacteria or other immunogens from the gut into the bloodstream, or the alteration of the immune response toward a more immune-activated state.

Type 2, or atrophic, Alzheimer's disease, is associated with a reduction in trophic, hormonal, or nutritive support. These patients often present with a relatively pure amnestic syndrome, are often ApoE4+, and their symptoms often initiate later than those of type 1. The microbiome may play a key role in type 2 Alzheimer's through its absorption and metabolism of critical nutrients and hormones. Furthermore, specific gut microorganisms may be associated with increases in BDNF (O'Sullivan et al., 2011), offering yet another mechanism through which the composition of the human microbiome is likely to be critical in Alzheimer's disease pathogenesis.

Type 1.5, or glycotoxic, Alzheimer's disease is so named because it shares features of both inflammatory and atrophic Alzheimer's disease: the non-enzymatic glycation of proteins induces immune recognition and inflammation, thus inducing type 1 Alzheimer's disease. The insulin resistance creates an atrophic effect due to the important trophic effect exerted by insulin through its tyrosine kinase receptor and related downstream signaling pathways, mediated by IRS-1. Glycotoxic Alzheimer's disease features both a pro-inflammatory effect and an atrophic effect. These patients may also have additional features of metabolic syndrome, are often ApoE4+, and typically present with an amnestic syndrome. The microbiome may contribute to type 1.5 Alzheimer's disease through its microbiota-dependent obesity and insulin resistance, its role in inflammation and immune responses, and potentially, as for all subtypes, through its role in amyloidogenesis.

Type 3, or toxic, Alzheimer's disease, differs markedly from canonical Alzheimer's disease (Bredesen, 2016). Presentation is often non-amnestic, and instead may feature executive dysfunction or cortical symptoms, most of which are parietal cortical functions, such as dyscalculia, visual perception abnormalities (as observed with posterior cortical atrophy), dyspraxias, agnosias, or aphasia (typically primary progressive aphasia). Interestingly, the executive dysfunction is usually of the parietal type, without behavioral abnormalities, unlike the dysfunction seen with frontotemporal lobar degeneration (Mendez, 2012). Depression is a common early feature and is associated with HPA (hypothalamic-pituitary-adrenal axis) dysfunction. The symptom onset is very early, typically in the 50s or even late 40s, often in association with menopause or with a major life stressor, and the symptoms are usually markedly exacerbated by stress and often progress rapidly. These patients are often ApoE4-negative, and virtually all of these patients have had significant toxic exposures—metallotoxins, organic toxins, and/or biotoxins—and successful treatment requires detoxification (Bredesen, 2016). The microbiome may contribute to type 3 Alzheimer's disease through its role in detoxification as well as via its role in trophic support.

As our conception of Alzheimer's disease is evolving, medicine itself is undergoing a revolution as well. The 20th-century idea of medicine that so many of us studied concerned itself primarily with the *what* of disease—making the appropriate diagnosis, in order to determine what the optimal treatment would be. Medical treatments were largely limited to monotherapies, typically pharmacological ones, but these have proven largely ineffectual in treating the many complex chronic conditions that limit our health spans today. By contrast, 21st-century medicine concerns itself with the *why* of disease, and therefore requires much larger data sets to understand the often numerous contributors to complex chronic illnesses like Alzheimer's disease, multiple sclerosis, lupus erythematosus, and cardiovascular disease. Appropriately, the optimal treatment protocols for these complex chronic conditions typically involve personalized, targeted therapy programs—precision medicine that involves both pharmacological and non-pharmacological therapeutics.

This individualized therapeutic approach requires a deep understanding of the personalized pathophysiology of each patient. In patients with cognitive decline— or those at risk for cognitive decline—due to Alzheimer's, the microbiome has been implicated repeatedly. The human gut microbiome plays an important role in virtually all of the major risk factors and drivers of cognitive decline: inflammation, auto-immunity, insulin resistance, lipid metabolism, obesity, nutrient absorption, amyloidogenesis, neurochemistry, sleep, stress response, and detoxification. Furthermore, the bi-directional connection between the gut and the brain is becoming as clear and as fundamental as the connection between the central and peripheral nervous systems. Therefore, it is highly likely that future development of the most effective prevention and therapeutic strategies for Alzheimer's disease will rely heavily on microbiome optimization.

Comparison of the microbiomes of patients with dementia due to Alzheimer's disease versus age-matched controls showed a marked difference in both the complexity and distribution of microbiota, as shown by Vogt et al. (Vogt et al., 2017) and noted in this book's chapter by Dr. Zhang. The phyla Firmicutes and Actinobacteria were reduced in patients with Alzheimer's disease, a finding that parallels results from patients with obesity and type 2 diabetes. Within Firmicutes, the families *Ruminococcaceae*, *Turicibacteraceae*, *Peptostreptococcaceae*, *Clostridiaceae*, and *Mogibacteriaceae* were reduced, and within Actinobacteria, the family *Bifidobacteriaceae* was reduced. In contrast, members of the phylum Bacteroidetes were found to be increased in patients with Alzheimer's disease, reflected at the family level by an increase in *Bacteroidaceae* and *Rikenellaceae*. This reduction led the authors to speculate that the insulin resistance associated with all three conditions (Alzheimer's, obesity, and type 2 diabetes) may actually be a microbiome-driven mechanism. Furthermore, the degree of abnormality in the cerebrospinal fluid (CSF) samples from Alzheimer's patients tended to correlate with the microbiome alterations, such that those individuals with more exaggerated microbiome changes tended to also have more severe CSF abnormalities.

Beyond the correlation of microbiome changes in patients with Alzheimer's disease, studies in germ-free mice suggest both causation and a bi-directional influence. Using a mouse model of Alzheimer's disease (APPPS1) based on mutations present in some cases of familial Alzheimer's disease (FAD, which represents about 5% of Alzheimer's disease patients), Harach and colleagues (Harach et al., 2017) found that these mutations are associated with an alteration in the microbiome. Just as Vogt et al. found, there was a decrease in Firmicutes and Actinobacteria, with a concomitant increase in Bacterioidetes. This alteration preceded the deposits of amyloid-β plaques in the mouse model. Furthermore, when the same mutations were present in germ-free mice (i.e., mice lacking a microbiome), the amyloid-β plaque deposits were strikingly mitigated (about 70% at 8 months). Repopulation of the microbiome with microbiota from Alzheimer's model mice increased amyloid deposits, whereas repopulation with microbiota from control mice produced a lesser effect on amyloid deposition.

These results suggest that, even when the Alzheimer's phenotype is genetically induced in mice—as opposed to sporadic Alzheimer's, which makes up about 95% of human Alzheimer's disease—there is an alteration in the microbiome that parallels, at least at the phylum level, the alteration observed in human patients with sporadic Alzheimer's disease. The mutations introduced into the mouse genomes apparently cooperate with the microbiome alterations to generate the Alzheimer's phenotype, since lacking the mutations leads to a non-Alzheimer's phenotype, but lacking a microbiome also markedly retards the amyloid deposition. Furthermore, the phenotype is more severe when the Alzheimer's-associated microbiota are used to recolonize the gut, again implicating the microbiome as an important causal contributor to the Alzheimer's pathotype. These results parallel those obtained in Parkinson's model mice, in which the effect of an α-synuclein mutation associated with familial Parkinson's disease was mitigated by a germ-free endogenous environment (Sampson et al., 2016). These results reinforce the notion that both diseases actually represent protective responses—specifically the antimicrobial peptides amyloid-β and α-synuclein—to insults that in at least some cases involve alterations to the microbiome, regardless of whether those alterations are induced sporadically or genetically.

Since the majority of Alzheimer's and Parkinson's cases are sporadic rather than familial, it is relevant to ask what factors generate changes in gut bacteria, recognizing that, as with the mouse studies, cause and effect may be bi-directional. Cesarean birth, stress, antibiotics, alcohol, reduced fiber consumption, refined carbohydrates, aging, inflammation, and parasites are among the many factors that can affect the intestinal microbiome (Wen and Duffy, 2017; Belkaid and Hand, 2014). Therefore, all of these factors represent potential risk factors for microbiome-driven contributions to neurodegeneration. On the flip side, probiotics, prebiotics, gut healing (e.g., with bone broth or colostrum or deglycyrrhizinated licorice or butyrate), and fecal transplants all offer promise as potential therapeutics for the beneficial manipulation of the gut microbiome.

There are multiple mechanisms through which microbiome alterations may contribute to the pathophysiology of Alzheimer's disease, as can be expected given the remarkably multi-factorial functioning of the human microbiome. For example, species of *Lactobacillus* and *Bifidobacteria* are involved in the production of GABA from glutamate, and an imbalance in this ratio occurs in Alzheimer's disease (Bhattacharjee and Lukiw, 2013). Cyanobacteria, another type of bacteria populating the microbiome, may produce the excitotoxin L-BMAA (β-N-methylamino L-alanine), which is shown to be elevated in Alzheimer's disease and other neurodegenerative conditions such as amyotrophic lateral sclerosis (ALS). Therefore, direct neurochemical effects may play a role in the gut-brain connections driving cognitive decline.

Inflammation caused by "leaky gut," systemic inflammation that plays a prominent role in type 1 Alzheimer's disease, provides a second potential mechanism through which the microbiome could drive neurodegenerative conditions like Alzheimer's (Bredesen, 2015). The gut mucosal immune system is comprised of lymph nodes, epithelial cells, and the lamina propria, and it provides a protective barrier for the intestinal tract (Shi et al., 2017). The microbiome includes commensals, which support normal immune function, and pathogenic organisms, which mediate immune dysfunction. Microbiome alterations that reduce commensals in favor of pathogenic organisms are associated with abnormal immune responses, inflammation, and failure of the normal gut barrier, promulgating systemic inflammation. As a specific example, when *Bacteroides fragilis* is present in the human microbiome it produces a lipopolysaccharide that is neurotoxic, associated with nuclei in Alzheimer's disease, and induces the inflammatory mediator NF-κB (nuclear factor kappa light chain enhancer of B-cells) via pro-inflammatory microRNAs 9, 34a, 125b, 146a, and 155 (Zhao and Lukiw, 2018). This may have implications for one of the biggest questions pondered by those in the neurodegenerative field: why do these diseases often begin in late adulthood even when an associated mutation has been present throughout life? One potential explanation for at least some cases is the increasing leakiness of the gut with age, which can lead to systemic inflammation caused by body-wide exposure to lipopolysaccharides and other inflammagens. A parallel increase in blood–brain barrier permeability is likely to be an amplifying factor in the exposure of the central nervous system (CNS) to a host of cytokines, bacterial fragments, ingested protein fragments, and other potential contributors to CNS inflammation. The resulting activation of the innate immune system would then include the formation, reduced degradation, and reduced clearance, of β-amyloid peptides. Inflammation plays a critical role in Alzheimer's disease and appears to be a critical determinant of the presence or absence of cognitive decline in the large fraction of elderly people that develop amyloid deposition in the brain. In other words, those with amyloid deposits but no inflammation may avoid cognitive decline, whereas those with amyloid deposits and inflammation typically suffer from reduced cognitive abilities.

A related but distinct mechanism through which the microbiome may contribute to Alzheimer's disease pathophysiology involves the intimate relationship between the microbiome and immune system function. Alterations in the microbiome are associated with optimal immunological responses to pathogens and biotoxins, as well as the induction of autoimmunity (Ball et al., 2013; Douglas-Escobar et al., 2013; Hornig, 2013). In particular, developmental aspects of the adaptive immune system are dependent on the microbiome (Round and Mazmanian, 2009), and this may have important implications for the role of the microbiome in Alzheimer's disease. In one sense, Alzheimer's disease itself may represent a chronic activation of the innate immune system without effective adaptive immune system activation and removal of the offending pathogens. Such a view coincides with the proposal by Shoemaker that the chronic inflammatory response syndrome (CIRS) that occurs in response to mycotoxins and other biotoxins involves innate immune system activation with insufficient adaptive immune response (Shoemaker and House, 2006). Supporting this notion is the fact that there is a substantial overlap in patients with CIRS and cognitive decline due to Alzheimer's disease, and these Alzheimer's patients have been described as type 3, or toxic, Alzheimer's disease patients (Bredesen, 2016). Thus the relationship between innate immune system function and adaptive immune system response, which is substantially impacted by the microbiome, may play a critical role in Alzheimer's and other inflammatory diseases. Optimizing this relationship via the assessment and enhancement of the microbiome may therefore represent an effective strategy for mollifying cognitive decline.

A fourth mechanism through which the microbiome may play an important mediating role in Alzheimer's disease is its effect on the coordinated system dysfunction referred to as metabolic syndrome: insulin resistance, hyperglycemia, hypertension, dyslipidemia, and obesity with visceral fat accumulation. It has been estimated that 20–25% of the adult population suffers from metabolic syndrome (Mazidi et al., 2016), and this syndrome has been strongly linked to Alzheimer's risk (Razay et al., 2007), especially type 1.5 (glycotoxic) Alzheimer's disease. Although the mechanism(s) through which the gut microbiome affects metabolic syndrome are incompletely understood, some of the suggested pathways include energy homeostasis, modulation of inflammatory signaling pathways, immune system alterations, nutrient effects, and interference with the renin–angiotensin system (Mazidi et al., 2016).

A fifth mechanism through which the microbiome could influence Alzheimer's disease pathophysiology is via its effects on trophic signaling, which are especially important in the progression of type 2 (atrophic) Alzheimer's disease. Brain-derived neurotrophic factor (BDNF), for example, exerts a powerful anti-Alzheimer's effect, and its production is increased with exercise (Griffin et al., 2011). The gut microbiome affects both the production and signaling of BDNF (Maqsood and Stone, 2016). Degradation of the microbiome is associated with a reduction in BDNF, inhibiting the maintenance of NMDA receptors and in turn altering glutamatergic output to the GABAergic inhibitory neurons—neurons that are affected early on in the progression of Alzheimer's disease. Just like the mechanisms through which the microbiome impacts metabolic syndrome, the bio-chemical mechanisms are incompletely understood. However, these may include the effects of short-chain fatty acids (SCFA), kynurenine pathway effects, or other neurochemical modulatory effects.

Nutrient absorption and production represent a sixth mechanism through which the microbiome may impact Alzheimer's disease risk and pathophysiology, espe-cially type 2 (atrophic) Alzheimer's disease. Approximately 85% of carbohydrates, 65–95% of proteins, and virtually 100% of fats are absorbed in the upper gut (mostly the proximal small intestine) after being consumed; following this initial digestion, the remaining 10–30% of total ingested caloric potential enters the large intestine (Krajmalnik-Brown et al., 2012). These indigestible carbohydrates and proteins are acted upon by the colonic microbiota, which ferment both resistant and non-resistant starches, unabsorbed sugars, polysaccharides, and mucins, producing short-chain fatty acids (SCFA) such as butyrate, propionate, and acetate, and gases like car-bon dioxide, methane, and molecular hydrogen. Branched-chain amino acids add formate, valerate, caproate, isobutyrate, 2-methylbutyrate, and isovalerate to these metabolites (Krajmalnik-Brown et al., 2012). The specifics of SCFA production depend on numerous factors such as age, diet, microbiome, gut transit time, colonic segment, and colonic pH (Ho et al., 2018). Ho noted that specific SCFAs potently interfered with the formation of amyloid-β aggregates, and therefore suggested that these SCFAs may be inhibitory to Alzheimer's disease pathogenesis. Obesity, another risk factor for Alzheimer's disease, is also affected by microbiome-associated nutri-ents and metabolism: molecular hydrogen is produced by the microbiota, and then oxidized by specific microorganisms (methanogens, acetogens, and sulfate reduc-ers), which are overabundant in obese individuals (Krajmalnik-Brown et al., 2012).

A crucial role in detoxification represents the seventh mechanism through which the microbiome composition and function may impact risk and pathogenesis of Alzheimer's disease, especially type 3 (toxic) Alzheimer's disease. The gut microbi-ome exerts a major effect on metabolomics and detoxification (Wikoff et al., 2009). Furthermore, probiotic "feeding" of the microbiome affects transit time and excre-tion of toxins. In a reciprocal fashion, specific toxins alter the microbiome, such as triclosan, pesticides, glyphosate, plasticizers, heavy metals, and some drugs (e.g., antibiotics, proton pump inhibitors, and synthetic estrogens) (Christensen, 2017).

Beyond the above-referenced metabolic, immunological, and toxic effects of the microbiome and its effects on cognitive decline, the microbes of the gut may actu-ally produce their own amyloids (also noted in Chapter 3), and these may impact amyloid-β production, degradation, and clearance (Pistollato et al., 2016). It has been hypothesized that bacterial-derived amyloids may indeed deposit in the CNS and affect overall amyloidogenesis (Zhao and Lukiw, 2018). Furthermore, prions such as PrP are capable of aggregating and producing amyloids, and they are capable of migration/transport along neural pathways, such as those that link the enteric nervous system (ENS) and the CNS.

LOOKING FORWARD

The potential for using microbiome analysis and manipulation in the prevention and treatment of Alzheimer's disease and its precursors, SCI (subjective cognitive impairment) and MCI (mild cognitive impairment), offers both exciting opportunities and significant challenges. In one study using probiotics in a transgenic mouse model of Alzheimer's disease (Bonfili et al., 2017), cognitive decline was reduced, inflammatory cytokines were inhibited, and proteolysis was restored. Probiotic treatment was shown to activate the SirT1 pathway, inducing antioxidant and neuroprotective effects (Bonfili et al., 2018).

Another promising therapeutic approach is to identify specific bacterial taxa that are associated with ameliorative biochemical and cognitive effects: for example, in one study, an increase in brain-derived neurotrophic factor (BDNF) was associated with one species of *Bifidobacterium* (O'Sullivan et al., 2011). In another study, *Mycobacterium vaccae* immunization was associated with a reduction in the stress response and microglial activation, inducing an anti-inflammatory response in the central nervous system (Frank et al., 2018). Although this result was accomplished using standard immunization techniques, analogous approaches using various microbial species to alter microbiome-related immunity may be feasible. Given the large number of potential species, there are almost limitless opportunities for therapeutic neurochemical and immunological effects in neurodegeneration, and indeed this approach is highly promising.

However, if microbiome manipulation is to be optimized for the treatment of Alzheimer's disease and other neurodegenerative conditions, several critical research topics will need to be addressed. For example, we will need rapid analysis, both quantitative and qualitative, of the extremely complex microbiomes of individual patients. We will need the ability to generate accurate, reliable predictions of the specific effects of individual microbiome manipulations and the potential side effects of these manipulations. We may need better surviving probiotics, computer-based algorithms to identify the optimal treatment program for each patient, and more efficient methods to heal the gut and prevent chronic "leaky gut." We will certainly need more information on the genomic-probiotic-prebiotic interactions likely to occur for each patient and the potentially therapeutic and potentially pathogenic microbiota. Clearly, the complexity of obtaining accurate analysis and optimizing microbiome therapeutics is staggering. However, the promise of this approach in the successful treatment of Alzheimer's disease, or as part of an overall personalized program of therapy, is arguably greater than any other avenue of inquiry into therapeutics for neurodegenerative diseases.

Interestingly, 1907 was both the year that Alzheimer described the disease that bears his name and the year that the beneficial effects of human microbiota were described by Metchnikoff (Bhattacharjee and Lukiw, 2013). Hopefully, these two observations will increasingly intersect in a successful, microbiome-driven therapeutic program for Alzheimer's disease.

REFERENCES

Ball, M., et al., 2013. Intracerebral propagation of Alzheimer's disease: Strengthening evidence of a herpes simplex virus etiology. *Alzheimer's & Dementia* 9(2):169–175.

Belkaid, Y., and Hand, T., 2014. Role of the microbiota in immunity and inflammation. *Cell* 157(1):121–141.

Bhattacharjee, S., and Lukiw, W., 2013. Alzheimer's disease and the microbiome. *Frontiers in Cellular Neuroscience* 7:153.

Bonfili, L. et al., 2017. Microbiota modulation counteracts Alzheimer's disease progression influencing neuronal proteolysis and gut hormones plasma levels. *Scientific Reports* 7(1):2426. https://www.nature.com/articles/s41598-017-02587-2.

Bonfili, L. et al., 2018. SLAB51 probiotic formulation activates SIRT1 pathway promoting antioxidant and neuroprotective effects in an AD mouse model. *Molecular Neurobiology* Feb. 28. https://link.springer.com/article/10.1007%2Fs12035-018-0973-4.

Bredesen, D., 2014. Reversal of cognitive decline: A novel therapeutic program. *Aging* 6(9):707–717.

Bredesen, D., 2015. Metabolic profiling distinguishes three subtypes of Alzheimer's disease. *Aging* 7(8):595–600.

Bredesen, D., 2016. Inhalational Alzheimer's disease: An unrecognized – and treatable – epidemic. *Aging* 8(2):304–313.

Bredesen, D. et al., 2016. Reversal of cognitive decline in Alzheimer's disease. *Aging* 8(6):1250–1258.

Christensen, L., 2017. Are environmental toxins disrupting your gut bacteria? *Ascent2health. com.* https://www.ascent2health.com/blog/are-environmental-toxins-disrupting-your-gut-bacteria.

Douglas-Escobar, M., Elliott, E., and Neu, J., 2013. Effect of intestinal microbial ecology on the developing brain. *JAMA Pediatrics* 167(4):374–379.

Famenini, S. et al., 2017. Increased intermediate M1-M2 macrophage polarization and improved cognition in mild cognitive impairment patients on ω-3 supplementation. *FASEB Journal* 31(1):148–160.

Frank, M. et al., 2018. Immunization with *Mycobacterium vaccae* induces an anti-inflammatory milieu in the CNS: Attenuation of stress-induced microglial priming, alarmins and anxiety-like behavior. *Brain, Behavior, and Immunity* May 2018. https://www.sciencedirect.com/science/article/pii/S088915911830196X?via=ihub.

Griffin, E. et al., 2011. Aerobic exercise improves hippocampal function and increases BDNF in the serum of young adult males. *Physiology and Behavior* 104(5):934–941.

Harach, T. et al., 2017. Reduction of Abeta amyloid pathology in APPPS1 transgenic mice in the absence of gut microbiota. *Scientific Reports* 7:41802. https://www.nature.com/articles/srep41802.

Ho, L. et al., 2018. Protective roles of intestinal microbiota derived short chain fatty acids in Alzheimer's disease-type beta-amyloid neuropathological mechanisms. *Expert Review of Neurotherapeutics* 18(1):83–90.

Hornig, M., 2013. The role of microbes and autoimmunity in the pathogenesis of neuropsychiatric illness. *Current Opinion in Rheumatology* 25(4):488–795.

James, B. et al., 2014. Contribution of Alzheimer disease to mortality in the United States. *Neurology* 82(12):1045–1050.

Krajmalnik-Brown, R. et al., 2012. Effects of gut microbes on nutrient absorption and energy regulation. *Nutrition in Clinical Practice* 27(2):201–214.

Kumar, K. et al., 2016. Amyloid-β peptide protects against microbial infection in mouse and worm models of Alzheimer's disease. *Science Translational Medicine* 8(340):1–15.

Maqsood, R., and Stone, T., 2016. The gut-brain axis, BDNF, NMDA and CNS disorders. *Neurochemical Research* 41(11):2819–2835.

Mazidi, M. et al., 2016. Gut microbiome and metabolic syndrome. *Diabetes & Metabolic Syndrome: Clinical Research and Reviews* 10(2 Suppl 1):S150–S157.

Mendez, M., 2012. Early-onset Alzheimer's disease: Nonamnestic subtypes and type 2 AD. *Archives of Medical Research* 43(8):677–685.

Ngandu, T. et al., 2015. A 2 year multidomain intervention of diet, exercise, cognitive training, and vascular risk monitoring versus control to prevent cognitive decline in at-risk elderly people (FINGER): A randomised controlled trial. *Lancet* 385(9984):2255.

O'Sullivan, E. et al., 2011. BDNF expression in the hippocampus of maternally separated rats: Does Bifidobacterium breve 6330 alter BDNF levels? *Beneficial Microbes* 2(3):199–207.

Pistollato, F. et al., 2016. Role of gut microbiota and nutrients in amyloid formation and pathogenesis of Alzheimer disease. *Nutrition Reviews* 74(10):624–634.

Razay, G., Vreugdenhil, A., and Wilcock, G., 2007. The metabolic syndrome and Alzheimer disease. *Archives of Neurology* 64(1):93–96.

Round, J., and Mazmanian, S., 2009. The gut microbiota shapes intestinal immune responses during health and disease. *Nature Reviews Immunology* 9(5):313–323.

Sampson, T. et al., 2016. Gut microbiota regulate motor deficits and neuroinflammation in a model of Parkinson's disease. *Cell* 167(6):1469–1480.

Shi, N. et al., 2017. Interaction between the gut microbiome and mucosal immune system. *Military Medical Research* 4:14. https://mmrjournal.biomedcentral.com/articles/10.1186/s40779-017-0122-9.

Shinto, L. et al., 2014. A randomized placebo-controlled pilot trial of omega-3 fatty acids and alpha lipoic acid in Alzheimer's disease. *Journal of Alzheimer's Disease* 28(1):111–120.

Shoemaker, R., and House, D., 2006. Sick building syndrome (SBS) and exposure to water-damaged buildings: Time series study, clinical trial and mechanisms. *Neurotoxicology and Teratology* 28(5):573–588.

Vogt, N. et al., 2017. Gut microbiome alterations in Alzheimer's disease. *Scientific Reports* 7(1):13537. https://www.nature.com/articles/s41598-017-13601-y.

Wen, L., and Duffy, A., 2017. Factors influencing the gut microbiota, inflammation, and type 2 diabetes. *The Journal of Nutrition* 147(7):1468S–1475S.

Wikoff, W. et al., 2009. Metabolomics analysis reveals large effects of gut microflora on mammalian blood metabolites. *PNAS* 106(10):3698–3703.

Zhao, Y., and Lukiw, W., 2018. *Bacteroidetes* neurotoxins and inflammatory neurodegeneration. *Molecular Neurobiology* April 10. https://link.springer.com/article/10.1007/s12035-018-1015-y.

7 Microbial Involvement in Alzheimer's Disease

Can (Martin) Zhang

CONTENTS

INTRODUCTION: AD AND HUMAN MICROBIOME

Alzheimer's disease is an irreversible and progressive neurodegenerative disorder. It is the primary cause of dementia in the elderly, affecting approximately 5.3 million Americans. Diagnosis, management and research of Alzheimer's and other forms of dementia cost the United States $226 billion annually [1, 2]. *The State of US Health:1990–2010* placed on Alzheimer's the unenviable title of the fastest-growing incidence rate among the most burdensome diseases over a period of 20 years [3]. When you consider the fact that aging is the first risk factor for Alzheimer's and Americans are enjoying increasing lifespans, the number of Alzheimer's patients may nearly triple to 13.8 million by 2050, with the associated costs rising to as high as $1.1 trillion in the US [2, 4]. At present there are no therapies that can modify disease progression. The current pharmacological interventions for Alzheimer's include acetylcholinesterase inhibitors and N-methyl-D-aspartate (NMDA) receptor partial antagonists, but these agents are only palliative and may provide temporary and modest symptomatic relief. They have no impact on the underlying pathology of Alzheimer's, nor can they halt the progression of the disease [2]. Therefore, there is an urgent medical need to develop therapeutic agents that can modify the pathology or decrease the risk of Alzheimer's [2, 3].

Alzheimer's is a genetically complex and heterogeneous disorder. It has two primary forms: early- or late-onset Alzheimer's, a distinction which is drawn based on the patient's age at the onset of the disease. More than 200 fully penetrant mutations in the amyloid β protein precursor (*APP*), presenilin 1 (*PSEN1*), and presenilin 2 (*PSEN2*) have been identified as causing inherited, early-onset familial Alzheimer's disease (FAD) (<60 years old; 5–10% cases). Several genetic variants, including those encoding the apolipoprotein E (*APOE*) [5, 6] and the triggering receptor expressed on myeloid cells 2 (*TREM2*) [7, 8], have been identified as being associated with the late-onset of Alzheimer's (>60 years old; 90–95% cases). Although the molecular mechanisms underlying Alzheimer's have not been completely elucidated, the pathology of Alzheimer's is well known. The disease is characterized by a build-up of β-amyloid plaques comprised of a small protein, amyloid-β (Aβ), and neurofibrillary tangles composed of the phosphorylated tau protein in the brain. Aβ is produced by serial cleavage of the transmembrane APP protein by the β- and γ-secretase. Considerable genetic, biochemical, molecular biological, and pathological evidence supports the "*Aβ hypothesis*," which posits that the excessive accumulation of Aβ is the primary pathological event of Alzheimer's, as this build-up of Aβ precipitates phosphorylated tau levels and neurofibrillary tangle formation. This process may fundamentally change the neuro-inflammatory status in the brain, ultimately leading to synaptic dysfunction, neurodegeneration and, finally, the clinical manifestations of dementia [9–12].

Numerous studies, ranging back decades, have identified the critical pathological and physiological role of the microbiome in human health and disease [13–18]. The human microbiome is a term used to represent all of the microbial cells and their products as well as their genetic material that live on, in, or around humans. It functions by shaping and regulating the structure and molecular profile of our immune system and systems-level inflammatory and metabolic status [14, 15]. The human microbiome interacts directly with its host and presents a source for human genetic and metabolic diversity. It evolves alongside lifelong developmental stages in humans and varies across different locations of the world; there are even perceptible changes in different tissues and organs of the same body [15]. Furthermore, increasing evidence suggests that the human microbiome, particularly the gut microbiota, impacts not only the immune diseases of the gastrointestinal (GI) tract, but also neurodegenerative disorders, including Alzheimer's disease. This chapter will review the role microbes play in the pathophysiology of Alzheimer's, with a focus on the microbiome–host and gut–brain relationships, as well as the potential for developing microbiome-targeted therapies for this disease.

GUT MICROBIOTA AND ALZHEIMER'S

Colonization, or the "seeding" of gut microbiota (commensal flora), occurs immediately following birth. The gut microbiome plays major and lifelong roles in the development, maturation, and functioning of the gastrointestinal, immune, neuroendocrine, and metabolic systems, as well as the central nervous system (CNS) [16]. Regulation of the microbiome–gut–brain axis is essential for maintaining homeostasis and allowing these systems to fulfill their physiological roles [16]. Several animal models with a deficiency or perturbed composition of microbiota have been characterized for their roles in the cognitive functions and pathological changes related to Alzheimer's.

Germ-free (GF) animals provide an effective tool for functional analysis and modeling of the effects of a deficiency in the microbiome [19–22]. One study using germ-free animals demonstrated that the microbiome is related to hippocampus-dependent memory formation [19]. Specifically, Gareau and co-authors investigated the effects of microbiota on hippocampus-dependent memory formation in germ-free mouse models using exposure to water-deprived stress [19]. The T-maze test was utilized to analyze the hippocampus-dependent working memory that represents animals' natural tendency toward exploring a novel environment, in favor of a familiar one [20]. In this study, working memory was impaired in the germ-free mice, with or without exposure to stress, in contrast to the control animals with normally developed gut microbiota. Moreover, the water avoidance-based stress model showed affected working memory formation in *Citrobacter rodentium*-infected mice, as expected, and this deficit could be restored by the probiotics. The mechanisms are related to hippocampal expression of brain-derived neurotrophic factor (BDNF) and c-Fos proteins [20]. In other studies, germ-free animals were characterized by anxiety-like behavior that could be normalized through the restoration of the gut microbiota [21], while presenting neurochemical changes in the brain [21, 23], including altered levels of the NMDA receptor subunit NR2B in the central amygdala and the serotonin receptor 1A (5HT1A) in the hippocampal dentate granule cells [23]. Furthermore, the serotonergic system is associated with aging and the development of Alzheimer's and has been further investigated in germ-free animals [24]. Clarke and co-authors found that, early in life, the microbiome regulates the hippocampal serotonergic system in a sex-dependent manner in germ-free animals. Specifically, male germ-free animals had a significant elevation in the hippocampal concentration of the 5-hydroxytryptamine (5-HT) and a decrease in BDNF levels, compared with conventionally colonized control male animals. Moreover, the changes in the 5-HT and BNDF levels were not observed in female mice, while the immunological and neuroendocrine changes were present in both sexes [21]. The sex-dependent mechanism by which the microbiome regulates neurobiology remains unclear and requires further study to be fully understood. Collectively, these results highlight the importance of the gut microbiota in CNS development and hippocampal memory formation.

Recently, gut microbiota have been manipulated in several animal-based studies to better understand its impact on Alzheimer's and other neurological disorders. First, Minter et al. utilized transgenic Alzheimer's animals demonstrating that gut-administrated antibiotics attenuated Alzheimer's pathology in the brain [25, 26]. In the first study, Minter and co-authors examined the role of the host microbiome in regulating cerebral amyloidosis using an APP[Swedish]/PS1[ΔE9] mouse model of Alzheimer's. Long-term exposure to broad-spectrum, combinatorial antibiotics led to prolonged shifts in gut microbial composition and diversity, as well as altered circulating cytokine levels and chemokine signatures in the blood. Interestingly, the gut microbial changes and blood cytokine changes are related to decreased amyloid plaque deposition and elevated soluble Aβ proteins, as well as altered microglial morphology and attenuated plaque-localized glial reactivity in the brain [26]. Because the postnatal period is critical to the development of neuro-immunity and microbiota–host interactions, Minter et al. investigated whether acute exposure of the antibiotics during this critical period (P14-P21) could have long-term effects on Alzheimer's pathogenic events using APP[Swedish]/PS1[ΔE9] mice [25]. Indeed, the authors found that early exposure to antibiotics resulted in long-term altered gut microbial composition (predominantly

Lachnospiraceae and S24-7), elevated levels of blood- and brain-resident Foxp3[+] T-regulatory cells, and an altered inflammatory milieu of the blood and cerebrospinal fluid (CSF) [25]. These changes were related to reduced amyloid deposition, and down-regulated plaque-localized microglia and astrocytes in the brain [25]. Notably, treatment using gut antibiotics in early life resulted in robust and long-lasting effects on Alzheimer's pathology in the brain in later life [25].

These findings, using gut-administrated antibiotics, [25, 26] are in agreement with the aforementioned [21] study, along with several others, in pinpointing the importance of the microbiome on physiology in early developmental stages. For example, one study by Cox and co-authors showed that altering intestinal microbiota during early developmental stages led to long-term metabolic consequences in mice [27]. Specifically, low-dose penicillin delivered from infancy affected intestinal expression of immunity-related genes and induced lasting changes in host metabolism and adiposity. Furthermore, the microbiota phenotypes induced by low-dose penicillin are transferrable to germ-free animals, indicating they have roles other than antibiotics per se in the pathogenetic events [27]. Taken together, these findings suggest that the structure and diversity of gut microbiota impact Aβ amyloidosis and amyloid pathology by regulating host immunity and neuroinflammation [25, 26].

Other studies have further characterized the role of gut microbial involvement in the progression of Alzheimer's using animal models. Harach et al. utilized an APP transgenic mouse model and sequenced fecal bacterial 16S rRNA compared to non-transgenic wild-type mice and discovered a gut microbiota population shift [28]. The authors also found that germ-free APP transgenic mice displayed a reduction of amyloid pathology in the brain compared to the mice with normal composition of microbiota. Intriguingly, when germ-free APP transgenic mice were colonized with microbiota from normal microbiota-containing APP transgenic mice, amyloid pathology was restored in the brain. In contrast, wild-type mice were less effective in driving cerebral Aβ levels when colonized with normal microbiota-containing mice [28].

Furthermore, the importance of gut microbiota in Alzheimer's has been characterized in humans [29]. Vogt and co-investigators studied the bacterial taxonomic composition of fecal samples and found that Alzheimer's patients demonstrated distinct composition and decreased microbial diversity when compared to age- and sex-matched controls [29]. Furthermore, this study reported differences in bacterial abundance as represented by decreased *Firmicutes* and *Bifidobacterium* and increased *Bacteroidetes* in the microbiome of Alzheimer's patients. Furthermore, levels of differentially abundant genera were correlated with CSF biomarkers of Alzheimer's [29]. Taken together, these studies evidence the idea that gut microbiota may not only affect innate immunity in the gut [30, 31], but also regulate the systemic immune and metabolic status through the gut-brain crosstalk and, by extension, neuroinflammation [32, 33].

Our understanding of the role of the human microbiome in Alzheimer's began several decades ago with studies identifying microbes in the brain. These studies have recently evolved to focus specifically on the human microbiome–host relationship at the systems levels. A considerable number of microbes have been identified in the brain, including *Borrelia spirochetes* [34], *Chlamydia pneumonia* [35], and herpes simplex virus type 1 [36, 37], among others. These microbes may lie dormant for many years and may be associated with Alzheimer's by regulating the host immune system in response to the microbes. These studies suggest that there may be microbial reactivation and neuronal damage present during aging or other conditions associated with decreased immunity and pathological host–microbiome interaction. Overall, these findings highlight the importance of microbial involvement in the development of amyloid pathology in the brains of patients with Alzheimer's.

IMPAIRED MICROBIOTA AND ALZHEIMER'S

The gut microbiota and the gut-brain axis play critical roles in maintaining healthy local and systemic immunological status and are responsible for certain pathological conditions and diseases, including Alzheimer's. The mechanisms by which gut microbial activity changes Alzheimer's pathology in the brain and neurobehavior have not been fully understood, but may involve several lines of action. We have already discussed the idea that a deficiency or perturbation of the microbiome composition appears to be related to Alzheimer's due those pathways' ability to regulate host immunity and neuroinflammation [25, 26, 28]. Below, we will provide more evidence that impaired microbiota may lead to the phenotypical changes seen in Alzheimer's.

Impaired gut microbiota, also known as gut dysbiosis, can first occur in the local tissues of the gut. This impairment can then expand beyond the gut itself to a generalized systemic response with functional immune changes and subsequent neuroinflammatory responses [38–40]. The immune system may contribute to and drive the pathogenesis of Alzheimer's and thus could also provide strategies for developing novel therapeutic approaches [38–40]. Immune cells include phagocytes or macrophages in the peripheral system and the resident microglia and astrocytes in the brain and spinal cord [41]. Recently, Wu et al. showed that the effector cells/molecules in the gut dysbiosis are the hemocytes [41], also known as the phagocytes of invertebrates. They studied the roles of enteric dysbiosis in Alzheimer's using a Drosophila Alzheimer's model, in which enterobacteria infection increased immune hemocyte recruitment to the brain and elevated oxidative stress levels in the brain, while triggering TNF-JNK mediated neurodegeneration and exacerbating the progression of Alzheimer's phenotype. Interestingly, the authors also found that genetic depletion of hemocytes attenuated neuroinflammation and alleviated neurodegeneration [41]. Furthermore, this work was in line with other studies showing the role of microglia cells and astrocytes in the brain in response to changes in gut microbiota [25, 26, 28]. In future studies, the relationship of gut microbiota and neuroinflammation in Alzheimer's needs to be more precisely defined to identify Alzheimer's-specific microbial species and molecules.

Increasingly, studies suggest that unbalanced gut microbiota and pathogenic metabolites act on the brain in the following way. A dysfunctional gastrointestinal tract system, also known as a "leaky gut," will influence local and systemic neurochemical and immunological changes in the host. This is followed by blood–brain barrier (BBB) penetration and functional defects in the brain [42, 43]. The gut microbiome may produce secretory products, some of which have been identified in Alzheimer's brains. For example, lipopolysaccharide (LPS) has been detected in the hippocampus of Alzheimer's patients [44] and gram-negative bacterial molecules were identified in Alzheimer's brains [45]. Furthermore, one study showed that viral proteins, independent of pathogen replication, may predispose hosts to environmental stress associated with Alzheimer's risk [46]. Furthermore, neuroimmune interactions occur in other tissues and organs (e.g. the skin and respiratory tract) in addition to the gut [47]. These results suggest that modulation of neuroimmunological signaling may provide effective approaches to treating infections in these tissues [47]. Further characterization is required to determine how these primarily gastrointestinal tract-residing molecules were transported and identified in Alzheimer's brains, and the precise mechanisms of neuroimmunological signaling remain to be fully elucidated.

Notably, microbiota also generate and form amyloid fibers which are distinct from the Alzheimer's Aβ proteins that form in the brain and cause neurotoxicity, neurodegeneration, and dementia [48, 49]. On the other hand, Alzheimer's Aβ species display anti-microbial activities [50–54] that may be related to Alzheimer's pathogenesis. These anti-microbial activities have been demonstrated in cell-free and different model systems and can be independent of the immune activity of the host [52, 53]. Alzheimer's Aβ species and microbial amyloid may display both pathological impacts and physiological functions [52]. Therefore, a more complete understanding of the pathological and physiological roles of the human and microbial amyloid may provide new insights for the treatment of Alzheimer's and other amyloid diseases.

HUMAN MICROBIOME AND RISK FACTORS OF AD

Because the human microbiome affects host physiology, health status, and disease, it is vitally important to fully understand the relationship between the human microbiome and the risk factors for Alzheimer's. One's risk of developing Alzheimer's is determined by multiple factors, with aging and genetic inheritance being the two most important risk factors. Over the past century, drastic improvements in biomedical science, medical care, standard of living, and environmental conditions have rapidly increased our average life expectancy. By extension, these positive developments have also increased both the population of the elderly as a whole and the number of Alzheimer's patients [55]. As discussed below, studies and explored the association between age-related changes in gut microbiota and Alzheimer's risk in the elderly.

Considerable evidence suggests that gut microbiota changes can be driven by the aging process and influences the overall risk of developing Alzheimer's [56–58] alongside the other known aging-related changes in the immune and both the peripheral and central nervous systems. The microbiota structure and resulting inflammatory molecules have been identified as potential biological markers to represent the aging processes and/or potential longevity [55, 59–62]. For example, one study showed an increase of the *Firmicutes/Bacteroidetes* ratio from 0.4 in infancy to 10.9 in adulthood (25–45 years), followed by a decrease to 0.6 in the elderly (70– 90 years) [63]. Another study investigated the structure of the human gut microbiota and its homeostasis with the host's immune system by comparing young adults, elderly over 70 years old, and centenarians over 100 years old [64]. The authors observed that the young adults and the elderly displayed similar gut microbial composition and diversity, but both groups differed greatly when compared to the centenarians. Interestingly, the centenarians contained microbiota remodeling that featured several properties: (1) the compromised microbiota with notable pathobionts, that is, rearranged *Firmicutes* population and enriched facultative anaerobes, (2) a marked decrease in *Faecalibacterium prauznitzii* and relatives that are known as anti-inflammatory and beneficial symbiotic species; (3) a ten-fold increase in *Eubacterium limosum* and relatives as signature bacteria of long life; and (4) an increased inflammatory status with a range of peripheral blood inflammatory markers (e.g. increased IL-6 and IL-8). The causes of the pro-inflammatory status in the centenarians may have been counterbalanced by other physiological events that are related to an exceptional lifespan. This study warrants more research to define the roles of microbiota in the aging process. Collectively, this study supports the notion that the structure of the gut microbiota is relatively stable through adulthood, and that the aging process starts to impact gut microbiota at or after 70 years of age, a period that represents increased Alzheimer's incidence.

Studying Alzheimer's risk factors provides more precise and integrative information to help us understand the pathogenesis of Alzheimer's. Furthermore, the underlying mechanisms of these risk-conferring components as they relate to the human microbiome and Alzheimer's are only beginning to be understood in an integrative approach. In addition to inheritance and aging, the other risk factors for Alzheimer's are comprised of metabolic diseases (e.g. diabetes [65–67]), gender, sleep [68, 69], diet [70], medications, and psychological conditions (e.g. stress), among others. For example, medical and dietary exposures (folate, vitamin E and C, and coffee) are protective factors that are related to decreased risk of Alzheimer's [66]. Furthermore, using non-steroidal anti-inflammatory drugs (NSAIDs) is a medical exposure that relates to a decreased risk of Alzheimer's, although its potential as a useful therapeutic for Alzheimer's remains to be confirmed [66]. Evidence shows that treatments using NSAIDs lead to changes in the gut microbial population while modulating neuroinflammatory events [71]. Because sleep and diet may be major lifestyle components related to a decreased risk of Alzheimer's, leading a healthy life with balanced sleep and diet may be useful for the prevention of disease. These findings suggest that the human microbiome may interact with and react to our changing lifestyle, the aging process and other environmental factors [15], and then may expose us to a disease-protective or susceptible condition and function as a risk factor for Alzheimer's.

Metabolic conditions/disorders [72] and stress [73, 74] are also important risk factors of Alzheimer's that interact closely with the microbiome. Notably, the obesity caused by high-fat-diet consumption is related to altered gut microbiota, represented by a decrease in *Bacteroidetes* and an increase in *Firmicutes*, as well as inflammatory changes in the blood and neurons [75–77]. Elucidating the mechanisms by which high-fat diets lead to changes in gut microbiota and disease-related pathological and functional defects is critical in helping regulate the dysbiosis status, ensure the anti-obesity effects, and avoid chronic diseases. Furthermore, exposure to antibiotics in early life may alter the gut microbiome and adiposity in mice [78]. Moreover, postnatal germ-free animals have altered hypothalamic-pituitary-adrenal (HPA) axis, which is the stress response system, resulting in impaired stress-related response in these animals, compared to control specimens. These results underscore the role of gut microbiota in programming the HPA system and systemic immune response, as well as neuroinflammation and stress-related neurobehaviors. Collectively, the microbiome is related to the biological processes of Alzheimer's-related risk factors and collectively highlight the importance of microbiome-gut-brain crosstalk as a fundamental regulatory system in modulating Alzheimer's pathology in the brain and potentially the risk of the disease altogether.

TARGETING GUT MICROBIOTA FOR AD INTERVENTIONS

Uncovering the mechanisms by which the human microbiome affects the pathophysiology of Alzheimer's may help identify and develop effective gut microbiota-based therapeutics for the disease. Dr. Bredesen's chapter in this book has provided a discussion of the underlying mechanisms that may relate the microbiome to Alzheimer's disease. Maintaining a healthy commensal population and microbiome–host interaction may promote certain immune system functions, overall wellbeing, and longevity [18]. Below, we will provide evidence and perspectives for modulating gut microbial molecules and activity for Alzheimer's therapeutics.

Developing gut microbiota-based therapeutics began with a focus on immune system-related gastrointestinal disorders and metabolic syndromes, which resulted in the development of interventions that effectively modulate the gut microbiota for these conditions and diseases. These microbiome-based interventions are primarily probiotics, prebiotics, antibiotics, and fecal microbiota transplantation [72]. Due to the role of Aβ proteins and amyloid pathology in Alzheimer's pathogenesis and interventions [79–83], it will be interesting to study whether these microbiome-based molecules can affect Aβ levels and amyloid pathology and neurobehavioral functions. In turn, this area of study may facilitate our understanding of these microbial entities so as to better translate them into interventions for Alzheimer's.

One such study investigated whether or not probiotics may slow down the progression of Alzheimer's using animal models. Specifically, Bonfili et al. utilized 3xTg-AD mice that were treated with SLAB51 probiotic formulation in the early stages of Alzheimer's-like pathology [84]. The treatment cascaded an array of events that were suggested to relate to reduced Alzheimer's risk, including changes in (1) gut microbiota composition and metabolites; (2) plasma levels of inflammatory cytokines and hormones; (3) neuronal proteolytic pathways (the ubiquitin proteasome system and autophagy); (4) reduced brain damage with decreased Aβ aggregates; and most importantly, (5) decreased cognitive decline [84]. Moving forward, it will be useful to evaluate the roles of probiotics in the prevention and treatment of Alzheimer's patients through clinical trials [85].

A study reported earlier this year by Ma et al. investigated whether a ketogenic diet intervention in early life could alter the gut microbiome and enhance neurovascular functions [86]. Indeed, young healthy mice (12–14 weeks old) treated with a ketogenic diet for 16 weeks showed increased putatively beneficial gut microbiota (*Akkermansia muciniphila* and *Lactobacillus*) and reduced putatively pro-inflammatory taxa (*Desulfovibrio* and *Turicibacter*) compared to a control diet. Furthermore, the microbiota changes were related to upregulated neurovascular functions, as shown by increased cerebral blood flow and P-glycoprotein transports on BBB. The treatment also led to an improved metabolic profile as shown by reduced blood glucose levels and body weight, and increased blood ketone levels. Another study demonstrated that a diet rich in non-digestible carbohydrates reduced the phenotype of a human genetic obesity known as Prader-Willi syndrome, while changing the gut microbiota composition and alleviating inflammation [87]. Taken together, these studies provide evidence linking the association of diet and increased beneficial gut microbiota to reduced risk for Alzheimer's.

Importantly, the underlying pathway and microbial molecules/analogs that are responsible for disease-related pathophysiology have been explored and characterized. For example, one study investigated the role of the gut microbiota on intestinal gluconeogenesis, a critical process for glucose and energy homeostasis and metabolic conditions [16]. Gut microbiota ferment soluble fiber to generate short-chain fatty acids like propionate and butyrate that may utilize a gut–brain neural circuit involving the fatty acid receptor FFAR3 to activate the expression of genes responsible for intestinal gluconeogenesis [16]. Another study focused on trimethylamine (TMA) N-oxide (TMAO), which is a gut-microbiota-dependent dietary metabolite that is generated from the intestinal and hepatic metabolism of dietary choline and carnitine [88]. Related to the formation of atherosclerotic lesions and cardiometabolic diseases, TMAO also exists in human CSF and has potential pathophysiological roles in the CNS [89]. The study showed that a choline analog, 3,3-dimethyl-1-butanol (DMB), can non-lethally inhibit TMA formation and reduce TMAO levels that resulted in a decrease in the formation of atherosclerotic lesions [88]. Furthermore, a new pathway has been identified through which the gut microbiota generates the metabolites of dietary tryptophan and controls CNS inflammation, microglial activation, and the transcriptional program of astrocytes involving the aryl hydrocarbon receptor [32, 33]. This pathway may in turn guide new interventions for multiple sclerosis and other neurodegenerative disorders, including Alzheimer's. In future studies, it will be useful to thoroughly characterize the roles of reputed microbiome modulators, including DMB, on Alzheimer's-related pathology and neurobehavioral functions.

In summary, the complex interactions of lifestyle and microbial metabolites and their potential impacts on human pathophysiology have rapidly become an important field of study [90]. Nascent gut microbiota-based therapeutics have shown promising results for influencing both the safety and effectiveness of overall human health and diseases, including Alzheimer's. These early findings suggest that further investigations in this area will be helpful in capitalizing on both the potential for modulating the gut microbiota-mediated host in health and disease and the potential for improving Alzheimer's management.

FUTURE DIRECTIONS

In the future, it will be critical to identify and elucidate the systems-level molecular events that modulate the role of the microbiome in Alzheimer's in relationship to the condition's genetic and environmental risk factors [79]. As suggested in Dr. Bredesen's chapter, characterizing the microbiome may be useful to further stratifying different types of Alzheimer's. Overall, these studies require an integrative effort informed by multiple areas of expertise. Specifically, the genomes, proteomes, and metabolomes and microbiome, as well as the systems-level studies on the gut–brain system, will produce a superior level of understanding specifically how the microbiome affects the pathophysiologic aspects of Alzheimer's. Regarding pathogenesis, it will be interesting to study the effects of genetic variants of Alzheimer's, including the FAD mutations and the ε4 risk allele of APOE, on gut microbial activity in animals and human. The findings discussed in this chapter and others suggest that microbial involvement may act as an inevitable environmental factor that can help control the outcome of human health and disease, alongside other factors. Therefore, its relationship to other Alzheimer's risk factors needs to be further characterized. Furthermore, it is unknown how transferring microbiota from non-Alzheimer's subjects to Alzheimer's patients may impact Alzheimer's-related pathophysiology in humans (and in animals). In the end, human microbiome sequencing and composition may ultimately be used as a biomarker for the detection and diagnosis of this disease.

The ability to study the human microbiome and its relationship to human pathophysiology has been greatly improved by high-throughput microbiome sequencing and other technologies. Microbiome sequencing has primarily been studied by 16S gene profiling that is focused on the highly conserved 16S rRNA gene in the bacterial and archaeal ribosome [91]. It has been advanced with large-scale metagenomic studies that can sequence the entire microbiome community. For example, the metagenomics of the human intestinal tract (MetaHIT) consortium [92] and the human microbiome project (HMP) [93] and their methods for functional analyses [94] have been publicly reported and provide an increased and richer functional understanding of the human microbiome. The human microbiome may be used as a molecular biomarker that is unique to different individuals or disease stages. The results from the human microbiome project will be useful to stratify human subjects based on disease risks and stages, which can be further evaluated together with data from other clinical approaches, including the human genome project, cognitive scores, and Alzheimer's-related PET imaging for amyloid or tau proteins. Ultimately, these findings will provide useful and unprecedented resources to identify the role of the microbiome in human pathophysiology for Alzheimer's and other diseases or conditions.

CONCLUSIONS

In this chapter, we have reviewed the role of microbial involvement in the pathophysiology of Alzheimer's, with a focus on the microbiome–host interaction and the gut-brain axis. We first introduced the molecular pathogenesis and risk factors of Alzheimer's, and then discussed the microbial involvement and the potential mechanisms underlying Alzheimer's, with a focus on the pathological events and risk factors of the disease. Microbial involvement may act as an inevitable environmental factor that can predict or determine the outcome of Alzheimer's, along with aging and other risk factors. We then went on to discuss the potential for using the human microbiome as a biomarker, as well as modulating microbial molecules as a strategy to develop useful therapeutics for Alzheimer's. Importantly, an integrative and multidisciplinary analysis of the human microbiome, combined with the human genome data, amyloid or tau-based PET imaging, cognitive scores and other clinical approaches, may provide a complete view for the roles of human microbiome in Alzheimer's. In conclusion, investigation of microbial involvement in Alzheimer's has helped broaden our knowledge of disease pathogenesis and has provided possible avenues for using microbiome-based molecules in Alzheimer's therapeutics. We envision that studying the human microbiome will continue to not only advance our understanding of Alzheimer's, but also may open new avenues for developing microbiome-based interventions for this condition.

REFERENCES

1. Cummings, J.L., Alzheimer's disease. *N Engl J Med*, 2004. **351**(1): p. 56–67.
2. 2015 Alzheimer's disease facts and figures. *Alzheimers Dement*, 2015. **11**(3): p. 332–84.
3. Murray, C.J., et al., The state of US health, 1990–2010: Burden of diseases, injuries, and risk factors. *JAMA*, 2013. **310**(6): p. 591–608.
4. Hebert, L.E., et al., Alzheimer disease in the United States (2010–2050) estimated using the 2010 census. *Neurology*, 2013. **80**(19): p. 1778–83.
5. Strittmatter, W.J., et al., Apolipoprotein E: High-avidity binding to beta-amyloid and increased frequency of type 4 allele in late-onset familial Alzheimer disease. *Proc Natl Acad Sci U S A*, 1993. **90**(5): p. 1977–81.
6. Corder, E.H., et al., Gene dose of apolipoprotein E type 4 allele and the risk of Alzheimer's disease in late onset families. *Science*, 1993. **261**(5123): p. 921–3.
7. Wang, Y., et al., TREM2 lipid sensing sustains the microglial response in an Alzheimer's disease model. *Cell*, 2015. **160**(6): p. 1061–71.
8. Guerreiro, R., et al., TREM2 variants in Alzheimer's disease. *N Engl J Med*, 2013. **368**(2): p. 117–27.
9. Hardy, J., and D.J. Selkoe, The amyloid hypothesis of Alzheimer's disease: Progress and problems on the road to therapeutics. *Science*, 2002. **297**(5580): p. 353–6.
10. Bertram, L., and R.E. Tanzi, Thirty years of Alzheimer's disease genetics: The implications of systematic meta-analyses. *Nat Rev Neurosci*, 2008. **9**(10): p. 768–78.
11. Gandy, S., The role of cerebral amyloid beta accumulation in common forms of Alzheimer disease. *J Clin Invest*, 2005. **115**(5): p. 1121–9.
12. Choi, S.H., et al., A three-dimensional human neural cell culture model of Alzheimer's disease. *Nature*, 2014. **515**(7526): p. 274–8.
13. Morgan, X.C., N. Segata, and C. Huttenhower, Biodiversity and functional genomics in the human microbiome. *Trends Genet*, 2013. **29**(1): p. 51–8.
14. Lee, Y.K., and S.K. Mazmanian, Has the microbiota played a critical role in the evolution of the adaptive immune system? *Science*, 2010. **330**(6012): p. 1768–73.
15. Yatsunenko, T., et al., Human gut microbiome viewed across age and geography. *Nature*, 2012. **486**(7402): p. 222–7.
16. De Vadder, F., et al., Microbiota-generated metabolites promote metabolic benefits *via* gut-brain neural circuits. *Cell*, 2014. **156**(1–2): p. 84–96.
17. Muszer, M., et al., Human microbiome: When a friend becomes an enemy. *Arch Immunol Ther Exp (Warsz)*, 2015. **63**(4): p. 287–98.

18. Mazmanian, S.K., J.L. Round, and D.L. Kasper, A microbial symbiosis factor prevents intestinal inflammatory disease. *Nature*, 2008. **453**(7195): p. 620–5.

19. Gareau, M.G., et al., Bacterial infection causes stress-induced memory dysfunction in mice. *Gut*, 2011. **60**(3): p. 307–17.

20. Deacon, R.M., and J.N. Rawlins, T-maze alternation in the rodent. *Nat Protoc*, 2006. **1**(1): p. 7–12.

21. Clarke, G., et al., The microbiome-gut-brain axis during early life regulates the hippocampal serotonergic system in a sex-dependent manner. *Mol Psychiatry*, 2013. **18**(6): p. 666–73.

22. Sudo, N., et al., Postnatal microbial colonization programs the hypothalamic-pituitary-adrenal system for stress response in mice. *J Physiol*, 2004. **558**(Pt 1): p. 263–75.

23. Neufeld, K.M., et al., Reduced anxiety-like behavior and central neurochemical change in germ-free mice. *Neurogastroenterol Motil*, 2011. **23**(3): p. 255–64, e119.

24. Rodriguez, J.J., H.N. Noristani, and A. Verkhratsky, The serotonergic system in ageing and Alzheimer's disease. *Prog Neurobiol*, 2012. **99**(1): p. 15–41.

25. Minter, M.R., et al., Antibiotic-induced perturbations in microbial diversity during post-natal development alters amyloid pathology in an aged APPSWE/PS1DeltaE9 murine model of Alzheimer's disease. *Sci Rep*, 2017. **7**(1): p. 10411.

26. Minter, M.R., et al., Antibiotic-induced perturbations in gut microbial diversity influences neuro-inflammation and amyloidosis in a murine model of Alzheimer's disease. *Sci Rep*, 2016. **6**: p. 30028.

27. Cox, L.M., et al., Altering the intestinal microbiota during a critical developmental window has lasting metabolic consequences. *Cell*, 2014. **158**(4): p. 705–21.

28. Harach, T., et al., Reduction of Abeta amyloid pathology in APPPS1 transgenic mice in the absence of gut microbiota. *Sci Rep*, 2017. **7**: p. 41802.

29. Vogt, N.M., et al., Gut microbiome alterations in Alzheimer's disease. *Sci Rep*, 2017. **7**(1): p. 13537.

30. Ahuja, M., et al., Orai1-mediated antimicrobial secretion from pancreatic acini shapes the gut microbiome and regulates gut innate immunity. *Cell Metab*, 2017. **25**(3): p. 635–46.

31. An, D., et al., Sphingolipids from a symbiotic microbe regulate homeostasis of host intestinal natural killer T cells. *Cell*, 2014. **156**(1–2): p. 123–33.

32. Rothhammer, V., et al., Microglial control of astrocytes in response to microbial metabolites. *Nature*, 2018. **557**(7707): p. 724–8.

33. Rothhammer, V., et al., Type I interferons and microbial metabolites of tryptophan modulate astrocyte activity and central nervous system inflammation via the aryl hydrocarbon receptor. *Nat Med*, 2016. **22**(6): p. 586–97.

34. MacDonald, A.B., and J.M. Miranda, Concurrent neocortical borreliosis and Alzheimer's disease. *Hum Pathol*, 1987. **18**(7): p. 759–61.

35. Balin, B.J., et al., Identification and localization of *Chlamydia pneumoniae* in the Alzheimer's brain. *Med Microbiol Immunol*, 1998. **187**(1): p. 23–42.

36. Itzhaki, R.F., et al., Herpes simplex virus type 1 in brain and risk of Alzheimer's disease. *Lancet*, 1997. **349**(9047): p. 241–4.

37. Ball, M.J., et al., Intracerebral propagation of Alzheimer's disease: Strengthening evidence of a herpes simplex virus etiology. *Alzheimers Dement*, 2013. **9**(2): p. 169–75.

38. Morales, I., et al., Neuroinflammation in the pathogenesis of Alzheimer's disease. A rational framework for the search of novel therapeutic approaches. *Front Cell Neurosci*, 2014. **8**: p. 112.

39. Heneka, M.T., et al., Neuroinflammation in Alzheimer's disease. *Lancet Neurol*, 2015. **14**(4): p. 388–405.

40. Heppner, F.L., R.M. Ransohoff, and B. Becher, Immune attack: The role of inflammation in Alzheimer disease. *Nat Rev Neurosci*, 2015. **16**(6): p. 358–72.

41. Wu, S.C., et al., Intestinal microbial dysbiosis aggravates the progression of Alzheimer's disease in Drosophila. *Nat Commun*, 2017. **8**(1): p. 24.
42. Hu, X., T. Wang, and F. Jin, Alzheimer's disease and gut microbiota. *Sci China Life Sci*, 2016. **59**(10): p. 1006–23.
43. Jiang, C., et al., The gut microbiota and Alzheimer's disease. *J Alzheimers Dis*, 2017. **58**(1): p. 1–15.
44. Zhao, Y., V. Jaber, and W.J. Lukiw, Secretory products of the human GI tract microbiome and their potential impact on Alzheimer's disease (AD): Detection of lipopolysaccharide (LPS) in AD hippocampus. *Front Cell Infect Microbiol*, 2017. **7**: p. 318.
45. Zhan, X., et al., Gram-negative bacterial molecules associate with Alzheimer disease pathology. *Neurology*, 2016. **87**(22): p. 2324–32.
46. Chow, J., et al., Environmental stress causes lethal neuro-trauma during asymptomatic viral infections. *Cell Host Microbe*, 2017. **22**(1): p. 48–60.e5.
47. Baral, P., et al., Nociceptor sensory neurons suppress neutrophil and gammadelta T cell responses in bacterial lung infections and lethal pneumonia. *Nat Med*, 2018. **24**(4): p. 417–26.
48. Hufnagel, D.A., C. Tukel, and M.R. Chapman, Disease to dirt: The biology of microbial amyloids. *PLOS Pathog*, 2013. **9**(11): p. e1003740.
49. Fowler, D.M., et al., Functional amyloid–From bacteria to humans. *Trends Biochem Sci*, 2007. **32**(5): p. 217–24.
50. Bourgade, K., et al., Protective effect of amyloid-beta peptides against herpes simplex virus-1 infection in a neuronal cell culture model. *J Alzheimers Dis*, 2016. **50**(4): p. 1227–41.
51. Bourgade, K., et al., beta-Amyloid peptides display protective activity against the human Alzheimer's disease-associated herpes simplex virus-1. *Biogerontology*, 2015. **16**(1): p. 85–98.
52. Kumar, D.K., et al., Amyloid-beta peptide protects against microbial infection in mouse and worm models of Alzheimer's disease. *Sci Transl Med*, 2016. **8**(340): p. 340ra72.
53. Soscia, S.J., et al., The Alzheimer's disease-associated amyloid beta-protein is an antimicrobial peptide. *PLOS ONE*, 2010. **5**(3): p. e9505.
54. Little, C.S., et al., *Chlamydia pneumoniae* induces Alzheimer-like amyloid plaques in brains of BALB/c mice. *Neurobiol Aging*, 2004. **25**(4): p. 419–29.
55. Larbi, A., et al., Aging of the immune system as a prognostic factor for human longevity. *Physiology*, 2008. **23**: p. 64–74.
56. Woodmansey, E.J., et al., Comparison of compositions and metabolic activities of fecal microbiotas in young adults and in antibiotic-treated and non-antibiotic-treated elderly subjects. *Appl Environ Microbiol*, 2004. **70**(10): p. 6113–22.
57. Woodmansey, E.J., Intestinal bacteria and ageing. *J Appl Microbiol*, 2007. **102**(5): p. 1178–86.
58. Hopkins, M.J., and G.T. Macfarlane, Changes in predominant bacterial populations in human faeces with age and with *Clostridium difficile* infection. *J Med Microbiol*, 2002. **51**(5): p. 448–54.
59. Ng, T.P., et al., Markers of T-cell senescence and physical frailty: Insights from Singapore Longitudinal Ageing Studies. *NPJ Aging Mech Dis*, 2015. **1**: p. 15005.
60. Ouwehand, A.C., et al., *Bifidobacterium* microbiota and parameters of immune function in elderly subjects. *FEMS Immunol Med Microbiol*, 2008. **53**(1): p. 18–25.
61. Biagi, E., et al., Gut microbiota and extreme longevity. *Curr Biol*, 2016. **26**(11): p. 1480–5.
62. Kong, F., et al., Gut microbiota signatures of longevity. *Curr Biol*, 2016. **26**(18): p. R832–3.
63. Mariat, D., et al., The *Firmicutes/Bacteroidetes* ratio of the human microbiota changes with *age*. *BMC Microbiol*, 2009. **9**: p. 123.

64. Biagi, E., et al., Through ageing, and beyond: Gut microbiota and inflammatory status in seniors and centenarians. *PLOS ONE*, 2010. **5**(5): p. e10667.

65. Niedowicz, D.M., et al., Obesity and diabetes cause cognitive dysfunction in the absence of accelerated beta-amyloid deposition in a novel murine model of mixed or vascular dementia. *Acta Neuropathol Commun*, 2014. **2**: p. 64.

66. Xu, W., et al., Meta-analysis of modifiable risk factors for Alzheimer's disease. *J Neurol Neurosurg Psychiatry*, 2015. **86**(12): p. 1299–306.

67. Li, J.Q., et al., Risk factors for predicting progression from mild cognitive impairment to Alzheimer's disease: A systematic review and meta-analysis of cohort studies. *J Neurol Neurosurg Psychiatry*, 2016. **87**(5): p. 476–84.

68. Kang, J.E., et al., Amyloid-beta dynamics are regulated by orexin and the sleep-wake cycle. *Science*, 2009. **326**(5955): p. 1005–7.

69. Xie, L., et al., Sleep drives metabolite clearance from the adult brain. *Science*, 2013. **342**(6156): p. 373–7.

70. Shakersain, B., et al., Prudent diet may attenuate the adverse effects of Western diet on cognitive decline. *Alzheimers Dement*, 2016. **12**(2): p. 100–9.

71. Rogers, M.A.M., and D.M. Aronoff, The influence of non-steroidal anti-inflammatory drugs on the gut microbiome. *Clin Microbiol Infect*, 2016. **22**(2): p. 178.e1–178.e9.

72. Marchesi, J.R., et al., The gut microbiota and host health: A new clinical frontier. *Gut*, 2016. **65**(2): p. 330–9.

73. Soderholm, J.D., et al., Neonatal maternal separation predisposes adult rats to colonic barrier dysfunction in response to mild stress. *Am J Physiol Gastrointest Liver Physiol*, 2002. **283**(6): p. G1257–63.

74. Gareau, M.G., et al., Neonatal maternal separation causes colonic dysfunction in rat pups including impaired host resistance. *Pediatr Res*, 2006. **59**(1): p. 83–8.

75. Murphy, E.A., K.T. Velazquez, and K.M. Herbert, Influence of high-fat diet on gut microbiota: A driving force for chronic disease risk. *Curr Opin Clin Nutr Metab Care*, 2015. **18**(5): p. 515–20.

76. Zhang, C., et al., Structural resilience of the gut microbiota in adult mice under high-fat dietary perturbations. *ISME J*, 2012. **6**(10): p. 1848–57.

77. Zhang, C., et al., Cytokine-mediated inflammation mediates painful neuropathy from metabolic syndrome. *PLOS ONE*, 2018. **13**(2): p. e0192333.

78. Cho, I., et al., Antibiotics in early life alter the murine colonic microbiome and adiposity. *Nature*, 2012. **488**(7413): p. 621–6.

79. Zhang, C., Developing effective therapeutics for Alzheimer's disease – Emerging mechanisms and actions in translational medicine. *Discov Med*, 2017. **23**(125): p. 105–11.

80. Ward, J., et al., Mechanisms that synergistically regulate eta-secretase processing of APP and Aeta-alpha protein levels: Relevance to pathogenesis and treatment of Alzheimer's disease. *Discov Med*, 2017. **23**(125): p. 121–8.

81. Raven, F., et al., Soluble gamma-secretase modulators attenuate Alzheimer's beta-amyloid pathology and induce conformational changes in presenilin 1. *EBioMedicine*, 2017. **24**: p. 93–101.

82. Liang, F., et al., Nanoplasmonic fiber tip probe detects significant reduction of intracellular Alzheimer's disease-related oligomers by curcumin. *Sci Rep*, 2017. **7**(1): p. 5722.

83. Yu, J.T., and C. Zhang, Pathogenesis and therapeutic strategies in Alzheimer's disease: From brain to periphery. *Neurotox Res*, 2016. **29**(2): p. 197–200.

84. Bonfili, L., et al., Microbiota modulation counteracts Alzheimer's disease progression influencing neuronal proteolysis and gut hormones plasma levels. *Sci Rep*, 2017. **7**(1): p. 2426.

85. Akbari, E., et al., Effect of probiotic supplementation on cognitive function and metabolic status in Alzheimer's disease: A randomized, double-blind and controlled trial. *Front Aging Neurosci*, 2016. **8**: p. 256.
86. Ma, D., et al., Ketogenic diet enhances neurovascular function with altered gut microbiome in young healthy mice. *Sci Rep*, 2018. **8**(1): p. 6670.
87. Zhang, C., et al., Dietary modulation of gut microbiota contributes to alleviation of both genetic and simple obesity in children. *EBioMedicine*, 2015. **2**(8): p. 968–84.
88. Wang, Z., et al., Non-lethal inhibition of gut microbial trimethylamine production for the treatment of atherosclerosis. *Cell*, 2015. **163**(7): p. 1585–95.
89. Del Rio, D., et al., The gut microbial metabolite trimethylamine-*N*-oxide is present in human cerebrospinal fluid. *Nutrients*, 2017. **9**(10): p. 1–4.
90. Clemente, J.C., J. Manasson, and J.U. Scher, The role of the gut microbiome in systemic inflammatory disease. *BMJ*, 2018. **360**: p. j5145.
91. Tringe, S.G., and P. Hugenholtz, A renaissance for the pioneering 16S rRNA gene. *Curr Opin Microbiol*, 2008. **11**(5): p. 442–6.
92. Qin, J., et al., A human gut microbial gene catalogue established by metagenomic sequencing. *Nature*, 2010. **464**(7285): p. 59–65.
93. The Human Microbiome Project Consortium. Structure, function and diversity of the healthy human microbiome. *Nature*, 2012. **486**(7402): p. 207–14.
94. Cai, Y., H. Gu, and T. Kenney, Learning microbial community structures with supervised and unsupervised non-negative matrix factorization. *Microbiome*, 2017. **5**(1): p. 110.

8 The Role of the Microbiome in Mood

Kirsten Tillisch and Arpana Gupta

CONTENTS

INTRODUCTION

Mood disorders like anxiety and depression are complex heterogeneous disorders (Fajemiroye, Silva et al. 2016) that represent an enormous health burden and are responsible for some of the highest levels of disability worldwide (Collins, Patel et al. 2011). Despite an increased neurobiological understanding of these disorders and the corresponding development of pharmacological and behavioral treatments for anxiety and depression, full remission remains elusive and strategies for prevention are not well established (Fajemiroye, Silva et al. 2016).

Recently, however, the underlying pathophysiological mechanisms of anxiety and depression have been associated with alterations in the bidirectional brain-gut-microbiota axis (BGMA) (Cryan and Dinan 2012; Foster and McVey Neufeld 2013; Park, Collins et al. 2013). To date, the clinical evidence for this connection is still tenuous, but the preclinical work is compelling. Driven by the exciting new mechanistic possibilities the BGMA provides for prevention and treatment of psychiatric disorders, a large number of review articles have extrapolated preclinical findings to explain human neuropsychiatric disease (Borre, Moloney et al. 2014; Mayer, Knight et al. 2014; Evrensel and Ceylan 2015; Mayer, Tillisch et al. 2015; Petra, Panagiotidou et al. 2015). Despite the growing evidence and enthusiasm, controversy still exists regarding the sites, pathways, and molecular mechanisms that are responsible for the BGMA alterations that contribute to anxiety and depression. However, a better understanding of the underlying pathways contributing to the pathophysiology of mood disorders will have direct implications for the development and implementation of appropriate and effective therapeutic strategies for anxiety and depression (Borre, Moloney et al. 2014). Therefore, an understanding of the basic physiology of the BGMA is essential to evaluate the putative role of microbes in mood.

This chapter will first briefly describe the gut microbiota and its gastrointestinal environment, the presumed pathways and molecules by which the microbes communicate with the brain, and the key features of the brain and its development that are relevant to the BGMA. It will then describe potential environmental factors that influence the brain-gut microbiota pathways, including those of potential therapeutic value. Finally, the chapter will critically review the current clinical literature on the role of the gut microbiota in modulating the brain-gut axis as it relates to anxiety and depression, explore how preclinical findings contribute to our understanding, and identify future directions of translational research.

THE GUT AND ITS MICROBIOTA

The gastrointestinal microbiota is a diverse and dynamic ecosystem (Ursell, Haiser et al. 2014; Mayer, Tillisch et al. 2015). The gut, which is essentially a long tube reaching from the mouth to the anus, is our largest connection to the external environment. It has a staggeringly large surface area, a sophisticated enteric nervous system, and the largest collection of immune and endocrine cells in the body. Each section of the gut harbors unique features, including differences in specialized mucosal lining, site-specific types of gastrointestinal motility, secretion, and luminal contents. The gut is also the most heavily colonized area of the human body, containing over a trillion bacteria, eukaryotes, viruses, and fungi; within the gut, the greatest concentration of organisms can be found in the colon (Sender, Fuchs et al. 2016). Bacteria dominate the gut microbiota and while enormous inter-individual variation exists, in health the majority of the gut bacteria are from the phyla *Bacteroidetes* and *Firmicutes* (Allaband, McDonald et al. 2019).

Unfortunately, most of these organisms cannot be identified using standard culture techniques (Biedermann and Rogler 2015; Kelly, Kennedy et al. 2015) so historically there was no ability to mine this vast source of data. However, recent advances in the analytic techniques (see Chapter 1) have allowed for objective measurement of the composition and potential function of the bacterial component of the gut microbiota. This has created the opportunity to test a vast number of fascinating hypotheses about microbiota-disease interactions. But despite these steps forward, much remains to be learned. Better accounting of the important contributions made by viruses and fungi and their roles beside the bacteria is needed. Furthermore, the methodology for collecting and analyzing gut microbiota samples has tended to be determined by cost and convenience but would certainly benefit from more careful consideration. Are stool samples sufficient to answer some questions but biopsies or small intestinal sampling required for others? How quickly and how often does the composition and function of the gut microbiota change over time and how can we take into consideration such important factors as diet, activity level, and medications? Finally, with a myriad of available analytic techniques and very little standardization, samples collected in an identical way can yield divergent results depending on the analytic approach taken (Allaband, McDonald et al. 2019). Moving forward, it is essential to keep these factors in mind as we examine human studies and extrapolate from preclinical models.

BRAIN-GUT MICROBIOTA AXIS

If microbes are to have an impact on mood, they must first make contact with the brain through the intestinal and the blood-brain barriers, both of which are designed to carefully control contact from the outside world. The main function of the intestinal barrier is to regulate the absorption of essential nutrients into the host and to prevent the uptake of external pathogens or toxins from the gut lumen (Kelly, Kennedy et al. 2015). When the intestinal barrier is impaired, a condition commonly referred to as a "leaky gut" (Mayer, Tillisch et al. 2015), there is evidence that systemic and neuroinflammation can occur, which can be associated with behavioral symptoms like those seen in neurologic and psychiatric disorders like major depression (Biedermann and Rogler 2015; Kelly, Kennedy et al. 2015; Mayer, Tillisch et al. 2015). Disruption in the epithelial wall, caused by environmental factors or by the lumen microbes themselves, can also lead to an imbalance or dysbiosis of the gut microbiota (Elamin, Masclee et al. 2013; Jakobsson, Rodriguez-Pineiro et al. 2015). Across this intestinal barrier, the gut and the brain maintain a communication stream that relays a continuous status report to the brain and allows the gut to receive moment to moment modulating input from the brain.

Despite our understanding of the bidirectional brain-gut axis, traditional investigation of the pathophysiology of mood disorders in humans has focused largely on the central nervous system (CNS) (Mayer, Knight et al. 2014). More recently, as better measurements and characterization of both the brain and the microbiome emerge, brain diseases and psychiatric disorders are now being linked to alterations in the gut microbiota (Mayer, Padua et al. 2014; Kelly, Kennedy et al. 2015). Increasingly, it is being acknowledged that brain-gut-microbe communication can impact the stress response and influence risk for disease (El Aidy, Stilling et al. 2016; Sherwin, Rea et al. 2016). This communication can occur via circulating factors between the gut microbiota and the central nervous system (CNS), or through the enteric nervous system (ENS), autonomic nervous system (ANS), hypothalamic-pituitary-adrenal axis (HPA), and/or through the immune system (Foster and McVey Neufeld 2013). The high comorbidity of mood disorders among individuals with gastrointestinal disorders, like irritable bowel syndrome (IBS) or inflammatory bowel disease (IBD), and the high frequency of visceral symptoms in mood disorders support the role of BGMA interactions (Moloney, Desbonnet et al. 2014; Mayer, Tillisch et al. 2015), though directionality is not always clear. The working theory is that through this bidirectional loop, individuals either have primary alterations at the gut microbial level that impact the brain (bottom-up effects) or have alterations at the brain level that lead to abnormal gut signaling pathways (top-down effects) that influence the microbiota (Mayer, Knight et al. 2014; Tillisch and Labus 2014).

BRAIN-GUT MICROBIOTA SIGNALING PATHWAYS AND MOLECULES

The primary pathways through which the brain can modulate the gut microbiota are the autonomic nervous system, the hypothalamic-pituitary-adrenal (HPA) axis, the immune system, and via circulating gut-derived metabolites (Sherwin, Rea et al. 2016; Huang, Lai et al. 2019).

Signaling Pathways

The Autonomic Nervous System (ANS). The ANS regulates gut function, mostly via the vagus nerve, by modulating acid secretion, bicarbonate production, gut motility, and pain sensation. This pathway also modulates mucus secretion, influencing the quality of the habitat where the gut microbiota resides, and mucosal immune responses, which can alter gut permeability. These changes in intraluminal environment then impact microbial colonization and metabolic behavior. This central modulation of the gut is one of the conduits through which environmental influences like quality of sleep and stress act on the BGMA (Mayer, Tillisch et al. 2015).

The HPA Axis. The HPA axis is the main route by which stress responses can be signaled from the brain to the gut, leading to increased intestinal permeability, inflammation, and altered microbial composition. Exemplifying the bidirectionality of the BGMA, manipulation of gut bacteria can work in a bottom-up fashion to change HPA function. For example, stress-sensitive rats raised without the normal gut microbiota develop exaggerated stress responses with greater anxiety behaviors, higher corticosterone secretion, and lower dopamine levels in the frontal cortex, hippocampus, and striatum (Nishino, Mikami et al. 2013; Crumeyrolle-Arias, Jaglin et al. 2014).

The Immune System. The immune system is influenced by the gut microbiota, including resident microbes, pathogens, or ingested probiotics (Cryan and Dinan 2012; Mayer, Tillisch et al. 2015). The increased expression of bacterial lipopolysaccharides (LPS) and activation of host toll-like receptors in response to gut microbes influences the expression of pro-inflammatory cytokines. This inflammatory state, in turn, increases the permeability of the intestinal and blood-brain barriers, influencing brain function and behavior (Round and Mazmanian 2009; Mayer, Tillisch et al. 2015; Petra, Panagiotidou et al. 2015) , Bercik and Collins 2014).

The Brain. Multiple brain regions have been implicated in mood disorders and these overlap with the regions found to be relevant in the BGMA. The most commonly discussed are those regions referred to as "limbic" brain regions, including the cingulate gyrus, basal ganglia, thalamus, hypothalamus, hippocampus, and amygdala. Acting alongside the modulatory prefrontal cortex, the insula, and other sensory areas, these regions work in networks to regulate homeostatic processes and to generate our conscious sense of mood.

Molecules

Catecholamines, serotonin, GABA, and cytokines are released into the gut lumen through the functional properties of neurons, immune cells, and enterochromaffin cells (Lyte and Freestone 2010; Lyte 2013). The release of these mediators is upregulated during the host stress response; for example, catecholamines are released into the circulating system and into the gut under stressful conditions (Mayer, Knight et al. 2014; Mayer, Tillisch et al. 2015) but the gut microbes can also produce many of these same metabolites themselves even in the absence of stress. In addition, other gut microbes produce anti-inflammatory products such as short-chain fatty acids, which can signal via gut epithelial receptors or can be released into circulation to influence the brain signaling system (Mayer, Tillisch et al. 2015). When they are in homeostasis, the gut microbes help the organism balance these key molecules to achieve health; however, when pro-inflammatory microbes out-produce those with anti-inflammatory profiles, the risk of illness increases.

INFLUENCE OF ENVIRONMENTAL FACTORS ON THE BRAIN-GUT MICROBIOTA AXIS IN HEALTH

Numerous environmental factors influence the brain-gut microbiota axis. Indeed, these pathways provide a potential explanation for observations that healthy lifestyle choices may reduce risk of mood disorder or help prevent relapse.

Infections and Antibiotics

Infections of the gut can lead to anxiety and depression behaviors through the signaling of pro-inflammatory cytokines and other mediators (Bercik, Collins et al. 2012). For example, an infection of the colon can produce accompanying decreases in brain-derived neurotropic factor (BDNF) in the hippocampus, increased levels of pro-inflammatory cytokines such as tumor necrosis factor-α (TNFα), and increased kynurenine, which together have been linked to anxiety-like phenotypes in mice (Bercik, Verdu et al. 2010). The treatment of infections can also trigger the BGMA, as antibiotic use induces intestinal dysbiosis with demonstrated changes in metabolism of neuroactive substances such as GABA and SCFA, which can affect brain function and behavior (Bercik and Collins 2014).

Prebiotics and Probiotics

Prebiotics are compounds, usually dietary fibers, that may have positive health benefits on the activity of certain species of the gut microbiota in the host. These effects are thought to occur through reduction of low-grade inflammation and improving metabolic function (Kelly, Kennedy et al. 2015). Clinical studies have demonstrated that prebiotic galacto-oligosaccharides improve intestinal barrier function and help reduce inflammatory and oxidative stress markers, cytokine levels, and plasma lipopolysaccharides (Cani, Possemiers et al. 2009). Prebiotic galacto-oligosaccharides have also shown influences on brain neurochemistry and attenuation in anxiety-like behaviors (Kelly, Kennedy et al. 2015).

Probiotics are bacteria, fungi, or other organisms with health benefits to humans. Probiotic-containing or fermented foods are found in the diets of most cultures, though the typical Western diet is less rich in them than others. Taken either as food or as dietary supplements, probiotics do appear to have positive health benefits in some health domains, including mood, metabolism, and immune function (Ford, Quigley et al. 2014; Mayer, Savidge et al. 2014). Recently, the term "psychobiotics" has been used to describe the potential positive effects of probiotics on the brain-gut axis in modulating mood, anxiety, and cognition (Dinan, Stanton et al. 2013).

Diet and Exercise

It is like that diet and exercise are primary drivers of gut metabolism and gut microbial composition, which may provide the mechanistic link between diet and mood. (Yuan, Ferreira Rocha et al. 2015; Aguirre, Eck et al. 2016). A diverse plant- and fiber-rich diet appears to be the most beneficial to maintaining a healthy microbiota, while diets rich in fat may have negative consequences on gut barrier function and increased inflammation (Zmora, Suez et al. 2019). While diets should definitely be individualized for maximum benefit, recent studies indicate that simple changes to shift towards a Mediterranean style diet can improve mood in depressed patients (Jacka, O'Neil et al. 2017).

Early Life Adversity and Stress

Increasingly, evidence has shown that early life adversity impacts brain structure and function, with associated increases in psychiatric disease (McCrory, De Brito et al. 2010). Most recently, evidence has emerged implying that the gut microbiota may be the missing piece of the puzzle that helps explain the underlying mechanisms behind the long-lasting effects of early adversity and stress on the brain (Cryan and O'Mahony 2011). Namely, as an individual's gut microbial signature is established in childhood and is programmed for adulthood, the impact of early life events on that signature has the potential to impact lifelong physical and mental health.

Sex Differences

The effect of sex on the BGMA has been widely overlooked. Potential dimorphic sex differences in brain-gut interactions could impact the factors involved in shaping the sex-based differences observed in mood disorders (Jasarevic, Morrison et al. 2016). Critical developmental periods like infancy, puberty, and aging occur in parallel in the brain and in the gut microbiota, and sex differences at these points in time may eventually lead to sex-specific risk for disease (Borre, Moloney et al. 2014). For example, exposure to specific microbial metabolites like butyrate and propionate during the prenatal stage can lead to sex-specific delays in neurodevelopment. Associated sex differences in behavior are observed during later development, where male rodents but not females show increased anxiety, decreased social interactions, and increased stress responses (MacFabe, Cain et al. 2011; Foley, Ossenkopp et al. 2014).

Another link between sex and stress is seen in a maternal stress model where decreased levels of *Lactobacillus* and corresponding increases in *Bacteroides* and *Clostridium* are observed during the postnatal phase after vaginal delivery of males only. This is also associated with corresponding sex-related shifts in the availability of gut nutrients such as histidine and glutamate, and in amino acids in the paraventricular nucleus of the hypothalamus (Jasarevic, Morrison et al. 2016). Sex differences in brain-gut microbiota processes can persist through adolescence and continue into adulthood via hormones and neurotransmitters like serotonin, which can impact the brain and the gut (Clarke, Grenham et al. 2013). In future studies, it will be essential to keep in mind that sex differences influence the brain-gut microbiota interactions that can impact disease and treatment outcomes.

THE ROLE OF GUT MICROBIOTA RELATED TO ANXIETY AND DEPRESSION

The evolving physiological understanding of the brain-gut-microbiota axis, has led to a variety of preclinical models being utilized to better understand its influence on mental health and disease. Early infection models modulated the gut microbes to show the impact on mood. Subclinical Campylobacter infections in mice, despite signs of a systemic inflammatory response, induce anxiety-like behavior. Furthermore, anxiety-associated brain regions are induced by Campylobacter infection, changes which appear to be mediated by gastrointestinal vagal afferents (Lyte, Varcoe et al. 1998; Goehler, Gaykema et al. 2005; Marshall, Thabane et al. 2006). While these models attempted to carefully control for potential symptom-based effects of the pathogen by utilizing subclinical infections, the suggestion that anxiety and depression behaviors might be related to the BGMA can also be seen in the germ-free animal model.

Animals raised in germ-free conditions have impaired immune function with increased HPA axis reactivity and stress responsiveness in some strains and reduced anxiety behaviors in others (Sudo, Chida et al. 2004; Clarke, Grenham et al. 2013; Desbonnet, Clarke et al. 2014). Some investigators have been able to "rescue" behavioral changes in germ-free animals using probiotics or fecal microbial transplantation (FMT). Even more suggestive of the power of the BGMA are studies in which behavioral traits can be transferred from one mouse strain to another—and even from depressed humans to animals—via fecal transplantation (Brinks, van der Mark et al. 2007; Zheng, Zeng et al. 2016). The results of these dramatic experiments have not been replicated in human fecal microbial transplants, but they nonetheless support the underlying importance of the BGMA, albeit in the much simpler system of an animal model.

While the preclinical studies have provided many elegant and convincing examples of how various aspects of brain-gut microbiota interactions can influence centrally driven behavior, there is still very limited data from human studies. This is primarily due to the complexity of influences from genetic and environmental factors in humans and to the large inter-individual differences in gut microbial composition. Furthermore, the effects of the gut microbiome on the limbic circuitry of the brain are likely most prominent in early development and are consequently more difficult to observe in adulthood. Finally, the strong influence of the prefrontal cortex on behavior and emotional regulation in humans may blunt the more modest effects of gut microbes.

Despite these challenges, initial proof-of-concept studies in healthy individuals support the presence of measurable associations between gut microbes and the brain. Most of these studies have utilized probiotics, and there is parallel emerging evidence that prebiotics may also play a role. Brain structure and function have been linked to gut microbial composition in a cross-sectional study, revealing correlations between brain regions' associated emotional, attentional, and sensory processing, response to negative emotional imagery, and specific 16s ribosomal RNS–based bacterial signatures in fecal samples (Tillisch, Mayer et al. 2017). One interventional study following healthy women who ingested a probiotic yogurt for four weeks observed changes in brain reactivity in similar emotional and sensory brain regions with decreased reactivity to negative affect faces in the treated women compared to placebo and no treatment arms (Tillisch, Labus et al. 2013). While no clear associations with mood symptoms were noted, these studies are supportive of the underlying hypothesis that gut microbes could impact mood disorders.

Depression

Evaluating gut microbial composition and metabolic function in depressed versus non-depressed individuals has been one popular method for investigating the relevance of the BGMA to depression. Several studies have looked for evidence of altered microbial diversity in depressed individuals, but most have shown no difference compared to controls; surprisingly, one study even showed increased diversity, a finding most often considered as a sign of health (Naseribafrouei, Hestad et al. 2014; Jiang, Ling et al. 2015; Zheng, Zeng et al. 2016; Chen, Zheng et al. 2018). Evaluation of the specific taxa of bacteria in depression has also been inconsistent. As *Bifidobacteria* and *Lactobacillus* are often considered the "good bacteria" and are most often included in probiotic interventions, many studies have evaluated their abundance in depression. One study showed lower abundance of Lactobacillus in depression. (Aizawa, Tsuji et al. 2016), and two studies showed increased levels of bacteria from the genus *Alistipes* in depression with one of them also showing correlation of depressive symptoms with this finding. *Alistipes* has previously been shown in preclinical studies to increase with stress and to be associated with inflammation, while in humans it has been associated with irritable bowel syndrome (IBS) (Naseribafrouei, Hestad et al. 2014).

Decreases in a family of bacteria in the Clostridiales order, *Lachnospiraceae*, have also been identified in depressed individuals (Naseribafrouei, Hestad et al. 2014). *Lachnospiraceae* are producers of short chain fatty acids and may have anti-inflammatory properties. A member of this bacterial family has been shown to correlate with key sensory and limbic brain regions in both healthy individuals and those with IBS, a disorder with high levels of both depression and anxiety. The authors of this study suggest that the role of Clostridiales is in stimulation of biosynthesis and release of serotonin from gut enterochromaffin cells (Labus, Osadchiy et al. 2019). Whether the significance of *Alistipes* and *Lachnospiraceae* abundance in depression is pathophysiologic or if they play a role in the vulnerability or persistence of depression will require longitudinal study.

At the phyla level, decreased levels of *Bacteroidetes* were observed among depressed individuals across multiple studies (Zheng, Zeng et al. 2016; Lin, Ding et al. 2017; Chen, Zheng et al. 2018; Chen, Li et al. 2018), with one study showing increased levels of *Bacteroidetes*. This phylum has been associated with obesity and other metabolic diseases, which can be comorbid with depression. However, interpretation of the relevance of such a complex taxon is difficult given the differences that likely exist at the genus, species, and strain level.

Interventional studies with probiotics have also provided support for a potential role for the BGMA in depression. Only a few probiotic studies have enrolled individuals with depression, all of which are small and of relatively short duration. Using a *Lactobacillus-* and *Bifidobacterium*-containing probiotic, patients with major depressive disorder had greater decreases in the Beck Depression Inventory after eight weeks of treatment compared to placebo-treated subjects. They also had reduced C-reactive protein and serum insulin levels (Akkasheh, Kashani-Poor et al. 2016). For individuals already using antidepressants but with persistent symptoms, a small open label trial showed greater improvements in depression after eight weeks with a *Clostridium butyricum* strain compared to no treatment. Consistent with this, a small pilot study evaluated depression symptoms in a small number of individuals with serotonin reuptake inhibitor treatment-resistant depression, using a probiotic intervention and found benefits, though the study was methodologically poor (Bambling, Edwards et al. 2017). In a study of individuals with IBS, the level of depression was evaluated along with fecal metabolomics, inflammatory mediations, and functional brain imaging before and after a probiotic intervention (Pinto-Sanchez, Hall et al. 2017). This study noted no improvements in IBS symptoms but depression symptoms did decrease, as did reactivity of limbic brain regions in response to negative emotional stimuli; the other measured biologic parameters were unchanged.

In a larger number of studies, mostly also small and with methodological limitations, symptoms of anxiety and depression have been evaluated in response to probiotic interventions with variable results. While some studies have studied the use of probiotics in depression with negative results, meta-analyses of the intervention studies for depression have generally interpreted the literature as a whole as showing a small potential benefit (Huang, Wang et al. 2016; Liu, Walsh et al. 2019). Clearly larger, well-designed studies in patients with well-characterized depression are still needed.

Anxiety

There has been far less study of anxiety in human studies than depression, despite the robust preclinic work. Most evaluations of probiotic interventions for anxiety have been performed in healthy subjects or in the setting of other clinical conditions, such as pregnancy, chronic fatigue syndrome, schizophrenia, or irritable bowel syndrome. Meta-analysis of probiotic benefit are cautiously optimistic but clear conclusions cannot yet be made as to whether or not a clinical population with generalized anxiety may benefit (Liu, Walsh et al. 2019).

BGMA-BASED TREATMENT IN MOOD DISORDERS: BEYOND PROBIOTICS

Prebiotics, dietary interventions, antibiotics, fecal microbial transplantation, and vaccination have all been raised as potential interventions targeted at the microbiota for improving mood. Utilizing microbiota modulation as an adjunct to traditional psychiatric therapies is an under-developed strategy to date. As the field advances, analyzing baseline microbiota characteristics of patients as predictors of mood disorder treatment outcome may also be a useful approach. For example, it is well described that cognitive behavioral therapy (CBT) can help both anxiety and depression, but not all individuals respond to this approach. In a recent report, baseline gut microbes in IBS were predictors of CBT treatment response (Jacobs, Lackner et al. 2018).

CONCLUSIONS

It is tempting to hypothesize that modulation of the microbiota-gut-brain axis with probiotics, prebiotics, and diet will provide a new paradigm for the treatment of anxiety and depression. To date, we have only weakly supportive data, but even at this early stage of a complex field, it seems clear that a bidirectional connection exists between the microbiota and mood. What remains to be discovered is the relative importance of this connection, and how we can harness it to improve health and wellbeing.

However, many key questions remain unanswered, chief among them:

1) What is the optimal timing of microbiota-mood interactions? Is the perinatal or preadolescent period the most important, or can we harness the power of the microbiota in adulthood?
2) How can we best measure the microbiota-mood interaction? Does measurement of specific microbial species provide useful information, or must we evaluate microbial function via fecal and circulating metabolites?
3) Can diet, probiotics, and antibiotics help us prevent and/or treat mood disorders as alternatives or adjunctive therapies to traditional medications and behavioral interventions?
4) Are the changes we see in the BGMA sex specific and are there other key genetic or environmental factors we must take into account as we design future studies?

The future of mood and the brain-gut-microbiota relationship is likely to be one of the most exciting and productive avenues of clinical research in the coming years. To successfully convert this research from bench to bedside, an increased push to understand the mechanisms of BGMA function in humans is essential, coupled with carefully designed longitudinal observational and interventional studies which control for sex, diet, medications, and disease activity. Given the challenges of studying mood and the microbiota in humans, preclinical studies will remain vital to guide and inform these human studies. After years of relatively stagnant development in the pharmacological treatment of mood disorders the future for microbiota-based treatment strategies for depression and anxiety is bright.

Conflict of Interest: The authors declare that no conflict of interest exists.

Acknowledgments: The authors thank E. Gelfer, C. Liu, K. Hamadani, and C. Paydar for invaluable editorial assistance.

REFERENCES

Aguirre, M., A. Eck, M. E. Koenen, P. H. Savelkoul, A. E. Budding and K. Venema (2016). "Diet drives quick changes in the metabolic activity and composition of human gut microbiota in a validated in vitro gut model." *Res Microbiol* **167**(2): 114–125.

Aizawa, E., H. Tsuji, T. Asahara, T. Takahashi, T. Teraishi, S. Yoshida, M. Ota, N. Koga, K. Hattori and H. Kunugi (2016). "Possible association of Bifidobacterium and Lactobacillus in the gut microbiota of patients with major depressive disorder." *J Affect Disord* **202**: 254–257.

Akkasheh, G., Z. Kashani-Poor, M. Tajabadi-Ebrahimi, P. Jafari, H. Akbari, M. Taghizadeh, M. R. Memarzadeh, Z. Asemi and A. Esmaillzadeh (2016). "Clinical and metabolic response to probiotic administration in patients with major depressive disorder: A randomized, double-blind, placebo-controlled trial." *Nutrition* **32**(3): 315–320.

Allaband, C., D. McDonald, Y. Vazquez-Baeza, J. J. Minich, A. Tripathi, D. A. Brenner, R. Loomba, L. Smarr, W. J. Sandborn, B. Schnabl, P. Dorrestein, A. Zarrinpar and R. Knight (2019). "Microbiome 101: Studying, analyzing, and interpreting gut microbiome data for clinicians." *Clin Gastroenterol Hepatol* **17**(2): 218–230.

Bambling, M., S. C. Edwards, S. Hall and L. Vitetta (2017). "A combination of probiotics and magnesium orotate attenuate depression in a small SSRI resistant cohort: An intestinal anti-inflammatory response is suggested." *Inflammopharmacology* **25**(2): 271–274.

Bercik, P. and S. M. Collins (2014). "The effects of inflammation, infection and antibiotics on the microbiota-gut-brain axis." *Adv Exp Med Biol* **817**: 279–289.

Bercik, P., S. M. Collins and E. F. Verdu (2012). "Microbes and the gut-brain axis." *Neurogastroenterol Motil* **24**(5): 405–413.

Bercik, P., E. F. Verdu, J. A. Foster, J. Macri, M. Potter, X. Huang, P. Malinowski, W. Jackson, P. Blennerhassett, K. A. Neufeld, J. Lu, W. I. Khan, I. Corthesy-Theulaz, C. Cherbut, G. E. Bergonzelli and S. M. Collins (2010). "Chronic gastrointestinal inflammation induces anxiety-like behavior and alters central nervous system biochemistry in mice." *Gastroenterology* **139**(6): 2102–2112 e2101.

Biedermann, L. and G. Rogler (2015). "The intestinal microbiota: Its role in health and disease." *Eur J Pediatr* **174**(2): 151–167.

Borre, Y. E., R. D. Moloney, G. Clarke, T. G. Dinan and J. F. Cryan (2014). "The impact of microbiota on brain and behavior: Mechanisms & therapeutic potential." *Adv Exp Med Biol* **817**: 373–403.

Brinks, V., M. van der Mark, R. de Kloet and M. Oitzl (2007). "Emotion and cognition in high and low stress sensitive mouse strains: A combined neuroendocrine and behavioral study in BALB/c and C57BL/6J mice." *Front Behav Neurosci* **1**: 8.

Cani, P. D., S. Possemiers, T. Van de Wiele, Y. Guiot, A. Everard, O. Rottier, L. Geurts, D. Naslain, A. Neyrinck, D. M. Lambert, G. G. Muccioli and N. M. Delzenne (2009). "Changes in gut microbiota control inflammation in obese mice through a mechanism involving GLP-2-driven improvement of gut permeability." *Gut* **58**(8): 1091–1103.

Chen, J. J., P. Zheng, Y. Y. Liu, X. G. Zhong, H. Y. Wang, Y. J. Guo and P. Xie (2018). "Sex differences in gut microbiota in patients with major depressive disorder." *Neuropsychiatr Dis Treat* **14**: 647–655.

Chen, Z., J. Li, S. Gui, C. Zhou, J. Chen, C. Yang, Z. Hu, H. Wang, X. Zhong, L. Zeng, K. Chen, P. Li and P. Xie (2018). "Comparative metaproteomics analysis shows altered fecal microbiota signatures in patients with major depressive disorder." *Neuroreport* **29**(5): 417–425.

Clarke, G., S. Grenham, P. Scully, P. Fitzgerald, R. D. Moloney, F. Shanahan, T. G. Dinan and J. F. Cryan (2013). "The microbiome-gut-brain axis during early life regulates the hippocampal serotonergic system in a sex-dependent manner." *Mol Psychiatry* **18**(6): 666–673.

Collins, P. Y., V. Patel, S. S. Joestl, D. March, T. R. Insel, A. S. Daar, Scientific Advisory Board and the Executive Committee of the Grand Challenges on Global Mental, W. Anderson, M. A. Dhansay, A. Phillips, S. Shurin, M. Walport, W. Ewart, S. J. Savill, I. A. Bordin, E. J. Costello, M. Durkin, C. Fairburn, R. I. Glass, W. Hall, Y. Huang, S. E.

Hyman, K. Jamison, S. Kaaya, S. Kapur, A. Kleinman, A. Ogunniyi, A. Otero-Ojeda, M. M. Poo, V. Ravindranath, B. J. Sahakian, S. Saxena, P. A. Singer and D. J. Stein (2011). "Grand challenges in global mental health." *Nature* **475**(7354): 27–30.

Crumeyrolle-Arias, M., M. Jaglin, A. Bruneau, S. Vancassel, A. Cardona, V. Dauge, L. Naudon and S. Rabot (2014). "Absence of the gut microbiota enhances anxiety-like behavior and neuroendocrine response to acute stress in rats." *Psychoneuroendocrinology* **42**: 207–217.

Cryan, J. F. and T. G. Dinan (2012). "Mind-altering microorganisms: The impact of the gut microbiota on brain and behaviour." *Nat Rev Neurosci* **13**(10): 701–712.

Cryan, J. F. and S. M. O'Mahony (2011). "The microbiome-gut-brain axis: From bowel to behavior." *Neurogastroenterol Motil* **23**(3): 187–192.

Desbonnet, L., G. Clarke, F. Shanahan, T. G. Dinan and J. F. Cryan (2014). "Microbiota is essential for social development in the mouse." *Mol Psychiatry* **19**(2): 146–148.

Dinan, T. G., C. Stanton and J. F. Cryan (2013). "Psychobiotics: A novel class of psychotropic." *Biol Psychiatry* **74**(10): 720–726.

El Aidy, S., R. Stilling, T. G. Dinan and J. F. Cryan (2016). "Microbiome to brain: Unravelling the multidirectional axes of communication." *Adv Exp Med Biol* **874**: 301–336.

Elamin, E. E., A. A. Masclee, J. Dekker and D. M. Jonkers (2013). "Ethanol metabolism and its effects on the intestinal epithelial barrier." *Nutr Rev* **71**(7): 483–499.

Evrensel, A. and M. E. Ceylan (2015). "The gut-brain axis: The missing link in depression." *Clin Psychopharmacol Neurosci* **13**(3): 239–244.

Fajemiroye, J. O., D. M. Silva, D. R. de Oliveira and E. A. Costa (2016). "Treatment of anxiety and depression: Medicinal plants in retrospect." *Fundam Clin Pharmacol.*

Foley, K. A., K. P. Ossenkopp, M. Kavaliers and D. F. Macfabe (2014). "Pre- and neonatal exposure to lipopolysaccharide or the enteric metabolite, propionic acid, alters development and behavior in adolescent rats in a sexually dimorphic manner." *PLoS One* **9**(1): e87072.

Ford, A. C., E. M. Quigley, B. E. Lacy, A. J. Lembo, Y. A. Saito, L. R. Schiller, E. E. Soffer, B. M. Spiegel and P. Moayyedi (2014). "Efficacy of prebiotics, probiotics, and synbiotics in irritable bowel syndrome and chronic idiopathic constipation: Systematic review and meta-analysis." *Am J Gastroenterol* **109**(10): 1547–1561; quiz 1546, 1562.

Foster, J. A. and K. A. McVey Neufeld (2013). "Gut-brain axis: How the microbiome influences anxiety and depression." *Trends Neurosci* **36**(5): 305–312.

Goehler, L. E., R. P. Gaykema, N. Opitz, R. Reddaway, N. Badr and M. Lyte (2005). "Activation in vagal afferents and central autonomic pathways: Early responses to intestinal infection with *Campylobacter jejuni*." *Brain Behav Immun* **19**(4): 334–344.

Huang, R., K. Wang and J. Hu (2016). "Effect of probiotics on depression: A systematic review and meta-analysis of randomized controlled trials." *Nutrients* **8**(8).

Huang, T. T., J. B. Lai, Y. L. Du, Y. Xu, L. M. Ruan and S. H. Hu (2019). "Current understanding of gut microbiota in mood disorders: An update of human studies." *Front Genet* **10**: 98.

Jacka, F. N., A. O'Neil, R. Opie, C. Itsiopoulos, S. Cotton, M. Mohebbi, D. Castle, S. Dash, C. Mihalopoulos, M. L. Chatterton, L. Brazionis, O. M. Dean, A. M. Hodge and M. Berk (2017). "A randomised controlled trial of dietary improvement for adults with major depression (the 'SMILES' trial)." *BMC Med* **15**(1): 23.

Jacobs, J. P., J. M. Lackner, V. Lagishetty, G. D. Gudleski, R. S. Firth, K. Tillisch, B. D. Naliboff, J. S. Labus and E. A. Mayer (2018). "915 – Intestinal microbiota predict response to cognitive behavioral therapy for irritable bowel syndrome." *Gastroenterology* **154**(6): S-181.

Jakobsson, H. E., A. M. Rodriguez-Pineiro, A. Schutte, A. Ermund, P. Boysen, F. Bemark, F. Sommer, F. Backhed, G. C. Hansson and M. E. Johansson (2015). "The composition of the gut microbiota shapes the colon mucus barrier." *EMBO Rep* **16**(2): 164–177.

Jasarevic, E., K. E. Morrison and T. L. Bale (2016). "Sex differences in the gut microbiome-brain axis across the lifespan." *Philos Trans R Soc Lond B Biol Sci* **371**(1688).

Jiang, H., Z. Ling, Y. Zhang, H. Mao, Z. Ma, Y. Yin, W. Wang, W. Tang, Z. Tan, J. Shi, L. Li and B. Ruan (2015). "Altered fecal microbiota composition in patients with major depressive disorder." *Brain Behav Immun* **48**: 186–194.

Kelly, J. R., P. J. Kennedy, J. F. Cryan, T. G. Dinan, G. Clarke and N. P. Hyland (2015). "Breaking down the barriers: The gut microbiome, intestinal permeability and stress-related psychiatric disorders." *Front Cell Neurosci* **9**: 392.

Labus, J. S., V. Osadchiy, E. Y. Hsiao, J. Tap, M. Derrien, A. Gupta, K. Tillisch, B. Le Neve, C. Grinsvall, M. Ljungberg, L. Ohman, H. Tornblom, M. Simren and E. A. Mayer (2019). "Evidence for an association of gut microbial Clostridia with brain functional connectivity and gastrointestinal sensorimotor function in patients with irritable bowel syndrome, based on tripartite network analysis." *Microbiome* **7**(1): 45.

Lin, P., B. Ding, C. Feng, S. Yin, T. Zhang, X. Qi, H. Lv, X. Guo, K. Dong, Y. Zhu and Q. Li (2017). "Prevotella and Klebsiella proportions in fecal microbial communities are potential characteristic parameters for patients with major depressive disorder." *J Affect Disord* **207**: 300–304.

Liu, R. T., R. F. L. Walsh and A. E. Sheehan (2019). "Prebiotics and probiotics for depression and anxiety: A systematic review and meta-analysis of controlled clinical trials." *Neurosci Biobehav Rev* **102**: 13–23.

Lyte, M. (2013). "Microbial endocrinology in the microbiome-gut-brain axis: How bacterial production and utilization of neurochemicals influence behavior." *PLoS Pathog* **9**(11): e1003726.

Lyte, M. and P. P. E. E. Freestone (2010). *Microbial Endocrinology: Interkingdom Signaling in Health and Disease*, Springer Publishers.

Lyte, M., J. J. Varcoe and M. T. Bailey (1998). "Anxiogenic effect of subclinical bacterial infection in mice in the absence of overt immune activation." *Physiol Behav* **65**(1): 63–68.

MacFabe, D. F., N. E. Cain, F. Boon, K. P. Ossenkopp and D. P. Cain (2011). "Effects of the enteric bacterial metabolic product propionic acid on object-directed behavior, social behavior, cognition, and neuroinflammation in adolescent rats: Relevance to autism spectrum disorder." *Behav Brain Res* **217**(1): 47–54.

Marshall, J. K., M. Thabane, A. X. Garg, W. F. Clark, M. Salvadori, S. M. Collins and Walkerton Health Study Investigators (2006). "Incidence and epidemiology of irritable bowel syndrome after a large waterborne outbreak of bacterial dysentery." *Gastroenterology* **131**(2): 445–450; quiz 660.

Mayer, E. A., R. Knight, S. K. Mazmanian, J. F. Cryan and K. Tillisch (2014). "Gut microbes and the brain: Paradigm shift in neuroscience." *J Neurosci* **34**(46): 15490–15496.

Mayer, E. A., D. Padua and K. Tillisch (2014). "Altered brain-gut axis in autism: Comorbidity or causative mechanisms?" *Bioessays* **36**(10): 933–939.

Mayer, E. A., T. Savidge and R. J. Shulman (2014). "Brain-gut microbiome interactions and functional bowel disorders." *Gastroenterology* **146**(6): 1500–1512.

Mayer, E. A., K. Tillisch and A. Gupta (2015). "Gut/brain axis and the microbiota." *J Clin Invest* **125**(3): 926–938.

McCrory, E., S. A. De Brito and E. Viding (2010). "Research review: The neurobiology and genetics of maltreatment and adversity." *J Child Psychol Psychiatry* **51**(10): 1079–1095.

Moloney, R. D., L. Desbonnet, G. Clarke, T. G. Dinan and J. F. Cryan (2014). "The microbiome: Stress, health and disease." *Mamm Genome* **25**(1-2): 49–74.

Naseribafrouei, A., K. Hestad, E. Avershina, M. Sekelja, A. Linlokken, R. Wilson and K. Rudi (2014). "Correlation between the human fecal microbiota and depression." *Neurogastroenterol Motil* **26**(8): 1155–1162.

Nishino, R., K. Mikami, H. Takahashi, S. Tomonaga, M. Furuse, T. Hiramoto, Y. Aiba, Y. Koga and N. Sudo (2013). "Commensal microbiota modulate murine behaviors in a strictly contamination-free environment confirmed by culture-based methods." *Neurogastroenterol Motil* **25**(6): 521–528.

Park, A. J., J. Collins, P. A. Blennerhassett, J. E. Ghia, E. F. Verdu, P. Bercik and S. M. Collins (2013). "Altered colonic function and microbiota profile in a mouse model of chronic depression." *Neurogastroenterol Motil* **25**(9): 733–e575.

Petra, A. I., S. Panagiotidou, E. Hatziagelaki, J. M. Stewart, P. Conti and T. C. Theoharides (2015). "Gut-microbiota-brain axis and its effect on neuropsychiatric disorders with suspected immune dysregulation." *Clin Ther* **37**(5): 984–995.

Pinto-Sanchez, M. I., G. B. Hall, K. Ghajar, A. Nardelli, C. Bolino, J. T. Lau, F. P. Martin, O. Cominetti, C. Welsh, A. Rieder, J. Traynor, C. Gregory, G. De Palma, M. Pigrau, A. C. Ford, J. Macri, B. Berger, G. Bergonzelli, M. G. Surette, S. M. Collins, P. Moayyedi and P. Bercik (2017). "Probiotic *Bifidobacterium longum* NCC3001 reduces depression scores and alters brain activity: A pilot study in patients with irritable bowel syndrome." *Gastroenterology* **153**(2): 448–459 e448.

Round, J. L. and S. K. Mazmanian (2009). "The gut microbiota shapes intestinal immune responses during health and disease." *Nat Rev Immunol* **9**(5): 313–323.

Sender, R., S. Fuchs and R. Milo (2016). "Revised estimates for the number of human and bacteria cells in the body." *PLoS Biol* **14**(8): e1002533.

Sherwin, E., K. Rea, T. G. Dinan and J. F. Cryan (2016). "A gut (microbiome) feeling about the brain." *Curr Opin Gastroenterol* **32**(2): 96–102.

Sudo, N., Y. Chida, Y. Aiba, J. Sonoda, N. Oyama, X. N. Yu, C. Kubo and Y. Koga (2004). "Postnatal microbial colonization programs the hypothalamic-pituitary-adrenal system for stress response in mice." *J Physiol* **558**(Pt 1): 263–275.

Tillisch, K., J. Labus, L. Kilpatrick, Z. Jiang, J. Stains, B. Ebrat, D. Guyonnet, S. Legrain-Raspaud, B. Trotin, B. Naliboff and E. A. Mayer (2013). "Consumption of fermented milk product with probiotic modulates brain activity." *Gastroenterology* **144**(7): 1394–1401, 1401 e1391–1394.

Tillisch, K. and J. S. Labus (2014). "Neuroimaging the microbiome-gut-brain axis." *Adv Exp Med Biol* **817**: 405–416.

Tillisch, K., E. A. Mayer, A. Gupta, Z. Gill, R. Brazeilles, B. Le Neve, J. E. T. van Hylckama Vlieg, D. Guyonnet, M. Derrien and J. S. Labus (2017). "Brain structure and response to emotional stimuli as related to gut microbial profiles in healthy women." *Psychosom Med* **79**(8): 905–913.

Ursell, L. K., H. J. Haiser, W. Van Treuren, N. Garg, L. Reddivari, J. Vanamala, P. C. Dorrestein, P. J. Turnbaugh and R. Knight (2014). "The intestinal metabolome: An intersection between microbiota and host." *Gastroenterology* **146**(6): 1470–1476.

Yuan, T. F., N. B. Ferreira Rocha, F. Paes, O. Arias-Carrion, S. Machado and A. S. de Sa Filho (2015). "Neural mechanisms of exercise: Effects on gut miccrobiota and depression." *CNS Neurol Disord Drug Targets* **14**(10): 1312–1314.

Zheng, P., B. Zeng, C. Zhou, M. Liu, Z. Fang, X. Xu, L. Zeng, J. Chen, S. Fan, X. Du, X. Zhang, D. Yang, Y. Yang, H. Meng, W. Li, N. D. Melgiri, J. Licinio, H. Wei and P. Xie (2016). "Gut microbiome remodeling induces depressive-like behaviors through a pathway mediated by the host's metabolism." *Mol Psychiatry* **21**(6): 786–796.

Zmora, N., J. Suez and E. Elinav (2019). "You are what you eat: Diet, health and the gut microbiota." *Nat Rev Gastroenterol Hepatol* **16**(1): 35–56.

9 The Microbiome in Multiple Sclerosis

Helen Tremlett and Emmanuelle Waubant

CONTENTS

INTRODUCTION

The recognition of the "multiple sclerosis microbiome" is an exciting and emerging addition to the research surrounding the condition. Although there is great promise and much hope that the microbiome will provide an opportunity to enhance our understanding of what causes multiple sclerosis and drives the disease process(es), much remains unknown. This chapter views the multiple sclerosis microbiome through the lens of an epidemiologist and neurologist who, like many who study multiple sclerosis, are intrigued by the potential for the microbiome to be harnessed toward improving health outcomes in multiple sclerosis. Here, we discuss the importance of multiple sclerosis not just to individual patients but to society at large, and highlight some of the major unmet needs surrounding the condition. We then outline the current evidence supporting the microbiome's role in multiple sclerosis, including work we have conducted specifically in pediatric multiple sclerosis.[1-7] The focus naturally is on humans—multiple sclerosis is thought to only affect *Homo sapiens*—and on the gut microbiome. To date, the most-studied gut microbes in multiple sclerosis are the *Bacteria* and, to some extent, *Archaea*. Finally, we briefly touch on additional gut microbes that remain largely unexplored in multiple sclerosis (e.g., *Fungi, Viruses*) and conclude with a look forward with *"What's next for MS and the gut microbiome?"*

THE EPIDEMIOLOGY AND IMPORTANCE OF MS

Multiple sclerosis is a chronic inflammatory and degenerative disease of the central nervous system, which includes the brain, optic nerves, and spinal cord. North America has among the world's highest prevalence of multiple sclerosis; recent estimates suggest that more than 700,000 North Americans live with the condition, and that number is expected to rise by 30% before 2030.[8–13] Multiple sclerosis is the most common cause of non-traumatic neurological disability in young adults in the Western world,[14] placing a significant burden on the individual, family, and society as a whole.[13] The disease afflicts women more often than men and, on average, a person will begin to experience their first symptoms in their early thirties. However, the pathogenesis of the disease exists along a vast spectrum, with children as young as three or four years old and adults in their seventies being diagnosed with the condition. Around 5% of people with multiple sclerosis will develop symptoms and are diagnosed in their childhood years,[15] but on a population level, the average age of a person living with multiple sclerosis today in the Western world is between 55 and 60 years.[8,11] The total economic burden of multiple sclerosis in the United States alone is estimated to be $2.5 billion annually, with lifetime costs exceeding $4 million for every individual living with the disease.[16–18] Clearly, multiple sclerosis is an expensive condition that impacts a great number of people, along with the individuals and communities caring for them.

THE MS DISEASE COURSES AND TRAJECTORIES

Multiple sclerosis is a highly variable disease; it is often said that no two people with multiple sclerosis are alike. People with the condition experience a vast spectrum of symptoms, ranging from fatigue to sensory disturbances like numbness and tingling to issues with vision, cognition, bowel or bladder control, and mobility. The long-term trajectory of the disease can also be highly variable.[19] Although life expectancy, on average, is not dramatically reduced—estimates suggest lifespan to be 6–12 years shorter than expected.[20] Many people live well into their seventies with multiple sclerosis, while some individuals do have their lives and livelihoods tragically cut short. One famous example of the condition's potential to aggressively shorten lifespan is the cellist Jacqueline du Pré, who died from multiple sclerosis at 42 years old after living with the condition for a mere 16 years. The speed with which the condition claimed her life is even more shocking when viewed in light of the fact that, on average, people live with multiple sclerosis for almost 50 years from the onset of first symptoms.[20]

Approximately 85–95% of patients present with a relapsing form of multiple sclerosis at the onset of the disease.[19] This initial phase is called "relapsing-remitting" multiple sclerosis and, with time, most people will transition to a progressive phase of the disease, termed secondary progressive multiple sclerosis at which time disease progression becomes insidious, occurring with or without further relapses. A minority of multiple sclerosis patients—approximately 5–15%—present with a primary progressive form of the disease, whereby disability progression occurs from the outset of the condition with no relapses.[21,22] The average person with a relapsing-remitting form of multiple sclerosis at onset will live for 30 plus years before requiring a cane to walk—a score of six on the Expanded Disability Status Scale (EDSS)—versus only 10–15 years for a person with primary progressive multiple sclerosis.[19]

There are more than ten disease-modifying drugs approved by the Food and Drug Administration to treat the 85–95% of individuals suffering from relapsing-remitting multiple sclerosis or secondary progressive multiple sclerosis with relapses. These disease-modifying drugs can reduce relapse rates, relative to placebo, anywhere from 30 to 70%. There is only one drug licensed for primary progressive MS (2017). However, because multiple sclerosis is more often than not a relatively slowly progressing disease, we do not yet fully understand how effective any of these drugs will be in impacting long-term disability outcomes.[23]

SUMMARY COMMENTS ON MAJOR UNMET NEEDS IN MS

Due to the relatively modest efficacy and limited understanding of the long-term effectiveness of the current pharmaceutical interventions, researching and developing novel and effective therapeutics to treat multiple sclerosis remains a top priority.[24] Furthermore, because the cause(s) of multiple sclerosis are so poorly understood,[25] there is a real need to pursue new avenues toward understanding the genetic and environmental contexts that might collectively and/or individually trigger the onset of the disease. Finally, understanding what factors might explain or predict the variability in disease progression between patients and drive relapses or disease progression are both fundamental goals. Whether or not the microbiome can be harnessed to facilitate the answering of any of these questions remains to be seen, but the preliminary evidence is very promising. Below, we seek to outline our current understanding of the (gut) microbiome in multiple sclerosis.

THE MICROBIOME AND MULTIPLE SCLEROSIS: EVIDENCE FROM ANIMAL MODELS

Animal models of multiple sclerosis provided the first intriguing evidence of the potential for the microbiome to play a substantial role as either a precipitating factor in triggering multiple sclerosis onset or as a facilitator of subsequent disease activity.[26,27] Although multiple sclerosis is not thought to occur naturally outside of humans in the animal kingdom, numerous animal models of the disease have been developed over the years in an attempt to mimic the multiple sclerosis phenotype, with a general focus on the relapsing-remitting phase. Experimental autoimmune encephalomyelitis (EAE) is one of the most commonly used animal models and is typically induced in mice through a noxious dose of chemicals. Using this model, researchers in Germany and California published complementary studies in 2011[27,28] and then again in 2017[29,30] that focused on the role of the microbiome in the pathogenesis of this condition. Taken together, their work demonstrated the difficulty of inducing EAE in mice raised without exposure to normal or non-pathogenic microbes (i.e., raised in a "germ-free" environment, including conception/pre-conception).[31] If EAE could be induced in the germ-free mice, the animals typically exhibited only a "mild" form of EAE with minimal disability. Furthermore, exposing the germ-free mice to feces from mice with a "normal" gut microbiota increased both their propensity to develop EAE and their overall disease activity as measured by a move-ment-based disability/ability score, relative to germ-free mice without exposure to "normal" mice feces.[29,30] Because mice partake in coprophagia (the eating of feces), it is possible to transfer gut microbes from one mouse to another simply by housing the animals together.

In 2017, the German- and California-based researchers elaborated on these find-ings by transferring stool from humans with and without multiple sclerosis into germ-free mice. The German study included five pairs of monozygotic twins discordant for relapsing-remitting multiple sclerosis (i.e., genetically identical twinsets in which one individual had multiple sclerosis and the other did not) while the California-based team included three individuals with multiple sclerosis and three household controls.[29,30] Most of the cases had not been exposed to a disease-modifying multiple sclerosis drug in the last three months, with the exception of two of the individuals in the twin study who were taking a beta-interferon. These studies found that the subsequent induction of EAE in mice was more severe when the transplanted stool came from a person with multiple sclerosis.[29,30] Although based on relatively small sample sizes, these findings are intriguing, particularly the monozygotic twin stud-ies, because they represent a unique scientific opportunity in which variability in fac-tors like genetics and environment—assuming the individuals were raised together in a similar manner—between cases and controls were minimized.

CIRCUMSTANTIAL OR INDIRECT EVIDENCE SUGGESTING A ROLE OF THE GUT MICROBIOME IN MULTIPLE SCLEROSIS

Although it is interesting to note that many of the potential risk factors for multiple sclerosis also have a profound impact on the gut microbiota,[32,33] these observations are non-specific, circumstantial, and provide little-to-no truly convincing evidence of a causal link. For instance, our best evidence to date suggests that the risk factors for multiple sclerosis onset include the following demographic, lifestyle, and genetic factors: obesity; smoking; exposure to viruses, particularly the Epstein-Barr virus; low serum vitamin D and diminished sunlight exposure;[25] the presence of the human leukocyte antigen (HLA) *DRB1*1501* allele; age; and female sex. All of these fac-tors can also conceivably affect the gut microbiota's composition.[34-41] Furthermore, the relationship between host genetics and the microbiome was underscored in the German multiple sclerosis twin study referenced above, in which a greater similar-ity in the gut microbiota composition was observed between the monozygotic twin siblings discordant for multiple sclerosis than between the unrelated twins.[29]

The influence of a so-called "leaky gut" has been explored in multiple sclerosis, but data remain very limited.[42] One study sought to compare the "intestinal permeabil-ity" of 22 people with relapsing-remitting multiple sclerosis versus controls using an oral lactulose/mannitol test.[42] When compared to the 18 controls, a higher prevalence of "leaky gut" was reported in those with multiple sclerosis.[42] However, some of the multiple sclerosis subjects had suffered from the disease for a very long time, up to 20 years, and the source of the controls was not clear. In addition, the two groups differed demographically, with more women in the control group, which may well have contributed to the differences observed.[42] Therefore, whether or not intestinal permeability is a relevant health issue or risk factor in multiple sclerosis remains to be determined.

The relationship between multiple sclerosis and small intestinal bacterial overgrowth has been investigated by Chinese researchers using a hydrogen glucose breath test.[43] In performing the hydrogen glucose breath test, participants fasted overnight and then the hydrogen content of their breath was assessed before and after ingestion of a glucose (50g) drink. This test is a screening rather than diagnostic test and has low sensitivity—but good specificity—for small intestinal bacterial overgrowth.[43] Overall, 118 multiple sclerosis cases and 118 age-sex matched controls were enrolled from the same geographic area. The multiple sclerosis cases were four times more likely to test positive for the presence of small intestinal bacterial overgrowth (45 of the 118 multiple sclerosis cases, 38% vs. 10 of the 118 controls, 8%, OR, 4.50; 95% CI, 2.38–8.50). After adjusting for potential confounders, including DMT exposure, disability—measured on either the EDSS or multiple sclerosis severity scale—was associated with the presence of small intestinal bacterial overgrowth (e.g., for the MSSS, OR, 2.8; 95% CI, 1.4–4.9). Furthermore, while participants were excluded if major gastrointestinal issues were present (including irritable bowel syndrome) or taking drugs affecting either gut motility or gut composition (including proton pump inhibitors), 102 (86%) of the multiple sclerosis cases had at least one gastrointestinal-related symptom, such as constipation or fecal incontinence. In particular, flatulence and bloating were associated with the presence of small intestinal bacterial overgrowth in the multiple sclerosis cases (no data were reported for the controls).[43] The authors hypothesized that higher multiple sclerosis disability might predispose an individual to small intestinal bacterial overgrowth via impairment of gastrointestinal motility.[43] If true, this finding would be a consequence rather than a catalyst of disability progression in multiple sclerosis.

DOES THE GUT MICROBIOTA DIFFER BETWEEN INDIVIDUALS WITH MULTIPLE SCLEROSIS AND CONTROLS?

Table 9.1 summarizes the studies conducted to date in which the gut microbiota composition of individuals with and without multiple sclerosis has been surveyed and compared. These studies address the fundamental question of whether or not a measurable difference in gut microbiota composition exists in individuals with and without multiple sclerosis. Clearly, these data do not provide evidence of causation; whether having a chronic condition such as multiple sclerosis caused the observed differences or if the variant gut microbiota themselves had a role in triggering multiple sclerosis is not known. Because the predominant multiple sclerosis phenotype is relapsing-remitting onset, the majority of studies have enrolled patients with this form of the disease. However, the data does include a few multiple sclerosis cases who had reached the secondary progressive phase of multiple sclerosis (see Table 9.1, footnotes). All studies to date have been rather modest in size, ranging from 7 to

TABLE 9.1
Summary of Original Studies Surveying the Gut Microbiota in Multiple Sclerosis (MS)

First, senior authors, year of publication, location of study subjects (country)	Study design, participant numbers, biological sample type(s)	Source, location(s) of participants	Sex (F/M); age (mean, unless otherwise stated)	Disease duration at baseline sample collection‡ (mean); EDSS (median unless otherwise stated) and IMD exposure	Sequencing platform; hypervariable region (for primer-based approaches)	Potential confounders considered	Main findings	Main conclusions, implications, strength/ limitation
Cosorich, Falcone[64] 2017 Italy	Case/control 7/7 (selected from a wider group of19/17, total) Small Intestinal tissue (mucosa)	Cases & controls: undergoing diagnostic EGD procedure [1] San Raffaele Hospital. Milan, Italy	NR [Based on the total group of 19/17: Cases: 11/8; 41 years Controls: 10/7; 48 years]	NR [Based on the total group of 19/17: NR; 2 (EDSS range: 1-5.5); all cases IMD exposed (9 GA. 7 IFNB, 3 fingolimod)]	16S rRNA: Roche 454 (V3–V5)	Yes, but limited, e.g., assessed correlation between characteristics for the 7/7 cases/ controls (age. disease duration. EDSS) and relative abundance of Prevotella and Streptococcus (all p>0.05)	1. Alpha diversity not significantly different for MS cases vs. controls (p>0.05) 2. Phylum & Genus-level: MS cases vs. controls—no differences 3. Subgroup analyses of 7 MS cases, 3 with vs. 4 without evidence of disease activity[2] a. Phylum-level: higher Firmicutes, lower Bacteroidetes abundances, p<0.05 b. Genus-level higher Streptococcus ['mostly' Strep.mitis and Strep. oralis], lower Prevotella p<0.05 Additional work included T-cell profiling on total group (19 cases, 17 controls)	Microbiota composition of the intestinal mucosa was similar between MS cases and controls (diversity, phylum ad genus-level). Subgroup analyses indicated differences in MS cases depending on disease activity. However, IMD exposure also differed between groups [2] Strength: sequenced mucosa of small intestine in MS (novel) Limitation: small study

(Continued)

TABLE 9.1 (CONTINUED)

Summary of Original Studies Surveying the Gut Microbiota in Multiple Sclerosis (MS)

First, senior authors, year of publication, location of study subjects (country)	Study design, participant numbers, biological sample type(s)	Source, location(s) of participants	Sex (F/M); age (mean, unless otherwise stated)	Disease duration at baseline sample collection‡ (mean); EDSS (median unless otherwise stated) and IMD exposure	Sequencing platform; hypervariable region (for primer-based approaches)	Potential confounders considered	Main findings	Main conclusions, implications, strength/ limitation
Cekanaviciute, Baranzini,[30] 2017 USA	Case/control 71/71 stool	Cases & controls: via two institutions (University of California, San Francisco and Icahn School of Medicine, Mt Sinai, New York), USA. Cases: 49/22 Controls: 50/21 A control could include a member of the case's household	Cases: 44/27: 40.7 years Controls: 28/39 (sex missing for 4); 44.6 years (age missing for 9) [3]	~10 years [3]; EDSS (NR); 0 IMD exposed within previous 3 months	16S rRNA; Illumina (V4); Earth Microbiome Project protocol	No – although no IMD exposure in last 3 months for all cases	1. Alpha & beta diversity (Chao1, UniFrac) not significantly different for MS cases vs. controls (p-values not shown) 2. Taxa-level differences for MS vs. healthy controls: Higher abundance of *Akkermansia muciniphila* and *Acinetobacter calcoaceticus*, Lower abundance of *Parabacteroides distasonis* 3. Further *in vitro* and *in vivo* (mice) studies, including 3 MS cases/3 household controls stool transferred to mice, demonstrated potential importance in immune response and triggering/ severity of EAE:	In adults with MS (not exposed to an IMD in prior 3 months), relative to controls, gross gut microbiota composition did not differ, but taxa-level specific differences found, e.g., *Akkermansia muciniphila* higher in MS vs. controls and induced pro-inflammatory response in mice & human blood (PBMCs). **Strength:** additional *in vitro* and *in vivo* (mice) work provided biological evidence of the microbiota's role in immune response and hence MS **Limitation:** age/sex of controls differed from MS cases, long disease duration *(Continued)*

TABLE 9.1   (CONTINUED)

Summary of Original Studies Surveying the Gut Microbiota in Multiple Sclerosis (MS)

First, senior authors, year of publication, location of study subjects (country)	Study design, participant numbers, biological sample type(s)	Source, location(s) of participants	Sex (F/M); age (mean, unless otherwise stated)	Disease duration at baseline sample collection‡ (mean); EDSS (median unless otherwise stated) and IMD exposure	Sequencing platform; hypervariable region (for primer-based approaches)	Potential confounders considered	Main findings	Main conclusions, implications, strength/limitation
Berer, Wekerle.[29] 2017 Germany	Case/control 34/34 stool	Cases & controls: monozygotic twin pairs discordant for MS recruited via national campaign, incl. TV/German MS Society	Cases: 26/8; 41.3 years Controls: identical to cases	13.2 years (range: 1–33); EDSS (NR); 19/34 (56%) IMD exposed within previous 3 months:[13 months, 4 IFNB, 4 natalizumab, 1 GA, 1 azathioprine]	16S rRNA: Roche 454 (V3-V5)and bacterial metagenomic shotgun sequencing	Yes Either stratified or adjusted, e.g., IMD exposure	1. Alpha & beta diversity (Faith's Phylogenetic Diversity, UniFrac) comparable between MS cases vs. controls (plots shown, not p-values) 2. Taxa-level findings (cases vs. controls): no differences (up to genera/OTU-level); in the 'untreated' subset [4] 'several' taxa differed, e.g., abundance of *Akkermansia muciniphila* higher (Mann-Whitney U-test, p<0.05) 3. Bacterial metagenomics (n=32 twins): no differences in bacterial species, families or genes/pathways, although discordant twins were more similar than unrelated twins 4. Further *in vitro* and *in vivo* (mice) studies, including 5 cases/5 controls stool transferred to mice, demonstrated potential role in triggering/severity of 'spontaneous' EAE model	Gross gut microbiota/bacterial community did not differ between monozygotic twins with and without MS but taxa-level specific differences found. E.g. *Akkermansia* higher in untreated MS twins vs. controls *Akkermansia* has potential to stimulate pro-inflammatory response: colonization of mice with MS donor microbiota exacerbated disease severity in induced and spontaneous EAE. Contribution of host genetics on the composition of the gut microbiota demonstrated **Strength**: study design—genetically identical twins discordant for MS **Limitation**: relatively modest sample size

(Continued)

TABLE 9.1 (CONTINUED)
Summary of Original Studies Surveying the Gut Microbiota in Multiple Sclerosis (MS)

First, senior authors, year of publication, location of study subjects (country)	Study design, participant numbers, biological sample type(s)	Source, location(s) of participants	Sex (F/M); age (mean, unless otherwise stated)	Disease duration at baseline sample collection‡ (mean); EDSS (median unless otherwise stated) and IMD exposure	Sequencing platform; hypervariable region (for primer-based approaches)	Potential confounders considered	Main findings	Main conclusions, implications, strength/limitation
Jangi, Weiner,[44] 2016 USA	Case/control 60/43 stool	*Cases:* Clinic-based *Controls:* enrolled in a genetic-related study at same institute where cases drawn	*Cases:* 41/19: 49.7 years *Controls:* 37/6: 42.2 years	12.8 years; EDSS:1.2 (mean); 32/60 IMD exposed >6 months	16S rRNA: Roche 454 (V3–V5) & Illumina Miseq (V4)	Yes: Age, sex, BMI: IMD exposure status explored at taxa-level (other demographics eg diet described)	1. Alpha & beta diversity (Shannon, UniFrac) not significantly different for MS cases vs. controls (no p-values) 2. Taxa-level findings (genera): a) MS vs. healthy controls: higher abundance of: *Methanobrevibacter (Archaea)* and *Akkermansia* and lower *Butyricimonas* (p <0.05, q<0.1)[15] b) IMD exposed >6 months vs. unexposed MS: higher *Prevotella* and *Sutterella*; decreased *Sarcina*. (p<0.05, q<0.1)[15]	In adults with long-standing MS, relative to controls, gross gut microbiota composition did not differ, but taxa-level specific differences found; suggestive of inflammation. Similar associations observed with other autoimmune disease. IMD exposure may also influence the gut microbiota **Strength:** MS cases well phenotyped **Limitation:** cases had longstanding MS; some findings (e.g., *Methanobrevibacter*) might relate to underlying comorbidity (e.g., constipation) in MS cases

(Continued)

TABLE 9.1 (CONTINUED)
Summary of Original Studies Surveying the Gut Microbiota in Multiple Sclerosis (MS)

First, senior authors, year of publication, location of study subjects (country)	Study design, participant numbers, biological sample type(s)	Source, location(s) of participants	Sex (F/M); age (mean, unless otherwise stated)	Disease duration at baseline sample collection‡ (mean); EDSS (median unless otherwise stated) and IMD exposure	Sequencing platform; hypervariable region (for primer-based approaches)	Potential confounders considered	Main findings	Main conclusions, implications, strength/limitation
Chen, Mangalam,[62] 2016 USA	Case/control 31/36 stool	Cases: Clinic-based Controls: Not stated	Cases: 21/10; 42.9 years Controls: (unclear[6]): 40.3 years	NR [approx. 7–8 years based on age onset=35.4 years and age at sample =42.9 years]; EDSS: 19/31 (61%) <3 (range: 1–6) 20/31 IMD exposed	16S rRNA; V3–V5: sequencer used NR	Yes: IMD status, smoking, vitamin D supplements (data not shown)	1. Alpha diversity (richness) did not differ for MS cases vs. controls (p=0.73); beta diversity (Bray-Curtis) differed by relapse status (≤1 vs. > month of a relapse) vs. controls (p<0.001, PERMANOVA) 2. Taxa-level findings. MS cases vs. controls: increased abundance of *Psuedomonas, mycoplana [Proteobacterial], Haemophilus, Blautia, Dorea [Firmicutes]* [general] and decreased *Parabacteroides, Adlercreutzia* (Actinobacteria), [general], p<0.0005 [6]	In adults with MS, relative to controls, gross gut microbiota composition did not differ, but specific taxa did. Suggestion that gut microbiota composition differed by relapse status requires confirmation in longitudinal study **Strength:** use of random forest plots **Limitation:** source of controls unclear, relatively long disease duration
Tremlett, Waubant,[1] 2016 USA	Longitudinal cohort 17 stool	Cases: Clinic-based Controls: N/A	Cases: 10/7; 12.5 years	10.3 months (range 2.3–23.1); EDSS: 2.0; 9/17 IMD exposed	16S rRNA; V4; Illumina Miseq	Yes: IMD status, age (other demographics, e.g., diet described)	*Fusobacteria* absence (vs. presence) associated with higher relapse risk (HR:3.2; 95% CI. 1.2–9.0, p=0.024) age. IMD exposure adjusted [7]	Gut microbiota composition in pediatric MS associated with risk of future MS relapse **Strength:** longitudinal study (stool samples collected prior to the outcome), short disease duration **Limitation:** pilot study/small samples size

(Continued)

TABLE 9.1 (CONTINUED)
Summary of Original Studies Surveying the Gut Microbiota in Multiple Sclerosis (MS)

First, senior authors, year of publication, location of study subjects (country)	Study design, participant numbers, biological sample type(s)	Source, location(s) of participants	Sex (F/M); age (mean, unless otherwise stated)	Disease duration at baseline sample collection‡ (mean); EDSS (median unless otherwise stated) and IMD exposure	Sequencing platform; hypervariable region (for primer-based approaches)	Potential confounders considered	Main findings	Main conclusions, implications, strength/limitation
Tremlett, Waubant,[2] 2016 USA	Case/control 18/17 stool	Cases & controls: Pediatric clinics within same geographical location	Cases: 10/8; 12.5 years Controls: 9/8; 13.5 years	10.6 months (range 2.3–23.1); EDSS: 2.0 9/18 IMD exposed	16S rRNA; V4; Illumina Miseq	Yes: IMD status (all analyses). Sex, age, race, ethnicity fad/fiber groups, breastfeeding, IMD exposure and for the MS cases only, EDSS, corticosteroid use or history of a recent relapse (diversity analyses only)	1. Alpha, beta diversity did not differ for cases/controls (Mann-Whitney or PERMANOVA p>0.2), but beta-diversity differed by IMD exposure (Canberra. PERMANOVA p<0.02). 2. Taxa-level findings (OTU): a) MS vs. controls: i)higher abundance of: *Bilophila* (RR=3.0; 95% CI, 2.9–3.2), & *Desulfovibrio* [genus] & *Christensenellaceae* [family]. p&q<0.000005 [8] ii)lower abundance family: *Lachnospiraceae*, *Ruminococcaceae*, p and q<0.00005 [8]	In children assessed close to MS onset, overall gut microbiota composition did not differ vs. controls. However, subtle taxa-level differences found. Differences suggestive of a pro-inflammatory milieu. MS drug exposure may also influence the gut microbiota **Strength**: pediatrics MS: cases sampled very close to onset of disease **Limitation**: pilot study/small samples size

(Continued)

TABLE 9.1 (CONTINUED)
Summary of Original Studies Surveying the Gut Microbiota in Multiple Sclerosis (MS)

First, senior authors, year of publication, location of study subjects (country)	Study design, participant numbers, biological sample type(s)	Source, location(s) of participants	Sex (F/M); age (mean, unless otherwise stated)	Disease duration at baseline sample collection‡ (mean); EDSS (median unless otherwise stated) and IMD exposure	Sequencing platform; hypervariable region (for primer-based approaches)	Potential confounders considered	Main findings	Main conclusions, implications, strength/limitation
Miyake. Yamamura.[51] 2015. Japan	Case/control 20/40[9] stool	*Cases:* National hospital *Controls:* University staff	*Cases:* 14/6; 35.6 years *Controls:* 20/20 28.5 years	8.8 years; EDSS: NR; 9/20 IMD exposed	16S rRNA; V1-2 region: Roche 454	Yes: Age, sex, disease duration, relapse frequency, medical treatment (for 'microbial species' analyses only)	1. Alpha diversity did not differ between cases and controls (no p-value); beta-diversity differed. UniFrac (ANOSIM. p<0.05) [but IMD status not explored] 2. Taxa-level findings. MS cases vs. controls: a) Genus: lower abundance of *Faecalibacterium. Prevotella.* and *Anaerostipes*; p<0.05 [10] b) Species (21 differed), e.g.. higher abundance of *Eggerthella lenta*; lower abundance of *Clostridia* clusters XIVa & IV & several *Bacteroidetes* p<0.05 [10]	Moderate differences between case and controls observed (mainly at the taxa-level); authors concluded that the *clostridial* species associated with MS might be distinct from other autoimmune conditions **Strength:** One of the few studies from Asia/Japan **Limitation:** controls sourced from different population than cases, relatively long disease duration

(Continued)

TABLE 9.1 (CONTINUED)
Summary of Original Studies Surveying the Gut Microbiota in Multiple Sclerosis (MS)

First, senior authors, year of publication, location of study subjects (country)	Study design, participant numbers, biological sample type(s)	Source, location(s) of participants	Sex (F/M); age (mean, unless otherwise stated)	Disease duration at baseline sample collection‡ (mean); EDSS (median unless stated) and IMD exposure	Sequencing platform; hypervariable region (for primer-based approaches)	Potential confounders considered	Main findings	Main conclusions, implications, strength/limitation
Cantarel, Mowry,[50] 2015, USA	Case/control 7/8[11] stool	Cases & controls: A convenience sample nested within a vitamin D intervention study (location not specified)	Cases: 7/0; median 42 years Controls: 8/0; median 38 years	Not stated: 5/7 IMD exposed (all GA)	16S rRNA Phylochip (akin to DNA micro-array)	Yes: IMD status, vitamin D supplementation	1. Beta-diversity similar for cases & controls, p=0.74[12]; but differed for GA-exposed vs. unexposed cases, p=0.007 [12] 2. Taxa-level (OTU) findings, MS vs. controls: higher abundance of *Ruminococcus* (genus), lower abundance of: *Faecalibacterium* (genus), *Bacteroidaceae* (family). Adonis test p<0.05 3. After 5000 IU/d vitamin D3 for 90 days: *Faecalibacterium* abundance increased for GA naïve MS relative to GA-treated MS and health controls (p-value stated as 'significant' [13])	Glatiramer acetate and vitamin D supplementation were associated with differences or changes in the microbiota: small study: preliminary results **Strength**: homogeneous population **Limitation**: pilot study/small samples size: older chip-based technology

Footnotes and Key: Studies published up until February 2018 included. Primary source: PubMed

ANOSIM = ANalysis Of SIMilarity; CI = confidence interval; EDSS = Expanded Disability Status Scale (ranges from 0 'no neurological deficits' to 10 'death due to MS');
EGD=esophagogastroduodenoscopy; GA=glatiramer acetate; MS=multiple sclerosis; HR=hazard ratio; IFNB=beta-interferon; IMD=immunomodulatory drug; N/
A=not applicable; NR=not reported; PERMANOVA=permutational multivariate analysis of variance; RR= rate ratios; RRMS=relapsing-remitting multiple scle-
rosis; SPMS= secondary-progressive multiple sclerosis

‡ at 'baseline' typically indicated the first sample collected, unless otherwise stated

TABLE 9.1 (CONTINUED)
Summary of Original Studies Surveying the Gut Microbiota in Multiple Sclerosis (MS)

Disease course: the majority of participants had relapsing-onset MS and were in the RRMS phase at the time of stool collection, except Berer, Wekerle 2017 Germany[29]: 7/29 had reached SPMS; 2 had PPMS

[1] EGD procedures included: dyspepsia, gastroesophageal reflux, altered bowel habits.

Exclusion criteria: history of gastroenteritis, gastric ulcer, irritable bowel disease, celiac disease, inflammatory bowel disease, and gastric and colorectal cancers

[2] Authors contacted to request which of the n=7 MS cases did or did not have evidence of disease activity (measured using MRI, disability and relapses over a 2-year period):

Three of 7 had evidence of disease-activity (RR-EDA): MS009, MS018, MS020; IMD exposure: 2/3 glatiramer acetate, 1/3 fingolimod

4 of 7 had no evidence of disease-activity (RR-NEDA): MS011, MS013, MS016, MS017; IMD exposure: 1/4 glatiramer acetate, 3/4 beta-interferon

[3] Derived from Supplementary Table 1[30], original article. Disease duration was estimated based on the year of onset provided and assuming that a) all samples were obtained end/2016 and b) those with 'onset' of 2016 (the most recent onset year) had a disease duration of 1 year.

[4] Original article (Table 9.1) indicated n=15 received no IMD/immunosuppressant drug in the prior 3 months, although n=17 were included in the 'untreated' analyses (definition of treatment/untreated for this n=17 unclear)

[5] Significance determined using the statistical package 'DESeq2' (model used to derive p-value not stated); Benjamini–Hochberg corrected p values of 0.05 with a false discovery rate threshold of 0.1 reported

[6] Sex ratio was unclear; article[62] stated 36 controls in total, but gave a sex-split of '36/14' indicating a total of 50 controls.

Wilcoxon rank-sum test; for taxa with prevalence >10% and maximum proportion >0.002 assessed; Bonferroni corrected, false discovery rate of 5%

[7] Hazard ratios and 95% confidence intervals derived from Cox regression models (as applied on select phyla after Bonferroni corrected p-values from Kaplan-Meier curves, using the log-rank test)

[8] Generalized linear models (GLM, negative binomial regression); findings expressed as rate ratios (RR), and 95% confidence intervals (95% CI), along with p and q values (false discovery rate adjusted p-values; <0.05 was considered significant)

[9] A further 18 controls provided repeated samples; findings not shown here as repeated samples not obtained from cases

[10] Welch's t-test, p-values corrected for multiple testing using the Benjamini–Hochberg method

[11] Case/control stool samples available as follows: pre-vitamin D supplementation 4/8; post-vitamin D supplementation: 7/8

[12] p-values derived from the Adonis test, using the Unifrac metric to assess beta-diversity. 5 glatiramer acetate exposed vs. 2 IMD naïve MS cases [samples from either the pre or post vitamin D supplementation intervention were included, as available]

[13] Wilcoxon rank sum test with a Bonferroni correction

71 individuals with multiple sclerosis and a similar number of controls. Most were cross-sectional, procuring samples at one point in time, and included individuals with stool samples obtained at various times during the course of the disease, from soon after multiple sclerosis symptom onset[2] to decades after the disease was diagnosed.[29,30,44] Intriguingly, despite these differences (see also "Comments on study design"), there have been broad parallels between study findings. However, whether there is a specific "signature" of multiple sclerosis or the microbiota differences observed are common to other immune-mediated conditions remains to be determined, as does the direction and exact nature of the association.[7]

When researchers have compared the diversity (alpha or beta) of the gut microbiota between individuals with and without multiple sclerosis, they generally have not observed remarkable differences. This broad method of surveying the gut microbiota includes metrics like the overall richness and evenness of the gut microbes present (see also Chapter 1: Assessing the Microbiome). Gut diversity has typically not differed significantly between multiple sclerosis cases and controls, including between monozygotic twin pairs discordant for the condition[29] (Table 9.1), although it is always possible that modest differences were missed in the smaller sized studies conducted to date. When differences in beta-diversity between multiple sclerosis cases and controls have been found, they appear to be most likely related to multiple sclerosis disease-modifying drug exposure rather than the condition itself (Table 9.1).

However, when evaluating the *types* of microbes present—typically at the taxa level (e.g., *Phylum, Family*, and below) grouped by so-called "operational taxonomic units" (OTUs)—the relative abundance of specific groups of microbes differ significantly between multiple sclerosis cases and controls. There are two research groups that have taken a rather different approach to this examination: instead of surveying the gut microbiota using techniques like 16S, they focused on specific microbes. One American research team applied polymerase chain reaction (PCR) analyses to measure one microbe—*Clostridium perfringens*, serotype A—which they reported as less prevalent in 30 multiple sclerosis cases versus 31 controls (found in 23% vs. 52%, respectively, Chi-squared test, p=0.023).[45]

Another team used fluorescence in situ hybridization (FISH) ribosomal RNA-based probes and focused on a finite number of microbes. They enrolled 25 relapsing-remitting multiple sclerosis cases from one city hospital in northern Germany, and 14 controls from a University in a different city further south.[46] The differences they observed included lower mean concentrations of *Bacteroides* and *Faecalibacterium prausnitzii* in the cases relative to controls (student t-test, p<0.05). However, it should be noted that multiple comparisons were conducted without adjustment and no demographic information was reported for the cases and controls, somewhat weakening the reliability of these results.[46]

The remaining studies applied 16S sequencing or metagenomics to survey the gut microbiota (Table 9.1). Although it is rather challenging to carefully compare all of the results reported across the different studies—which include comparisons made across hundreds of microbes grouped at different taxa-levels, from *Phylum, Class, Order, Family, Genus* to *Species*—some consistent patterns have emerged. Overall, it seems reasonable to conclude that subtle, discrete taxonomic enrichments and depletions can be observed in multiple sclerosis cases relative to controls, and that, taken together, these findings suggest the presence of a pro-inflammatory milieu in the guts of adults and children with multiple sclerosis alike (see also Table 9.1).[2] One example of a microbe that can stimulate a pro-inflammatory response is *Akkermansia muciniphila*, and a higher relative abundance of this microbe has been found in multiple sclerosis cases relative to controls (see below and Table 9.1).

However, whether there is a specific gut microbiota signature of multiple sclerosis still remains to be determined. Some findings concur, or overlap, with those observed in other autoimmune inflammatory conditions,[2] including inflammatory bowel disease (e.g., Crohn's)[2,47,48] and conditions not traditionally considered as gut-related, like rheumatoid arthritis.[49] For example, the relative abundance of *Faecalibacterium prausnitzii* was lower in pediatric multiple sclerosis cases relative to controls,[2] and similar findings have been observed in children newly diagnosed with the autoimmune condition Crohn's disease.[47,48] Furthermore, *Prevotella copri* was found to be higher in both pediatric multiple sclerosis cases and new-onset untreated rheumatoid arthritis compared to the relative controls.[2,49]

Some groups have highlighted or pursued, through additional work, specific groups of microbes thought to be of relevance in multiple sclerosis. For example, the enrichment of *Archaea (Methanobrevibacter [genus])* in some multiple sclerosis subjects has been reported relative to controls[44] as has a depletion of members of the *Firmicutes* (e.g., *Clostridium genera*) and *Bacteroidetes* phyla.[2,45,50,51] Prior studies using animal models of multiple sclerosis have demonstrated a biologically plausible link with, for instance, *Bacteroidetes,*[32] wherein colonization of *Bacteroides fragilis* in the gut can protect against EAE via polysaccharide A production and subsequent gut-derived IL-10 from CD4+ Foxp3+ regulatory T cells.[32] Mouse models have also shown that this species can ameliorate neurodevelopmental issues, evidence suggestive of a gut-microbiota-brain connection.[52]

Researchers in Germany and the United States demonstrated that the relative abundance of *Akkermansia muciniphila*, a gram-negative anaerobe, was elevated in multiple sclerosis cases relative to controls (see Table 9.1).[29,30] Given that *Akkermansia* had previously been shown to stimulate pro-inflammatory responses, both teams conducted a series of *in vivo* and *in vitro* animal and cell-based studies exploring this potential in multiple sclerosis. Taken together, their findings add to the biological evidence demonstrating the potential importance of the gut microbiota in immune responses in multiple sclerosis and in animal models of multiple sclerosis.[29,30]

COMMENT ON STUDY DESIGN

The vast majority of studies in multiple sclerosis have been of a case–control design (Table 9.1). This is a very cost-effective way to study a given disease, especially if it is relatively "rare." However, case-control studies are also very prone to selection bias; if the controls are not sourced from the same "at-risk" population as the cases, then differences between cases and controls might have very little to do with the actual disease being studied.[53] Unfortunately, from where cases and controls are sourced and how they were selected could either not be determined in some studies, or were quite different (e.g., cases from a hospital setting vs. controls being

University staff members, and/or from different cities, Table 9.1). The monozygotic twin study largely by-passes many of these shortcomings, as presumably most twins were raised together in a similar environment.[29] Nonetheless, all of the studies are modest in terms of the number of multiple sclerosis cases and controls enrolled.

Consequently, although the majority of studies attempted to deal with potential confounders, their ability to adequately do so was very limited. Most groups to date have either been unable to adjust for factors associated with both the "exposure" (the gut microbiota) and outcome (multiple sclerosis) or have only been able to select one or two possible confounders to include (Table 9.1). At best, stratified analyses have been done, and typically then only by a crude measure of multiple sclerosis disease-modifying drug exposure, with all drugs grouped together (e.g., "ever vs. never" or "used in the last few months vs. not"). Most studies explicitly stated an inclusion/exclusion criteria to minimize heterogeneity between cases and controls, for instance, by avoiding collecting samples from individuals with recent antibiotic use or certain gastrointestinal diseases.

Regardless, the microbiome field is rapidly evolving, and new exposures, which may have been overlooked in earlier studies, are being formally recognized as major factors influencing the gut microbiota. One example of this is exposure to commonly used drugs like proton pump inhibitors.[54,55] The potential importance of measuring aspects such as gut motility has also been highlighted,[56] which might be of particular relevance in multiple sclerosis where bowel issues like constipation or fecal incontinence/diarrhea can be common.[57,58] Multiple sclerosis is associated with a higher risk of comorbid conditions and polypharmacy; these characteristics are seldom reported in studies, but might contribute to some of the differences observed between cases and controls, especially where adults with longstanding multiple sclerosis are studied. Finally, the most consistently and commonly assessed factor which might impact findings was exposure to disease-modifying drugs. All multiple sclerosis drugs have immunomodulatory properties and could affect the gut microbiota composition, as inferred in some studies (Table 9.1). As the capacity for larger and more longitudinal studies develops, it will be of great value to determine if and how both disease-specific and broader factors (e.g., ethnicity, diet, exercise, lifestyle, comorbidity) contribute to variation in both the gut microbiota and host health. Most, but not all, studies made attempts to consider the influence of multiple comparisons, such as reporting false discovery rates (FDR, express as q-values).

Other fundamental methodological aspects, such as the sequencing platform (e.g., the older Roche 454 vs. newer Illumina), primer choice, hypervariable region sequenced (e.g., V3–V5 vs. the now more commonly used V4)[59] and bioinformatics pipeline differed across studies, which could contribute to some of the variation in findings. Finally, all study samples were from prevalent multiple sclerosis subjects; whether observed differences in the gut microbiota between cases and controls resulted from or preceded multiple sclerosis remains unknown.

SUMMARY REMARKS

The studies conducted to date address a general proof-of-concept, that microbes in the gut may have a role to play in neurological and immune-mediated diseases like multiple sclerosis. Ultimately, the function(s) of the microbes rather than their actual name or phylogenic classification might be the most relevant factor(s). Although methodological differences between studies, small sample sizes (lack of power), and an inability to address confounders could certainly contribute to differences observed across studies, it is not necessarily unexpected to find differences in the gut microbiome based on geographical location. For example, when building predictive models to differentiate women with vs. without type 2 diabetes, separate models had to be developed for women in Europe vs. China, as the metagenomics markers differed by geographical location.[60]

WHAT ARE THEY DOING? EXPLORING THE FUNCTIONAL CAPACITY OF THE GUT MICROBIOME

There have been few studies using metagenomics to directly interrogate the functional capacity of the gut microbiota in people with multiple sclerosis. To date, most studies have employed animal models or looked at the effects of specific gut microbes on cells grown in the laboratory to explore specific aspects of microbial function. The German-based twin study reported using "bacterial metagenomics," and found no differences between 32 monozygotic twin pairs discordant for multiple sclerosis. However, discordant twins were more similar than unrelated twins, potentially inferring what others have observed—that the host genetics influences the gut microbiome.[29] Metagenomics is a costly endeavor, creating vast quantities of data requiring intense bioinformatics and complex analyses. However, a proxy-measure of the bacterial metagenome has been validated using the "PICRUSt" algorithm ("Phylogenetic Investigation of Communities by Reconstruction of Unobserved States").[61] Key findings from the limited number of studies in multiple sclerosis to explore this "predicted metagenome" include significant differences between multiple sclerosis cases and controls for pathways involving fatty acid metabolism, lipopolysaccharide biosynthesis, and glycolysis/glutathione metabolism, with multiple sclerosis disease-modifying drug exposure affecting some findings.[2,62] A French team re-used publicly available raw 16S rRNA sequences from two US-based studies[44,62] and focused on the inferred relative abundance of the enzyme EC 2.4.1.87 (N-acetyllactosaminide 3-alpha-galactosyltransferase) via the PICRUSt algorithm.[63] This enzyme corresponds to the GGTA1 gene, which is not found in humans, but has been associated with autoimmune diseases. A lower abundance was found in the multiple sclerosis cases relative to controls, which the authors proposed could suggest a role for the enzyme in multiple sclerosis, possibly mediated via IgG.[63] These hypotheses-generating findings have yet to be validated.

IS THE GUT MICROBIOTA ASSOCIATED WITH SUBSEQUENT MULTIPLE SCLEROSIS ACTIVITY?

Two small cross-sectional studies reported differences in the gut microbiota composition dependent on disease activity (Table 9.1).[62,64] Beta-diversity differed by proximity to a relapse in one US-based study (stool samples collected ≤ 1 vs. >1 month of a relapse from 12 vs. 19 individuals, respectively, p=0.05 Bray–Curtis distance, PERMANOVA).[62] Phylum and genus-level differences in intestinal mucosa samples were observed in a very small study in which three relapsing-remitting multiple sclerosis cases with evidence of disease activity were compared to four without in Italy (determined via MRI, relapse, and disability data).[64] Differences between groups included higher relative abundances of *Firmicutes* and lower relative abundance of *Bacteroidetes*. However, in both studies there were demographic and multiple sclerosis disease-modifying drug exposure differences between the small group and these confounding factors may have contributed to the observations. We published one small longitudinal study involving pediatric multiple sclerosis subjects and found that the gut microbiota profile, assessed at the phylum level, was associated with future relapse risk.[1] Specifically, in 17 California-based children, absence (depletion) of the *Fusobacteria* was associated with a 76% (95% CI, 55–90) risk of an earlier relapse (HR=3.2 (95% CI, 1.2–9.0), p=0.024 age and multiple sclerosis disease-modifying drug exposure adjusted).[1] The idea of whether or not the gut microbiota might contribute to disease activity is intriguing, and clearly more work is needed. If a causal relationship does exist, it could offer new treatment strategies for patients suffering from the disease.

BEYOND THE GUT BACTERIA

We found few published studies assessing the microbiome in body sites other than the gut or for Kingdoms other than *Bacteria* and *Archaea* in people with multiple sclerosis or at risk of developing multiple sclerosis. Briefly, groups are actively pursuing these areas by sampling from the mouth, nasal passages, cerebrospinal fluid[65] (which "bathes" the brain and spinal cord) and autopsied brain tissue.[66] Animal studies have also included lung tissue samples to assess the microbiome, as lung tissue may be an important site of immune activation.[67] Because smoking in adults and passive smoking in children is a potential risk factor for the onset of multiple sclerosis,[25] combined with some animal studies,[67] there is a biological rationale for further exploration of the lung microbiome, even though it is a challenging site from which to harvest samples for study.

Furthermore, very little is known about the mycobiome (*Fungi*) in multiple sclerosis. One Spanish group assayed serum samples from people with multiple sclerosis and compared the results to blood donors, reporting higher odds of serum antigen presence (vs. absence) to specific *Candida* spp., in multiple sclerosis participants.[68] However, the source of the *Fungi* and its role in multiple sclerosis could not be determined. The role of specific viruses, such as the Epstein–Barr virus, in triggering multiple sclerosis onset or relapses has long been of interest to people studying the disease.[25,69] However, no original study involving comprehensive interrogation of the virome in multiple sclerosis is, as of yet, available. Finally, the interaction between helminths ("macrobiota") and the gut microbiota and their potential to benefit those with multiple sclerosis through modulating the immune system is another active area of research,[70] but beyond the scope of this "microbiota" discussion.

MANIPULATING THE MULTIPLE SCLEROSIS MICROBIOME

Few studies were found for which the primary goal was to shift the gut microbiome in multiple sclerosis to assess whether or not there were any measurable health benefits, although there are anecdotal reports of fecal transplants performed in people with multiple sclerosis for other reasons (e.g., presence of *Clostridium difficile*).[71,72] See also Chapter 11: *The Role of Fecal Microbiota Transplantation in Neurological Diseases.* However, there are two small clinical trials (Phase II and 1b) exploring the role of orally or rectally administered fecal microbial transplant in multiple sclerosis (ClinicalTrials.gov identifiers and NCT03594487). A small pilot study also suggested that vitamin D supplementation could influence the gut microbiota in multiple sclerosis.[50] The effects of a six-month ketogenic diet on select microbes in the gut, analyzed using fluorescence in situ hybridization (FISH) ribosomal RNA-based probes, was explored in ten relapsing-remitting multiple sclerosis cases from Germany.[46] Unfortunately, despite having access to longitudinally collected samples, the team analyzed the information as a series of cross-sectionally collected data points and did not adjust for the multiple comparisons made. Most of the microbes examined did not change significantly from prior to the dietary intervention to study end, although *Bifidobacterium* decreased (from a mean 5.7 (SD 4.9) to 2.1 (SD 3), Student t-test, p=0.0008).[46] Furthermore, the effects on multiple sclerosis itself or health-related outcomes were not measured. Another small pilot study placed ten relapsing-remitting multiple sclerosis subjects on a high-vegetable/low-protein diet for 12 months and compared them to ten relapsing-remitting multiple sclerosis individuals continuing on their "Western Diet."[73] However, no pre-diet microbiome samples were collected, making it difficult to draw any conclusions from this uncontrolled, small study. The role of caloric restriction on the gut microbiota in multiple sclerosis is also under investigation in the United States (https://clinicaltrials.gov/ct 2/show/NCT02411838). Another US-based research team conducted a pilot study to explore the impact of an oral probiotic on immune-mediated blood biomarkers. This small two-month study involved nine multiple sclerosis patients and 13 controls.[74] Unfortunately, it is too early to ascertain what the future might hold in this area.

Fundamentally, it remains unclear which probiotic, if any, might be the most beneficial to try, and at which dose and for how long and with the view of affecting which outcome(s) in multiple sclerosis. The role of antibiotics or phage treatment remains other theoretical possibilities to alter the gut microbiome in multiple sclerosis.[75] Minocycline (a broad-spectrum tetracycline antibiotic) may reduce the risk of conversion from a clinically isolated syndrome to multiple sclerosis over the short term (at six months, but not 24 months) although whether the effect is mediated via the gut microbiota was not explored.[76] Other small pilot studies in multiple sclerosis have suggested that vitamin D supplementation or exposure to a disease-modifying drug called glatiramer acetate may also result in shifts in the gut microbiota.[50]

WHAT'S NEXT FOR MULTIPLE SCLEROSIS AND THE GUT MICROBIOME?

The role of the gut microbiota in multiple sclerosis remains an emerging field of inquiry. Collaborative efforts between diverse disciplines—including epidemiology, biostatistics, bioinformatics, microbiology, immunology, neurology, and engineering—will be needed to fully realize the many therapeutic possibilities this "newly discovered organ" may hold. As sequencing costs continue to drop, more complex analyses of the microbiome's full genetic repertoire (metagenomics) will offer greater opportunity than marker-based sequencing such as 16S rRNA, although metagenomics also requires advanced skills in "big data" analytics. Furthermore, where or what part of the human body should be sampled and sequenced may develop with time.

Aside from one small study, the main focus of studies to date has been to study microbes present (i.e., expelled) in stool. This might overlook key factors or the environment further along the gut, such as in the ileum/parenchyma.[75] Minimally invasive techniques, like tiny consumable sensors capable of surveying aspects of the gut functions *in vivo* beyond the contents of the colon, are also emerging.[77] Fundamental aspects of study design still need to be addressed (see earlier *Comment on Study Design*) and larger studies are needed to enable a better understanding of confounding factors (e.g., sex, age, other medication use). Longitudinal studies, with appropriately applied statistical analyses taking into account the relatedness of repeated measures from the same individual, are needed to demonstrate a temporal relationship between the gut microbiota and health outcomes in multiple sclerosis or the risk of developing multiple sclerosis.

Assessing the role of the gut microbiota, with samples collected *before* the onset of disease, has been feasible for common childhood onset conditions such as asthma and allergy.[78] However for multiple sclerosis, while a relatively common neurological condition, the *lifetime* prevalence is still modest at approximately 1 in 500, even in "high risk" areas such as North America.[8,12] Further, while most people will be diagnosed with multiple sclerosis between the ages of 20–45 years, the disease may have actually started many years prior.[79]

In short, demonstrating a causative role of the gut microbiota on the risk of actually developing multiple sclerosis would require a very ambitious study with samples collected in a sizable population with subsequent follow-up spanning decades tracking for signs of multiple sclerosis symptoms. Conversely, targeting "at risk" populations (e.g., those with family members with multiple sclerosis) might be a useful approach.[80] Validation and replication of findings, ideally across geographical locations, will also be key in understanding the role of the gut microbiota in multiple sclerosis, including the potential to modulate health outcomes in multiple sclerosis. Further, as most studies have focused on relapsing-remitting multiple sclerosis, it remains to be seen if the primary progressive multiple sclerosis gut microbiota differs in any meaningful way. Regardless of these challenges, we hold hope that one day we can harness the gut microbiome to lower the risk or prevent multiple sclerosis from occurring at all.

REFERENCES

1. Tremlett H, Fadrosh DW, Faruqi AA, Hart J, Roalstad S, Graves J, Lynch S, Waubant E. Gut microbiota composition and relapse risk in pediatric MS: A pilot study. *J Neurol Sci.* 2016;363:153–7.
2. Tremlett H, Fadrosh D, Faruqi A, Zhu F, Hart J, Roalstad S, Graves J, Lynch S, Waubant E. Gut microbiota in early pediatric multiple sclerosis: A case-control study. *Eur J Neurol.* 2016;23(8):1308–21.
3. Tremlett H, Fadrosh DW, Faruqi AA, Hart J, Roalstad S, Graves J, Spencer CM, Lynch SV, Zamvil SS, Waubant E. Associations between the gut microbiota and host immune markers in pediatric multiple sclerosis and controls. *BMC Neurol.* 2016;16(1):182.

4. Tremlett H, Bauer KC, Appel-Cresswell S, Finlay BB, Waubant E. The gut microbiome in human neurological disease: A review. *Ann Neurol.* 2017;1:369–82.

5. Tremlett H, Waubant E. Gut microbiome and pediatric multiple sclerosis. *Mult Scler J.* 2018;24(1):64–8.

6. Tremlett H, Waubant E. The gut microbiota and pediatric multiple sclerosis: Recent findings. *Neurotherapeutics.* 2018;15:102–8.

7. Tremlett H, Waubant E. The multiple sclerosis microbiome? *Ann Transl Med.* 2017;53.

8. Kingwell E, Zhu F, Marrie RA, Fisk JD, Wolfson C, Warren S, Profetto-McGrath J, Svenson LW, Jette N, Bhan V, Tremlett H, Elliott L, Tremlett H. High incidence and increasing prevalence of multiple sclerosis in British Columbia, Canada: Findings from over two decades (1991–2010). *J Neurol.* 2015;262(10):2352–63.

9. Marrie RA, Fisk JD, Stadnyk KJ, Yu BN, Tremlett H, Wolfson C, Warren S, Bhan V. The incidence and prevalence of multiple sclerosis in Nova Scotia, Canada. *Can J Neurol Sci.* 2013;40(06):824–31.

10. Marrie R, Yu N, Blanchard J, Leung S, Elliott L. The rising prevalence and changing age distribution of multiple sclerosis in Manitoba. *Neurology.* 2010;74(6):465–71.

11. Wallin W, Culpepper WJ, Campbell JD, Nelson LN, Langer-Gould A, Marrie RA, Cutter GR, Kaye WE, Wagner L, Tremlett H, Buka SL, Dilokthornsakul P, Topol B, Chen LH, LaRocca NG, on behalf of the United States Multiple Sclerosis Prevalence Workgroup. The prevalence of MS in the United States: A population-based estimate using health claims data. *Neurology.* 2019;92(10):e1–ee12. doi:10.1212/WNL.0000000000007035

12. Evans C, Beland S-G, Kulaga S, Wolfson C, Kingwell E, Marriott J, Koch M, Makhani N, Morrow S, Fisk J, Dykeman J, Jetté N, Pringsheim T, Marrie RA. Incidence and prevalence of multiple sclerosis in the Americas: A systematic review. *Neuroepidemiology.* 2013;40(3):195–210.

13. Amankwah N, Marrie RA, Bancej C, Garner R, Manuel DG, Wall R, Finès P, Bernier J, Tu K, Reimer K. Multiple sclerosis in Canada 2011 to 2031: Results of a microsimulation modelling study of epidemiological and economic impacts. *Health Promot Chronic Dis Prev Can.* 2017;37:37–48.

14. Leary S, Porter B, Thompson A. Multiple sclerosis: Diagnosis and the management of acute relapses. *Postgrad Med J.* 2005;81(955):302–8.

15. Waubant E, Ponsonby A-L, Pugliatti M, Hanwell H, Mowry EM, Hintzen RQ. Environmental and genetic factors in pediatric inflammatory demyelinating diseases. *Neurology.* 2016;87(9 Supplement 2):S20–7.

16. Hartung DM. Economics and cost-effectiveness of multiple sclerosis therapies in the USA. *Neurotherapeutics.* 2017;14:1018–26.

17. Owens GM. Economic burden of multiple sclerosis and the role of managed care organizations in multiple sclerosis management. *Am J Manag Care.* 2016;22(6 Supplement):s151–8.

18. O'Brien JA, Ward AJ, Patrick AR, Caro J. Cost of managing an episode of relapse in multiple sclerosis in the United States. *BMC Health Serv Res.* 2003;3(1):17.

19. Tremlett H, Zhao Y, Rieckmann P, Hutchinson M. New perspectives in the natural history of multiple sclerosis. *Neurology.* 2010;74(24):2004–15.

20. Kingwell E, van der Kop M, Zhao Y, Shirani A, Zhu F, Oger J, Tremlett H. Relative mortality and survival in multiple sclerosis: Findings from British Columbia, Canada. *J Neurol Neurosurg Psychiatry.* 2012;83(1):61–6.

21. Lublin FD, Reingold SC. Defining the clinical course of multiple sclerosis results of an international survey. *Neurology.* 1996;46(4):907–11.

22. Lublin FD, Reingold SC, Cohen JA, Cutter GR, Sørensen PS, Thompson AJ, Wolinsky JS, Balcer LJ, Banwell B, Barkhof F, Bebo B, Calabresi PA, Clanet M, Comi G, Fox RJ, Freedman MS, Goodman AD, Inglese M, Kappos L, Kieseier BC, Lincoln JA, Lubetzki C, Miller AE, Montalban X, O'Connor PW, Petkau J, Pozzilli C, Rudick RA,

Sormani MP, Stüve O, Waubant E, Polman CH. Defining the clinical course of multiple sclerosis: the 2013 revisions. *Neurology.* 2014;83(3):278–86.

23. Tramacere I, Del Giovane C, Salanti G, D'Amico R, Filippini G. *Immunomodulators and Immunosuppressants for Relapsing-Remitting Multiple Sclerosis: A Network Meta-Analysis.* The Cochrane Library. 2015.

24. Curtin F, Hartung H-P. Novel therapeutic options for multiple sclerosis. *Expert Rev Clin Pharmacol.* 2014;7(1):91–104.

25. McKay KA, Jahanfar S, Duggan T, Tkachuk S, Tremlett H. Factors associated with onset, relapses or progression in multiple sclerosis: A systematic review. *Neurotoxicology.* 2016;61:189–212.

26. Wang Y, Kasper LH. The role of microbiome in central nervous system disorders. *Brain Behav Immun.* 2014;38:1–12.

27. Berer K, Mues M, Koutrolos M, Rasbi ZA, Boziki M, Johner C, Wekerle H, Krishnamoorthy G. Commensal microbiota and myelin autoantigen cooperate to trigger autoimmune demyelination. *Nature.* 2011;479(7374):538–41.

28. Lee YK, Menezes JS, Umesaki Y, Mazmanian SK. Proinflammatory T-cell responses to gut microbiota promote experimental autoimmune encephalomyelitis. *Proc Natl Acad Sci U S A.* 2011;108(Supplement 1):4615–22.

29. Berer K, Gerdes LA, Cekanaviciute E, Jia X, Xiao L, Xia Z, Liu C, Klotz L, Stauffer U, Baranzini SE, Kümpfel T, Hohlfeld R, Krishnamoorthy G, Wekerle H. Gut microbiota from multiple sclerosis patients enables spontaneous autoimmune encephalomyelitis in mice. *Proc Natl Acad Sci U S A.* 2017;114:10719–24.

30. Cekanaviciute E, Yoo BB, Runia TF, Debelius JW, Singh S, Nelson CA, Kanner R, Bencosme Y, Lee YK, Hauser SL, Crabtree-Hartman E, Sand IK, Gacias M, Zhu Y, Casaccia P, Cree BAC, Knight R, Mazmanian SK, Baranzini SE. Gut bacteria from multiple sclerosis patients modulate human T cells and exacerbate symptoms in mouse models. *Proc Natl Acad Sci U S A.* 2017;114:10713–8.

31. Goverman J, Woods A, Larson L, Weiner LP, Hood L, Zaller DM. Transgenic mice that express a myelin basic protein-specific T cell receptor develop spontaneous autoimmunity. *Cell.* 1993;72(4):551–60.

32. Mielcarz DW, Kasper LH. The gut microbiome in multiple sclerosis. *Curr Treat Options Neurol.* 2015;17(4):344.

33. Conlon MA, Bird AR. The impact of diet and lifestyle on gut microbiota and human health. *Nutrients.* 2014;7(1):17–44.

34. Hollister EB, Riehle K, Luna RA, Weidler EM, Rubio-Gonzales M, Mistretta T-A, Raza S, Doddapaneni HV, Metcalf GA, Muzny DM, Gibbs RA, Petrosino JF, Shulman RJ, Versalovic J. Structure and function of the healthy pre-adolescent pediatric gut microbiome. *Microbiome.* 2015;3(1):1.

35. Markle JG, Frank DN, Mortin-Toth S, Robertson CE, Feazel LM, Rolle-Kampczyk U, von Bergen M, McCoy KD, Macpherson AJ, Danska JS. Sex differences in the gut microbiome drive hormone-dependent regulation of autoimmunity. *Science.* 2013;339(6123):1084–8.

36. Goodrich JK, Waters JL, Poole AC, Sutter JL, Koren O, Blekhman R, Beaumont M, Van Treuren W, Knight R, Bell JT, Spector TD, Clark AG, Ley RE. Human genetics shape the gut microbiome. *Cell.* 2014;159(4):789–99.

37. Davenport ER, Mizrahi-Man O, Michelini K, Barreiro LB, Ober C, Gilad Y. Seasonal variation in human gut microbiome composition. *PLOS ONE.* 2014;9(3):e90731.

38. Ridaura VK, Faith JJ, Rey FE, Cheng J, Duncan AE, Kau AL, Griffin NW, Lombard V, Henrissat B, Bain JR, Muehlbauer MJ, Ilkayeva O, Semenkovich CF, Funai K, Hayashi DK, Lyle BJ, Martini MC, Ursell LK, Clemente JC, Van Treuren W, Walters WA, Knight R, Newgard CB, Heath AC, Gordon JI. Gut microbiota from twins discordant for obesity modulate metabolism in mice. *Science.* 2013;341(6150):1241214.

39. Biedermann L, Zeitz J, Mwinyi J, Sutter-Minder E, Rehman A, Ott SJ, Steurer-Stey C, Frei A, Frei P, Scharl M, Loessner MJ, Vavricka SR, Fried M, Schreiber S, Schuppler M, Rogler G. Smoking cessation induces profound changes in the composition of the intestinal microbiota in humans. *PLOS ONE*. 2013;8(3):e59260.

40. Norman JM, Handley SA, Baldridge MT, Droit L, Liu CY, Keller BC, Kambal A, Monaco CL, Zhao G, Fleshner P, Stappenbeck TS, McGovern DP, Keshavarzian A, Mutlu EA, Sauk J, Gevers D, Xavier RJ, Wang D, Parkes M, Virgin HW. Disease-specific alterations in the enteric virome in inflammatory bowel disease. *Cell*. 2015;160(3):447–60.

41. Kernbauer E, Ding Y, Cadwell K. An enteric virus can replace the beneficial function of commensal bacteria. *Nature*. 2014;516(7529):94–8.

42. Buscarinu MC, Cerasoli B, Annibali V, Policano C, Lionetto L, Capi M, Mechelli R, Romano S, Fornasiero A, Mattei G, Piras E, Angelini DF, Battistini L, Simmaco M, Umeton R, Salvetti M, Ristori G. Altered intestinal permeability in patients with relapsing–remitting multiple sclerosis: A pilot study. *Mult Scler J*. 2017;23(3):442–6.

43. Zhang Y, Liu G, Duan Y, Han X, Dong H, Geng J. Prevalence of small intestinal bacterial overgrowth in multiple sclerosis: A case-control study from China. *J Neuroimmunol*. 2016;301:83–7.

44. Jangi S, Gandhi R, Cox LM, Li N, von Glehn F, Yan R, Patel B, Mazzola MA, Liu S, Glanz BL, Cook S, Tankou S, Stuart F, Melo K, Nejad P, Smith K, Topçuolu BD, Holden J, Kivisäkk P, Chitnis T, De Jager PL, Quintana FJ, Gerber GK, Bry L, Weiner HL. Alterations of the human gut microbiome in multiple sclerosis. *Nat Commun*. 2016;7:12015.

45. Rumah KR, Linden J, Fischetti VA, Vartanian T. Isolation of *Clostridium perfringens* type B in an individual at first clinical presentation of multiple sclerosis provides clues for environmental triggers of the disease. *PLOS ONE*. 2013;8(10):e76359.

46. Swidsinski A, Dörffel Y, Loening-Baucke V, Gille C, Göktas Ö, Reißhauer A, Neuhaus J, Weylandt K-H, Guschin A, Bock M. Reduced mass and diversity of the colonic microbiome in patients with multiple sclerosis and their improvement with ketogenic diet. *Front Microbiol*. 2017;8:1141.

47. Gevers D, Kugathasan S, Denson LA, Vazquez-Baeza Y, Van Treuren W, Ren B, Schwager E, Knights D, Song SJ, Yassour M, Morgan XC, Kostic AD, Luo C, Gonzalez A, McDonald D, Haberman Y, Walters T, Baker S, Rosh J, Stephens M, Heyman M, Markowitz J, Baldassano R, Griffiths A, Sylvester F, Mack D, Kim S, Crandall W, Hyams J, Huttenhower C, Knight R, Xavier RJ. The treatment-naive microbiome in new-onset Crohn's disease. *Cell Host Microbe*. 2014;15(3):382–92.

48. Sokol H, Pigneur B, Watterlot L, Lakhdari O, Bermudez-Humaran LG, Gratadoux JJ, Blugeon S, Bridonneau C, Furet JP, Corthier G, Grangette C, Vasquez N, Pochart P, Trugnan G, Thomas G, Blottiere HM, Dore J, Marteau P, Seksik P, Langella P. Faecalibacterium prausnitzii is an anti-inflammatory commensal bacterium identified by gut microbiota analysis of Crohn disease patients. *Proc Natl Acad Sci U S A*. 2008;105(43):16731–6.

49. Scher JU, Sczesnak A, Longman RS, Segata N, Ubeda C, Bielski C, Rostron T, Cerundolo V, Pamer EG, Abramson SB, Huttenhower C, Littman DR. Expansion of intestinal Prevotella copri correlates with enhanced susceptibility to arthritis. *Elife*. 2013;2:e01202.

50. Cantarel BL, Waubant E, Chehoud C, Kuczynski J, DeSantis TZ, Warrington J, Venkatesan A, Fraser CM, Mowry EM. Gut microbiota in multiple sclerosis: Possible influence of immunomodulators. *J Investig Med*. 2015;63(5):729–34.

51. Miyake S, Kim S, Suda W, Oshima K, Nakamura M, Matsuoka T, Chihara N, Tomita A, Sato W, Kim S-W, Morita H, Hattori M, Yamamura T. Dysbiosis in the gut microbiota of patients with multiple sclerosis, with a striking depletion of species belonging to clostridia XIVa and IV clusters. *PLOS ONE*. 2015;10(9):e0137429.

52. Hsiao EY, McBride SW, Hsien S, Sharon G, Hyde ER, McCue T, Codelli JA, Chow J, Reisman SE, Petrosino JF, Patterson PH, Mazmanian SK. Microbiota modulate behavioral and physiological abnormalities associated with neurodevelopmental disorders. *Cell*. 2013;155(7):1451–63.
53. Wacholder S, Silverman DT, McLaughlin JK, Mandel JS. Selection of controls in case-control studies: II. Types of controls. *Am J Epidemiol*. 1992;135(9):1029–41.
54. Imhann F, Bonder MJ, Vich Vila A, Fu J, Mujagic Z, Vork L, Tigchelaar EF, Jankipersadsing SA, Cenit MC, Harmsen HJ, Dijkstra G, Franke L, Xavier RJ, Jonkers D, Wijmenga C, Weersma RK, Zhernakova A. Proton pump inhibitors affect the gut microbiome. *Gut*. 2016;65(5):740–8.
55. Le Bastard Q, Al-Ghalith G, Grégoire M, Chapelet G, Javaudin F, Dailly E, Batard E, Knights D, Montassier E. Systematic review: Human gut dysbiosis induced by non-antibiotic prescription medications. *Aliment Pharmacol Ther*. 2018;47(3):332–45.
56. Vandeputte D, Falony G, Vieira-Silva S, Tito RY, Joossens M, Raes J. Stool consistency is strongly associated with gut microbiota richness and composition, enterotypes and bacterial growth rates. *Gut*. 2016;65(1):57–62.
57. Cotterill N, Madersbacher H, Wyndaele JJ, Apostolidis A, Drake MJ, Gajewski J, Heesakkers J, Panicker J, Radziszewski P, Sakakibara R, Sievert KD, Hamid R, Kessler TM, Emmanuel A. Neurogenic bowel dysfunction: Clinical management recommendations of the Neurologic Incontinence Committee of the Fifth International Consultation on Incontinence 2013. *Neurourol Urodyn*. 2018;37(1):46–53.
58. Marrie RA, Cohen J, Stuve O, Trojano M, Sørensen PS, Reingold S, Cutter G, Reider N. A systematic review of the incidence and prevalence of comorbidity in multiple sclerosis: Overview. *Mult Scler J*. 2015;21(3):263–81.
59. Thompson LR, Sanders JG, McDonald D, Amir A, Ladau J, Locey KJ, Prill RJ, Tripathi A, Gibbons SM, Ackermann G, Navas-Molina JA, Janssen S, Kopylova E, Vázquez-Baeza Y, González A, Morton JT, Mirarab S, Zech Xu Z, Jiang L, Haroon MF, Kanbar J, Zhu Q, Jin Song S, Kosciolek T, Bokulich NA, Lefler J, Brislawn CJ, Humphrey G, Owens SM, Hampton-Marcell J, Berg-Lyons D, McKenzie V, Fierer N, Fuhrman JA, Clauset A, Stevens RL, Shade A, Pollard KS, Goodwin KD, Jansson JK, Gilbert JA, Knight R, Earth Microbiome Project Consortium. A communal catalogue reveals Earth's multiscale microbial diversity. *Nature*. 2017;551(7681).
60. Karlsson FH, Tremaroli V, Nookaew I, Bergström G, Behre CJ, Fagerberg B, Nielsen J, Bäckhed F. Gut metagenome in European women with normal, impaired and diabetic glucose control. *Nature*. 2013;498(7452):99.
61. Langille MG, Zaneveld J, Caporaso JG, McDonald D, Knights D, Reyes JA, Clemente JC, Burkepile DE, Vega Thurber RL, Knight R, Beiko RG, Huttenhower C. Predictive functional profiling of microbial communities using 16S rRNA marker gene sequences. *Nat Biotechnol*. 2013;31(9):814–21.
62. Chen J, Chia N, Kalari KR, Yao JZ, Novotna M, Soldan MMP, Luckey DH, Marietta EV, Jeraldo PR, Chen X, Weinshenker BG, Rodriguez M, Kantarci OH, Nelson H, Murray JA, Mangalam AK. Multiple sclerosis patients have a distinct gut microbiota compared to healthy controls. *Sci Rep*. 2016;6:28484.
63. Montassier E, Berthelot L, Soulillou J-P. Are the decrease in circulating anti-α1, 3-Gal IgG and the lower content of galactosyl transferase A1 in the microbiota of patients with multiple sclerosis a novel environmental risk factor for the disease? *Mol Immunol*. 2018;93:162–5.
64. Cosorich I, Dalla-Costa G, Sorini C, Ferrarese R, Messina MJ, Dolpady J, Radice E, Mariani A, Testoni PA, Canducci F, Comi G, Martinelli V, Falcone M. High frequency of intestinal TH17 cells correlates with microbiota alterations and disease activity in multiple sclerosis. *Sci Adv*. 2017;3(7):e1700492.
65. Perlejewski K, Bukowska-Ośko I, Nakamura S, Motooka D, Stokowy T, Płoski R, Rydzanicz M, Zakrzewska-Pniewska B, Podlecka-Piętowska A, Nojszewska M, Gogol A, Caraballo

Cortés K, Demkow U, Stępień A, Laskus T, Radkowski M. Metagenomic analysis of cerebrospinal fluid from patients with multiple sclerosis. *Adv Exp Med Biol.* 2016;935:89–98.

66. Branton W, Lu J, Surette M, Holt R, Lind J, Laman J, Power C. Multiple sclerosis lesions show perturbations in cerebral microbiota (S37. 005). *Neurology.* 2016;86(16 Supplement):S37.005.

67. Odoardi F, Sie C, Streyl K, Ulaganathan VK, Schläger C, Lodygin D, Heckelsmiller K, Nietfeld W, Ellwart J, Klinkert WE, Lottaz C, Nosov M, Brinkmann V, Spang R, Lehrach H, Vingron M, Wekerle H, Flügel-Koch C, Flügel A. T cells become licensed in the lung to enter the central nervous system. *Nature.* 2012;488(7413):675.

68. Benito-Leon J, Pisa D, Alonso R, Calleja P, Diaz-Sanchez M, Carrasco L. Association between multiple sclerosis and Candida species: Evidence from a case-control study. *Eur J Clin Microbiol Infect Dis.* 2010;29(9):1139–45.

69. Dreyfus DH. Gene sharing between Epstein–Barr virus and human immune response genes. *Immunol Res.* 2016:1–9.

70. Reynolds LA, Finlay BB, Maizels RM. Cohabitation in the intestine: Interactions among helminth parasites, bacterial microbiota, and host immunity. *J Immunol.* 2015;195(9):4059–66.

71. Borody TJ, Leis S, Campbell J, Torres M, Nowak A. Fecal microbiota transplantation (FMT) in multiple sclerosis (MS). *Am J Gastroenterol.* 2011;106:S352.

72. Makkawi S, Metz L. *Case Report: Fecal Microbiota Transplantation Associated with 10 Years of Disease Stability in a Patient with Secondary Progressive Multiple Sclerosis.* ECTRIMS Online Library. 2017; 200657.

73. Saresella M, Mendozzi L, Rossi V, Mazzali F, Piancone F, LaRosa F, Marventano I, Caputo D, Felis GE, Clerici M. Immunological and clinical effect of diet modulation of the gut microbiome in multiple sclerosis patients: A pilot study. *Front Immunol.* 2017;8:1391.

74. Tankou SK, Regev K, Healy BC, Cox LM, Tjon E, Kivisakk P, Vanande IP, Cook S, Gandhi R, Glanz B, Stankiewicz J, Weiner HL. Investigation of probiotics in multiple sclerosis. *Mult Scler J.* 2018;24(1):58–63.

75. Wekerle H. Brain autoimmunity and intestinal microbiota: 100 trillion game changers. *Trends Immunol.* 2017;38(7):483–97.

76. Metz LM, Li DK, Traboulsee AL, Duquette P, Eliasziw M, Cerchiaro G, Greenfield J, Riddehough A, Yeung M, Kremenchutzky M, Vorobeychik G, Freedman MS, Bhan V, Blevins G, Marriott JJ, Grand'Maison F, Lee L, Thibault M, Hill MD, Yong VW, Minocycline in MS Study Team. Trial of minocycline in a clinically isolated syndrome of multiple sclerosis. *N Engl J Med.* 2017;376(22):2122–33.

77. Kalantar-Zadeh K, Berean KJ, Ha N, Chrimes AF, Xu K, Grando D, Ou JZ, Pillai N, Campbell JL, Brkljača R, Taylor KM, Burgell RE, Yao CK, Ward SA, McSweeney CS, Muir JG, Gibson PR. A human pilot trial of ingestible electronic capsules capable of sensing different gases in the gut. *Nat Electron.* 2018;1(1):79.

78. Arrieta M-C, Stiemsma LT, Dimitriu PA, Thorson L, Russell S, Yurist-Doutsch S, Kuzeljevic B, Gold MJ, Britton HM, Lefebvre DL, Subbarao P, Mandhane P, Becker A, McNagny KM, Sears MR, Kollmann T, CHILD Study Investigators, Mohn WW, Turvey SE, Finlay BB. Early infancy microbial and metabolic alterations affect risk of childhood asthma. *Sci Transl Med.* 2015;7(307):307ra152.

79. Wijnands JMA, Kingwell E, Zhu F, Zhao Y, Högg T, Stadnyk K, Ekuma O, Lu X, Evans C, Fisk J, Marrie RA, Tremlett H. Health-care use before a first demyelinating event suggestive of a multiple sclerosis prodrome: A matched cohort study. *Lancet Neurol.* 2017;16(6):445–51.

80. Xia Z, Steele SU, Bakshi A, Clarkson SR, White CC, Schindler MK, Nair G, Dewey BE, Price LR, Ohayon J, Chibnik LB, Cortese IC, De Jager PL, Reich DS. Assessment of early evidence of multiple sclerosis in a prospective study of asymptomatic high-risk family members. *JAMA Neurol.* 2017;74(3):293–300.

10 Bacteriophage Involvement in Neurodegenerative Diseases

George Tetz and Victor Tetz

CONTENTS

INTRODUCTION

There are a variety of neurodegenerative diseases characterized by a progressive cognitive decline accompanied by memory loss, and Alzheimer's disease is the most common among them.[1] These cognitive symptoms and neurodegeneration are primarily related to neuronal death caused by deposits of misfolded proteins in the brain—β-amyloid and tau proteins in Alzheimer's, α-synuclein in Parkinson's disease, and SOD1 and TDP-43 in amyotrophic lateral sclerosis (ALS).[2,3] The appearance of these extracellular protein aggregates results in neuronal death and synapse loss. This degradation in turn contributes to neural atrophy that, at least in the initial stages of Alzheimer's disease, is localized within the hippocampus and the entorhinal cortex.[4,5]

Under normal conditions, all of the above-mentioned proteins play an important regulatory role in the central nervous system (CNS). Specifically, β-amyloid is a cleavage product of a large, transmembrane amyloid precursor protein (APP); tau protein plays a role in microtubule stabilization; and α-synuclein serves in a variety of undifferentiated roles in synapse function.[6–8] Unfortunately, why these proteins adopt a misfolded β-sheet structure and form aggregates is not fully understood. Certainly the role of genetics requires further research, as dozens of genes (*APP*,

PSEN1, PSEN2, APOE, SOD1, LRRK2, and *PARK7*) have been indicated as potential risk factors associated with an increased APP aggregation rate.[9–11]

However, neurodegenerative development even in individuals with genetic susceptibilities still requires specific environmental and epigenetic factors. In particular, recent studies have suggested the role of a microbial component in the pathogenesis and progression of neurodegeneration.[12] Over the past few decades, the development of new sequencing technologies has enabled scientists to extensively characterize the human microbiome. The microbiome consists of complex, polymicrobial communities of bacteria, archaea, fungi, and viruses that reside in human tissues and biofluids. Currently, microbiota of the gut, skin, lung, placenta, and even the brain—which was previously thought to be sterile—have been identified.[13–16]

The role of microbiota in the development and progression of neurodegeneration is most studied in Alzheimer's. Notably, the microorganisms implicated in Alzheimer's can be found not only in the brain or cerebrospinal fluid—like HHV-1, *Borrelia* spp., *Escherichia coli*, and *Candida* spp.—but also within the gut microbiota. This evidences the idea that even distinct microbiomes from different localizations can affect the central nervous system (CNS).[17–20] Today, it is clear that gut microbiota, the largest microbiome in the human organism, perform not only key functions associated with the gastrointestinal and immune systems, vitamin biosynthesis, and protection against pathogen overgrowth, but also affect brain function through the so-called gut-brain axis. Furthermore, it is through this gut–brain connection that they have been implicated in a variety of neurodegenerative diseases.[20] Moreover, the newly identified skin-gut axis was also recently shown to impact some of the processes associated with normal brain function and neurodegeneration.

These distinct microbiota–brain axes, through neural and endocrinal pathways, allow for bi-directional communication between the organs and the brain, as well as the release of pathogen-associated-molecular patterns (PAMPs) and immune mechanisms.[21,22] Within this framework, alterations in the gut microbial communities of patients with Alzheimer's—such as decreased abundances of Firmicutes, *Bifidobacterium,* and anti-inflammatory *Eubacterium rectale*, along with increased *Bacteroidetes* and pro-inflammatory *E. coli* and *Shigella* spp—were associated with the triggering and worsening of Alzheimer's.[23] The majority of reported gut microbiota alterations associated with neurodegeneration are thought to be driven by systemic inflammation via multiple pathways, such as leaky gut that in turn leads to pathophysiological changes in the brain, including protein misfolding and glial activation.[24]

However, the question of why these microbiota alterations occur in neurodegenerative diseases remains unanswered, as previous studies have not found a positive association with external factors, including antibiotic exposure or disease-specific microbiota alteration. Recently, we turned our attention to bacteriophages, as they are the least-studied microbiota component that is known to still play a primary role in homeostasis. Bacteriophages (phages) are viruses that uniquely infect bacteria. They are one of the most widespread non-living genetic elements in nature. There are over 10^{15} phages in the average human organism and over 10^{30} in the oceans of the world.[25]

There are two types of bacteriophages, which have been classified based on the nature of their interaction with the bacterial hosts they infect. The first, lytic phages, multiply inside the bacterial cell and synthesize new infectious phages during replication and viral particle biogenesis that kill the bacteria and release progeny viri-ons.[26,27] The ability of phages to infect and destroy bacterial cells, including antibiotic-resistant species, gave rise to the clinical application of lytic phages in the treatment of poorly curable bacterial infections.[27] Today, some bacteriophages are even considered promising antibiotic alternatives to combat multidrug-resistant bacteria.[28]

The second type of phage, known as lysogenic or temperate phages, can repro-duce within bacterial cells using both lytic and lysogenic cycles.[27] During the lyso-genic cycle, the bacteriophage integrates its nucleic acids into the host cell DNA and propagates vertically by bacterial division without producing progeny. However, upon induction, these lysogenic phages can transition to a lytic state, killing their bacterial host by progeny release and consequently impacting bacterial abundance.

We have recently proposed the idea that bacteriophages, individually and as a collective—known as the phagobiota—are potential human pathogens with a direct association to neurodegenerative diseases. We suggest that in humans, phagobiota possess multiple direct and indirect pathways through which they contribute to the development of a variety of diseases. The concept of bacteriophages as new human viral pathogens actually opens a discussion of the central, and previously unknown, role of bacteriophages in human health pathology, neurodegeneration in particular.[29] Furthermore, phages were recently described as an important non-living genetic ele-ment, whose increased circulation in biological fluids was associated with aging, neuroaging in particular.[30]

This chapter will review the role of bacteriophages in neurodegenerative diseases, with a focus on how phages contribute to the genesis, progression, and maintenance of neurodegenerative diseases. It will also discuss perspectives for future phagobi-ome research.

BACTERIOPHAGES AND NEURODEGENERATION

The existing research on the role of human pathogen phages is very limited, with even less data on their connection to neurodegenerative pathologies. However, phages contribute to both the genesis and progression of Alzheimer's and Parkinson's in dif-ferent ways that will be further discussed in this chapter. Given the prominent role of phagobiota as a regulator in the bacterial component of the microbiota, and the crucial role of the microbiota in human physiology, phages clearly can have a direct impact on human health.[31]

Recent discoveries have indicated a direct interplay between phagobiota and mac-roorganisms in the process of neurodegeneration.[29,32] The interaction of phages with their host macroorganisms leading to neurodegenerative-associated alterations can be observed through their interactions with human cells or proteins. However, the mechanisms behind their direct interaction with eukaryotic cells and proteomes are only in the initial stages of exploration.

BACTERIOPHAGES, EUKARYOTIC CELLS, AND AUTOIMMUNITY

Recently, bacterial viruses were shown to possess the ability to directly interact with eukaryotic cells. Nguyen et al. (2017) demonstrated that phages can be picked up from the surface of epithelial cells via endocytosis and transcytosed across cell barriers.[33] Another study from Lehti et al. (2017) demonstrated the direct interaction of phages and human cells, demonstrating that Escherichia coli phage PK1A2 can bind and penetrate live eukaryotic neuroblastoma cells.[34] The direct interaction of phages with eukaryotic cells is notable because they can travel beyond the gut and are found in many different parts of the human body, including the central nervous system.

It was recently demonstrated that bacterial viruses use different methods to cross physical barriers and thereby access different human organs and biological fluids. The first studies on this topic showed that, in people with increased intestinal permeability, phages from the gut can cross into systemic circulation and disseminate to different organs of the body.[31,35,36] For example, during experimental therapy in patients with bacterial infections, certain phages could be found in blood samples following oral phage administration.[33] A study by Gorsky et al. (2006) showed the presence of active phages in circulation following oral administration, phages that were not neutralized by stomach secretions.[37,38] The possibility for phage dissemination is also confirmed by their presence in urine and amniotic fluid.[39–41] Our data demonstrated that, following phage administration, different phages could be found in rodent biological fluids with subsequent dissemination to the spleen, an organ responsible for circulatory viral clearance. Moreover, in mouse models, phage dissemination to the cerebrospinal fluid could be observed (unpublished data).[41]

The ability of bacterial viruses to reach the cerebrospinal fluid was further evidenced by a microbiome-based study of patients with multiple sclerosis. Our core was the first to detect bacteriophages, Shigella phage SfIV and Staphylococcus phage StB2, in the cerebrospinal fluid of patients with this pathology (unpublished data). By analyzing how phages are able to reach the central nervous system, we noted that patients with multiple sclerosis have altered intestinal and blood–brain barriers, allowing bacteriophage traffic between the circulatory system and the cerebrospinal fluid.[42] Considering that Alzheimer's disease is also characterized by a disrupted blood–brain barrier, one could suggest that phage translocation also occurs in this condition and that it has only not been described yet because of the technical difficulties inherent in this type of monitoring. Indeed, the majority of metagenomic cerebrospinal fluid and brain studies do not use sequencing methods conducive to phage identification, so there are no data on phage presence in the cerebrospinal fluid or brains of Alzheimer's patients from these studies. Most studies rely on 16S RNA gene sequencing, which allows for the identification of bacterial species but not bacteriophages, which require shotgun sequencing to be identified.[43]

Our idea that many of the conditions that are characterized by a leaky gut can result in phagemia and the subsequent entrance of phages into the cerebrospinal fluid was recently confirmed by Pou et al. (2018).[41] By studying the cerebrospinal fluid of patients with neurological complications following stem cell transplantation, they identified significantly elevated levels of bacteriophages in the cerebrospinal fluid compared to controls. They identified Brucella, Burkholderia, Streptococcus, and Vibrio phages in cerebrospinal fluid. Although they concluded that higher phage abundance was indicative of bacterial infections, we suggest that under certain conditions, phages themselves could contribute to disease progression.

The presence of bacteriophages within the cerebrospinal fluid is supported by multiple studies showing the presence of other microorganisms within the central nervous system, and the existence of the brain microbiome.[16,44] Originally suggested to be sterile, increasing amounts of data show that healthy individuals and Alzheimer's patients alike present with a number of bacteria, fungi, and viruses in the cerebrospinal fluid and brain.[16,45] For example, HHV-1, *Candida, E. coli, Chlamydophila pneumoniae*, and spirochetes are strongly associated with Alzheimer's, as evidenced by their DNA and surface components being found within amyloid plaques, suggesting they might play a role in the formation of amyloid beta plaques.[44,45] The pathogenic mechanisms of the microbial presence in the cerebrospinal fluid and brain in neurodegenerative pathogenesis are multifaceted and include the development of an autoimmune cascade and an altered inflammatory response.[46] Notably, some similarly altered autoimmune reactions can be triggered by bacteriophages.

The immunogenic role of phages as it relates to phage development as a therapy has shown that systemic bacteriophage circulation leads to a humoral immune response and the secretion of phage-specific IgM and IgG, similar to what is observed in bacteremia and viremia. Notably, although elevated levels of IgG and IgM antibodies were shown to be triggered by different phages, different phage proteins possess different triggering potentials.[47] Gorsky et al. (2018) demonstrated that the presence of phages in the blood might interact with the CD40–CD40L system, promoting inflammatory and thrombotic responses by causing further platelet activation.[48,49] Furthermore, phages were shown to accelerate NF-κB activation, and the implications of NF-κB over-activation in Alzheimer's and Parkinson's is well described because it suppresses the hippocampal TREM2 expression required for microglial amyloid clearance, the decline of which is associated with plaque formation.[50,51]

The molecular mechanisms of bacteriophage–eukaryotic cell interactions, as well as phage immunomodulatory activity, are not completely understood. However, the great diversity of phages and their close physical coexistence with humans raises questions about the previously unknown direct effects of phages on human cells and disease progression. In particular, future attention should be paid to multifaceted neurodegenerative diseases, Alzheimer's in particular.

BACTERIOPHAGES AND PROTEIN MISFOLDING

Protein misfolding, which triggers the formation of neurotoxic aggregates, has become the leading theory for the recognition of Alzheimer's, Parkinson's, ALS, and other neurodegenerative pathologies as prion-mediated disorders.[2–4] Prions are formed when normal proteins change their conformation to β-sheet-like motifs, becoming self-propagating and leading to the creation of new, misfolded proteins.[52] One of the initiating events in Alzheimer's pathogenesis is the misfolding of β-amyloid (Aβ) peptides and tau-proteins in the brain, with the formation of amyloid plaques and intracellular NFTs. Many recent studies have proved that Aβ, tau, α-synuclein, and TDP-43 proteins possess prion-like activity, with neurotoxic misfolded protein aggregation in the brain leading to the formation of self-propagating aggregates that allow them to spread throughout the nervous system.[2,53] The cellular mechanisms of prion-mediated neurotoxicity are not completely understood;

however, it is clear that the formation of neurotoxic insoluble misfolded aggregates is associated with synaptic dysfunction and neuronal death.[54] It was recently shown that brain homogenates from Alzheimer's patients could act as a disease transmitter to relevant animal model Tg2576 mice seeded with mutant human APP.[55,56]

However, one of the most important, but poorly studied, questions is what causes proteins to misfold. The formation of prions requires a pathogenic "seed" that is believed to be another prion. Recent data from a study conducted by Chen et al. (2016) pointed out the possibility of the cross-kingdom seeding of eukaryotic prions and protein misfolding in humans with prion-producing *E. coli*. In our recent work, we identified over 5,000 different prion-like domains on the surface of different bacteriophages, including phages found within human microbiota.[57] We contributed to the working theory that if bacteriophages possessing surface prions reach the cerebrospinal fluid and brain, those prions could act as seeding molecules for protein misfolding. Analysis of the prion-like domains on the surface structures of bacteriophages from the brains of Alzheimer's patients revealed interesting regularities. We revealed 530 proteins with prion-like domains within the bacteriophages of *E. coli*—microorganisms frequently found in the cerebrospinal fluid and brain of Alzheimer's patients.[58] Twenty-five of these proteins had a prion-like amino acid composition score over 20, reflecting a high probability of these proteins being prions. Currently, the lowest value for a known budding yeast prion-forming protein is ~21.0.[59] Among proteins with prion-like domains (PrDs), there are a number of surface-located proteins implicated in viral attachment and penetration such as the "putative tail fiber," "Gp37," "tail collar domain protein," "baseplate subunit," and others. The allocation of PrDs on the virion surface demonstrates that they can interact not only with bacterial surface domains, but also with mammalian proteins, acting like seeds contributing to prion misfolding.

Interestingly, we have not identified the presence of PrDs within the phages of other bacteria, such as *Borrelia spp., Treponema spp., Chlamydophila spp.* and others, like *E. coli*, found in the cerebrospinal fluid and brains of Alzheimer's patients.[45] However, both bacteriophages and the brain microbiome are poorly explored, with a high number of currently unknown species. Therefore, these results could be revisited with the possibility of identifying additional PrDs in other currently unknown bacterial phages found in the brains of patients with neurodegenerative diseases.

NEURODEGENERATION AND PHAGE-INDUCED MICROBIOTA DISEASE

Neurodegenerative pathologies, and Alzheimer's, in particular, are known to be associated with alterations in gut microbiota that influence central nervous system function through the gut-brain axis. Previous studies have identified the number of gut bacteria that were differentially abundant between Alzheimer's and control patients. These studies showed that certain families—*Bifidobacteriaceae, Clostridiaceae, Erysipelotrichaceae, Mogibacteriaceae, Ruminococcaceae, Turicibacteraceae, Peptostreptococcaceae, Rikenellaceae*, the *Bifidobacterium* and *Adlercreutzia* genera, *SMB53, Dialister, Clostridium*, and *Turicibacter*—were all less abundant in Alzheimer's. Conversely, other kinds of bacteria were more abundant in Alzheimer's gut samples compared to controls, including *Alistipes, Bacteroides, Blautia, Phascolarctobacterium, Gemella,* and pro-inflammatory *E. coli* and *Shigella* spp.[20,60]

However, further analysis revealed that only some of these bacteria were correlated with Alzheimer's severity. The increased abundance of *Bacteroides* and *Blautia*, along with a greater amyloid burden in the brain, were positively correlated with disease severity. Conversely, a negative correlation was revealed for bacteria that were less abundant in Alzheimer's, such as *Turicibacter*, *SMB53*, and *Dialister*, and a more difficult Alzheimer's pathology. One thing that particularly attracted our attention was the decrease of the *Bifidobacterium* genus, whose actions are associated with an altered immune response, chronic inflammation, and impaired intestinal permeability.[61]

We agree with the findings of Vogt et al. (2017), which pointed out that increased *Bacteroides* and decreased *Bifidobacterium* levels in Alzheimer's patients may be suggested as a microbiota phenotype associated with chronic inflammation and increased intestinal permeability. Although identified differences in the gut microbiome are notable, the reason for these alterations in Alzheimer's patients, and whether they preceded disease development and glial activation or appeared after AD onset, is unclear. In any case, a better understanding of the cause of certain alterations in the microbiome is central to understanding the resulting changes. Because there was no association between microbiota alteration and antibiotics exposure, bacteriophages are the most likely reason for these alterations as the critical regulators of microbiota stability.[20]

As stated above, phages can cause bacterial population lysis, leading to the development of diseases associated with microbiota phenotype, which is in turn implicated as a triggering or worsening factor for certain pathologies.[31,62] Our previous studies implicated this mechanism of phage-induced microbiota in Parkinson's, which may share common features with Alzheimer's.[32,62] By studying the microbiota of Parkinson's patients, we found a significantly decreased abundance of neurotransmitter-producing *Lactococcus* bacteria due to lytic Lactococcus phages. This association was particularly notable as *Lactococcus* spp. are known to produce intestinal dopamine, the decrease of which is linked to the development of increased intestinal permeability and development of Parkinson's gastrointestinal symptoms and α-synuclein misfolding.[32,63,64]

We have also identified a commonality for microbiota diseases due to phage infection, the impaired intestinal permeability that is a hallmark for patients with neurodegeneration and can precede the disease.[31,62,65] In our experiments, phage-induced microbiotal shifts led to increased intestinal permeability and chronic inflammation, increasing pro-inflammatory cytokine levels.[62] Moreover, bacteriophage-induced gut barrier impairment can lead to the increased circulation of phages in serum and cerebrospinal fluid, allowing increased interaction with human cells and proteins that under normal conditions would not be exposed to phages.

BACTERIOPHAGES AND PATHOGEN-ASSOCIATED MOLECULAR PATTERN (PAMPs)

PAMPs are molecules or components of microorganisms that are released from disrupted bacteria, fungi, or viruses that are recognized by the immune system and can trigger inflammation. Different PAMPs—like LPS, components of bacterial cell walls, DNA, and RNA—are known to be implicated in neuroinflammation following the activation of different Toll-like receptors (TLRs). These TLRs include those located in the cell surface (e.g., TLR4, TLR2, and others), or those like TLR9, which are located intracellularly. Upon stimulation, TLRs induce the expression of inflammatory cytokines via both MyD88-dependent and MyD88-independent signaling pathways.[66,67] Other receptors that also recognize certain PAMPs and are associated with neuroinflammation are IL-1R, NOD-like receptors, and scavenger receptor RAGE.[68]

Scientists have extensively studied the role of PAMPs in neuroinflammation. We know that different neurodegenerative diseases are more common in patients with chronic systemic infections, resulting in continuous PAMP exposure.[69] Moreover, the rate of cognitive decline among these patients is more pronounced in those with higher systemic inflammation rates and increased blood plasma TNF levels.[70] Different factors can lead to PAMP release, and both lytic and lysogenic bacteriophages are contributors. By causing the death of large bacterial populations in the human gut, phages can contribute to a particularly significant release of PAMPs, which can subsequently trigger the pro-inflammatory cytokine cascade and cause neuroinflammation associated with Alzheimer's and Parkinson's.[71]

Our recent analyses have identified the role of phages in triggering another multifaceted disease, type 1 diabetes, through the phage-induced lysis of E. coli populations and the release of highly immunogenic amyloid-DNA composites, which act as PAMPs.[72] We used an algorithm to analyze public longitudinal microbiome data, paying close attention to gut amyloid-producing bacterial composition, and found a positive correlation between the total disappearance of E. coli and autoantibody appearance. All of the children who developed autoimmunity showed the total disappearance, or an episode of disappearance, of E. coli before the detection of autoantibodies. This trend was not noted in controls. Another notable observation was the significantly higher initial abundance of E. coli in type 1 diabetes and seroconverter children than in the control group. We analyzed the E. coli phage/E. coli bacterial cell ratio and showed that this ratio increased in subjects prior to the decrease in E. coli abundance, indicating that productive phage infection was the cause of E. coli depletion.

We next developed an in vitro model and determined that phage-induced alteration of E. coli abundance lead to PAMP release from E. coli biofilms. Using an amyloid-diagnostic dye, we noted the release of highly immunogenic amyloids (curli-DNA composites) from E. coli biofilms upon E. coli prophage induction. Combining these results with existing data on the immunogenic role of enterobacterial amyloids, these findings suggest that phages indirectly contribute to the release of biofilm PAMPs that could trigger β-cell autoimmunity in type 1 diabetes susceptible hosts.

Based on these findings, we propose that similar processes might occur in patients with neurodegeneration characterized by an altered gut microbiome. Furthermore, if these alterations were induced by phage-induced lysis, they might be accompanied by PAMP release, leading to the entry of released bacterial PAMPs into the bloodstream and cerebrospinal fluid, as patients with Parkinson's, Alzheimer's, and ALS are also characterized by an impaired gut barrier which causes chronic systemic and neuroinflammation. Given that increased gut permeability facilitates PAMP translocation in circulation, under certain conditions particular bacteriophages might have a dual role in these pathologies, inducing gut leakiness and causing bacterial lysis, leading to elevated PAMP levels in biological fluids.[73]

As we previously described, the majority of microorganisms carry prophage DNA in their genomes that, under certain conditions, can lead to productive phage infections and bacterial death; it is particularly important to note the possible interaction between *E. coli*, *E. coli* phages, and Alzheimer's. *E. coli* is known to harbor multiple temperate prophage genomes and is identified as a hallmark microorganism in the brain of Alzheimer's patients.[45] Therefore, it is highly likely that the E. coli present in Alzheimer's brains and cerebrospinal fluid would also carry prophages; death by prophage activation would result in PAMP release, including *E. coli* DNA to the cerebrospinal fluid, thereby triggering neuroinflammation.[66] *E. coli* DNA is known to be implicated in the formation of bacterial prions in biofilms and is associated with transkingdom triggering of misfolded protein deposition in the mammalian brain when susceptible animals are colonized with amyloid-producing *E. coli*.[57]

Further supporting the role of PAMP and phage release as a cause for neurodegeneration are the data from our latest experiment. We have recently shown that microbial DNA, including DNA released as a result of phage infection, can interact with human proteins and directly lead to Tau protein misfolding. This opens the discussion of new mechanisms for bacterial DNA as an Alzheimer's triggering factor, and also for phage release (unpublished data). We have shown that this direct release of PAMPs to the cerebrospinal fluid can not only lead to neuroinflammation, but can also result in protein misfolding due to bacterial DNA release. This supports our previous studies showing that DNase I enzyme, capable of cleaving bacterial cfDNA, can provide significant benefit to patients with late-stage Alzheimer's.[74]

CONCLUSIONS

In this chapter, we have reviewed the possible role of bacteriophages in the development of neurodegenerative diseases, focusing on the mechanisms by which these previously overlooked human pathogens could be associated with these pathologies. We were the first group to identify multiple, consistent pathways implicating bacteriophages in the triggering and progression of neurodegeneration in general, and Alzheimer's, Parkinson's and ALS in particular. We suggest that bacterial viruses have various direct and indirect methods of association with neurodegenerative pathologies by affecting eukaryotic cells and proteins, leading to protein misfolding, microbiota alterations, and the triggering of neuroinflammation.

Moreover, by understanding that microbiota play a primary role in neurodegeneration, it is possible to speculate that Alzheimer's, Parkinson's, or ALS could be contagious pathologies. Because phages can spread between humans under certain conditions, people with genetic susceptibility and those with microbiota-determined susceptibility to certain bacteriophages could develop these diseases by contracting phages from an external source. One of the reasons phages are not more frequently found in human stool samples is that the most economical and widely used 16s RNA sequencing method does not allow for the identification of bacterial viruses. Therefore, novel metagenomic approaches could be more helpful in exploring the phagobiome, but are not yet widely used due to their cost. Another problem is the absence of "normal" criteria for the microbiota. Mammalian microbiota is highly individualized and does not allow for the accurate analysis of clinical data. Finally, to resolve the primary difficulty in determining correlation versus causation of microbiota implicated in neurodegeneration, longitudinal microbiome considering phages as a primary factor for microbiota alteration studies should begin prior to disease onset. However, because neurodegeneration is a slowly developing process, this type of investigation will very time-consuming.[75] Based on these recent analyses and in vitro studies, we want to open a wider discussion around the role of bacteriophages as previously overlooked pathogenic factors in neurodegenerative pathologies, considering different pathways through which they could contribute to pathogenesis and progression.

ACKNOWLEDGMENTS

We would like to thank Stuart M. Brown and Yuhan Hao from the New York School of Medicine for the help with bioinformatics research.

REFERENCES

1. Angelucci, F., et al., Alzheimer's disease (AD) and Mild Cognitive Impairment (MCI) patients are characterized by increased BDNF serum levels. *Curr Alzheimer Res*, 2010. **7**(1): p. 15–20.
2. Goedert, M., F. Clavaguera, and M. Tolnay, The propagation of prion-like protein inclusions in neurodegenerative diseases. *Trends Neurosci*, 2010. **33**(7): p. 317–325.
3. Ballatore, C., V.M. Lee, and J.Q. Trojanowski, Tau-mediated neurodegeneration in Alzheimer's disease and related disorders. *Nat Rev Neurosci*, 2007. **8**(9): p. 663.
4. Shoghi-Jadid, K., et al., Localization of neurofibrillary tangles and beta-amyloid plaques in the brains of living patients with Alzheimer disease. *Am J Geriat Psychiat*, 2002. **10**(1): p. 24–35.
5. Conway, K., et al., Acceleration of oligomerization, not fibrillization, is a shared property of both α-synuclein mutations linked to early-onset Parkinson's disease: Implications for pathogenesis and therapy. *PNAS*, 2000. **97**(2): p. 571–576.
6. Pearson, H.A., and C. Peers, Physiological roles for amyloid β peptides. *J Physiol*, 2006. **575**(1): p. 5–10.
7. Bendor, J.T., T.P. Logan, and R.H. Edwards, The function of α-synuclein. *Neuron*, 2013. **79**(6): p. 1044–1066.
8. Bloom, G.S., Amyloid-β and tau: The trigger and bullet in Alzheimer disease pathogenesis. *JAMA Neurol*, 2014. **71**(4): p. 505–508.
9. Kaur, S.J., S.R. McKeown, and S. Rashid, Mutant SOD1 mediated pathogenesis of amyotrophic lateral sclerosis. *Gene*, 2016. **577**(2): p. 109–118.
10. Verstraeten, A., et al., Progress in unraveling the genetic etiology of Parkinson disease in a genomic era. *Trends Genet*, 2015. **31**(3): p. 140–149.
11. Karch, C.M., and A.M. Goate, Alzheimer's disease risk genes and mechanisms of disease pathogenesis. *Biol Psychiatry*, 2015. **77**(1): p. 43–51.
12. Quigley, E.M., Microbiota-brain-gut axis and neurodegenerative diseases. *Curr Neurol Neurosci Rep*, 2017. **17**(12): p. 94.
13. Collado, M.C., et al., Human gut colonisation may be initiated *in utero* by distinct microbial communities in the placenta and amniotic fluid. *Sci Rep*, 2016. **6**: p. 23129.
14. Erb-Downward, J.R., et al., Analysis of the lung microbiome in the "healthy" smoker and in COPD. *PLOS ONE*, 2011. **6**(2): p. e16384.
15. Grice, E.A., and J.A. Segre, The skin microbiome. *Nat Rev Microbiol*, 2011. **9**(4): p. 244.

16. Emery, D.C., et al., 16S rRNA next generation sequencing analysis shows bacteria in Alzheimer's post-mortem brain. *Front Aging Neurosci*, 2017. **9**: p. 195.
17. Bhattacharjee, S., and W.J. Lukiw, Alzheimer's disease and the microbiome. *Front Cell Neurosci*, 2013. **7**: p. 153.
18. Ghaisas, S., J. Maher, and A. Kanthasamy, Gut microbiome in health and disease: Linking the microbiome–gut–brain axis and environmental factors in the pathogenesis of systemic and neurodegenerative diseases. *Pharmacol Therap*, 2016. **158**: p. 52–62.
19. Pistollato, F., et al., Role of gut microbiota and nutrients in amyloid formation and pathogenesis of Alzheimer disease. *Nutr Rev*, 2016. **74**(10): p. 624–634.
20. Vogt, N.M., et al., Gut microbiome alterations in Alzheimer's disease. *Sci Rep*, 2017. **7**(1): p. 13537.
21. Fung, T.C., C.A. Olson, and E.Y. Hsiao, Interactions between the microbiota, immune and nervous systems in health and disease. *Nat Neurosci*, 2017. **20**(2): p. 145.
22. Cryan, J.F., and T.G. Dinan, Mind-altering microorganisms: The impact of the gut microbiota on brain and behaviour. *Nat Rev Neurosci*, 2012. **13**(10): p. 701.
23. Cattaneo, A., et al., Association of brain amyloidosis with pro-inflammatory gut bacterial taxa and peripheral inflammation markers in cognitively impaired elderly. *Neurobiol Aging*, 2017. **49**: p. 60–68.
24. Rhee, S., C. Pothoulakis, and E.A. Mayer, Principles and clinical implications of the brain–gut–enteric microbiota axis. *Nat Rev Gastroenterol Hepatol*, 2009. **6**: p. 306–314.
25. Suttle, C.A., Viruses in the sea. *Nature*, 2005. **437**(7057): p. 356.
26. Clokie, M.R., et al., Phages in nature. *Bacteriophage*, 2011. **1**(1): p. 31–45.
27. Hobbs, Z., and S.T. Abedon, Diversity of phage infection types and associated terminology: The problem with 'lytic or lysogenic'. *FEMS Microbiol Lett*, 2016. **363**: p. 1–8.
28. Payet, J.P., and C.A. Suttle, To kill or not to kill: The balance between lytic and lysogenic viral infection is driven by trophic status. *Limnol Oceanogr*, 2013. **58**(2): p. 465–474.
29. Tetz, G., and V. Tetz, Bacteriophages as new human viral pathogens. *Microorganisms*, 2018. **6**(2): p. 54.
30. Tetz, G., and V. Tetz, Tetz's theory and law of longevity. *Theory Biosci*, 2018. **137**(2): p. 145–154.
31. Tetz, G., and V. Tetz, Bacteriophage infections of microbiota can lead to leaky gut in an experimental rodent model. *Gut Pathog*, 2016. **8**(1): p. 33.
32. Tetz, G., et al., Parkinsons disease and bacteriophages as its overlooked contributors. *Sci Rep*, 2018. **8**(1): p. 10812.
33. Nguyen, S., et al., Bacteriophage transcytosis provides a mechanism to cross epithelial cell layers. *MBio*, 2017. **8**(6): p. e01874-17.
34. Lehti, T.A., et al., Internalization of a polysialic acid-binding *Escherichia coli* bacteriophage into eukaryotic neuroblastoma cells. *Nat Commun*, 2017. **8**(1): p. 1915.
35. Górski, A., et al., Bacteriophage translocation. *FEMS Immunol Med Microbiol*, 2006. **46**(3): p. 313–319.
36. Handley, S.A., et al., Pathogenic simian immunodeficiency virus infection is associated with expansion of the enteric virome. *Cell*. 2012. **151**(2): p. 253–266.
37. Górski, A., et al., Phage therapy: Combating infections with potential for evolving from merely a treatment for complications to targeting diseases. *Front Microbiol*, 2016. **7**: p. 1515.
38. Łusiak-Szelachowska, M., et al., Bacteriophages in the gastrointestinal tract and their implications. *Gut Pathog*, 2017. **9**(1): p. 44.
39. Barr, J.J., A bacteriophages journey through the human body. *Immunol Rev*, 2017. **279**(1): p. 106–122.

40. Srivastava, A.S., D.P. Chauhan, and E. Carrier, *In utero* detection of T7 phage after systemic administration to pregnant mice. *Biotechniques*, 2004. **37**(1): p. 81–83.

41. Pou, C., et al., Virome definition in cerebrospinal fluid of patients with neurological complications after hematopoietic stem cell transplantation. *J Clin Virol*, 2018. **108**: p. 112–120.

42. Minagar, A., and J.S. Alexander, Blood-brain barrier disruption in multiple sclerosis. *Mult Scler J*, 2003. **9**(6): p. 540–549.

43. Garrido-Cardenas, J.A., and F. Manzano-Agugliaro, The metagenomics worldwide research. *Curr Genet*, 2017. **63**(5): p. 819–829.

44. Pisa, D., et al., Polymicrobial infections in brain tissue from Alzheimer's disease patients. *Sci Rep*, 2017. **7**(1): p. 5559.

45. Mawanda, F., and R. Wallace, Can infections cause Alzheimer's disease? *Epidemiol Rev*, 2013. **35**(1): p. 161–180.

46. Fasano, A., Leaky gut and autoimmune diseases. *Clin Rev Allergy Immunol*, 2012. **42**(1): p. 71–78.

47. Dąbrowska, K., et al., Immunogenicity studies of proteins forming the T4 phage head surface. *J Vir*, 2014. **88**: p. 12551–12557.

48. Freedman, J.E., CD240-CD40L and platelet function: beyond hemostasis. *Circ Res*, 2003. **92**(9): p. 944–946.

49. Górski, A., et al., Perspectives of phage–eukaryotic cell interactions to control Epstein–Barr virus infections. *Front Microbiol*, 2018. **9**: p. 630.

50. Zhao, Y., et al., Regulation of TREM2 expression by an NF-κB-sensitive miRNA-34a. *Neuroreport*, 2013. **24**(6): p. 318.

51. Jones, S.V., and I. Kounatidis, Nuclear factor-kappa B and Alzheimer disease, unifying genetic and environmental risk factors from cell to humans. *Front Immunol*, 2017. **8**: p. 1805.

52. Prusiner, S.B., Biology and genetics of prions causing neurodegeneration. *Annu Rev Genet*, 2013. **47**: p. 601–623.

53. Guo, J.L., and V.M. Lee, Cell-to-cell transmission of pathogenic proteins in neurodegenerative diseases. *Nat Med*, 2014. **20**(2): p. 130.

54. Nakamura, T., and S.A. Lipton, Cell death: Protein misfolding and neurodegenerative diseases. *Apoptosis*, 2009. **14**(4): p. 455–468.

55. Rosen, Rebecca F., et al., Exogenous seeding of cerebral β-amyloid deposition in βAPP-transgenic rats. *J Neurochem*, 2012. **120**(5): p. 660–666.

56. Soto, C., et al., Transmission of Alzheimer's disease by seeding and cross-seeding. *Alzheimer's Dement*, 2009. **5**(4): p. 115.

57. Chen, S.G., et al., Exposure to the functional bacterial amyloid protein curli enhances alpha-synuclein aggregation in aged Fischer 344 rats and *Caenorhabditis elegans*. *Sci Rep*, 2016. **6**: p. 34477.

58. Tetz, G., and V. Tetz, Prion-like domains in phagobiota. *Front Microbiol*, 2017. **8**: p. 2239.

59. An, L., D. Fitzpatrick, and P.M. Harrison, Emergence and evolution of yeast prion and prion-like proteins. *BMC Evol Biol*, 2016. **16**(1): p. 24.

60. Marizzoni, M., et al., Microbiota and neurodegenerative diseases. *Curr Opin Neurol*, 2017. **30**(6): p. 630–638.

61. Tlaskalová-Hogenová, H., et al., The role of gut microbiota (commensal bacteria) and the mucosal barrier in the pathogenesis of inflammatory and autoimmune diseases and cancer: Contribution of germ-free and gnotobiotic animal models of human diseases. *Cell Mol Immunol*, 2011. **8**(2): p. 110.

62. Tetz, G.V., et al., Bacteriophages as potential new mammalian pathogens. *Sci Rep*, 2017. **7**(1): p. 7043.

63. Asano, Y., et al., Critical role of gut microbiota in the production of biologically active, free catecholamines in the gut lumen of mice. *Am J Physiol Gastrointest Liver Physiol*, 2012. **303**(11): p. G1288–G1295.

64. Braak, H., et al., Idiopathic Parkinson's disease: Possible routes by which vulnerable neuronal types may be subject to neuroinvasion by an unknown pathogen. *J Neural Transm*, 2003. **110**(5): p. 517–536.

65. Bischoff, S.C., et al., Intestinal permeability–a new target for disease prevention and therapy. *BMC Gastroenterol*, 2014. **14**(1): p. 189.

66. West, A.P., A.A. Koblansky, and S. Ghosh, Recognition and signaling by toll-like receptors. *Annu Rev Cell Dev Biol*, 2006. **22**: p. 409–437.

67. Zhang, B., et al., TLR4 signaling mediates inflammation and tissue injury in nephrotoxicity. *J Am Soc Nephrol*, 2008. **19**(5): p. 923–932.

68. Salminen, A., et al., Inflammation in Alzheimer's disease: Amyloid-β oligomers trigger innate immunity defence *via* pattern recognition receptors. *Prog Neurobiol*, 2009. **87**(3): p. 181–194.

69. Perry, V.H., C. Cunningham, and C. Holmes, Systemic infections and inflammation affect chronic neurodegeneration. *Nat Rev Immunol*, 2007. **7**(2): p. 161.

70. Clark, I.A., and B. Vissel, Amyloid β: One of three danger-associated molecules that are secondary inducers of the proinflammatory cytokines that mediate Alzheimer's disease. *Br J Pharmacol*, 2015. **172**(15): p. 3714–3727.

71. Chen, W.W., X. Zhang, and W.J. Huang, Role of neuroinflammation in neurodegenerative diseases (Review). *Mol Med Rep*, 2016. **13**(4): p. 3391–3396.

72. Tetz, G., et al., Type 1 diabetes: An association between autoimmunity the dynamics of gut amyloid-producing *E. coli* and their phages. *bioRxiv*, 2018. **1**: p. 433110.

73. Wang, L., et al., Methods to determine intestinal permeability and bacterial translocation during liver disease. *J Immunol Methods*, 2015. **421**: p. 44–53.

74. Tetz, V., and G. Tetz, Effect of deoxyribonuclease I treatment for dementia in end-stage Alzheimer's disease: A case report. *J Med Case Rep*, 2016. **10**(1): p. 131.

75. Chatterjee, A., and B.A. Duerkop, Beyond bacteria: Bacteriophage-eukaryotic host interactions reveal emerging paradigms of health and disease. *Front Microbiol*, 2018. **9**: p. 1–8.

11 The Role of Fecal Microbiota Transplantation in Neurological Diseases

Thomas Borody and John Bienenstock

CONTENTS

INTRODUCTION

The last 20 years have generated unprecedented interest in the field of microbiology, due in large part to advancements in molecular biological approaches. One result of this growing interest in microbiology is the realization that we can no longer study the functioning of individual components and pathways in animals and plants without also examining them in the context of their associated microbiota. The complex community of host and total microbial content, known as an individual's microbiome, has been referred to as the "holobiont."[1] Therefore, when studying metabolic, endocrine, immune, and nervous system pathways, we must now consider the involvement of the microbiota and their largest domain, the gut. Interest in this type of research has increased exponentially in recent years, particularly in relation to the role of gut microbiota in the etiology and modulation of many human physiological functions and disease processes. However, most of the biological research to date in this area has been performed in animal models, with relatively little translation to clinical practice.

The bacterial communities that comprise the gut microbiome represent a continuum that increases both in number and complexity as you move through the gastrointestinal (GI) tract. The largest and most diverse microbial population is found in the colon, so most of the extant research has focused on the fecal microbiota. However, it is important to remember that the composition of gut microbiota, while predominantly bacterial, also contains vast amounts of viruses (predominantly bacteriophages [virome]), fungi (mycobiome), and also archaea. Therefore, feces and fecal extracts contain diverse microbial categories and a varying amount of bacterial products and components, including products of fermentation and digestion.

The microbiome–gut–brain axis (MGBA) is an umbrella term that has been loosely used to describe the effects and interactions of microbes in modulating the function of the enteric and peripheral nervous system, including the brain.[2,3,4,5,6,7] We offer the following as a concise introduction to the field and its numerous complexities.

ENTERIC VIROME

We are only beginning to characterize the gut virome, defined as the total population of viruses and their associated genetic material in the gut microbiome.[8] The majority of viruses are bacteriophages, or virus-infecting bacteria, which are intimately involved in the maintenance of host community stability. Although the importance of phages in the ecology of the gut is well established, we are only beginning to understand their role in the modulation of the MGBA.[9] Furthermore, the notion that enteric viruses may offer therapeutic benefits has only recently been explored. In recent models of experimental colitis, a murine norovirus demonstrated the ability to replace the beneficial function of commensal bacteria, including restoration of intestinal morphology and lymphocyte function.[10,11]

GUT MYCOBIOME

The gut mycobiome, which encompasses all fungal strains within the gut, is an often-neglected component of the gut microbiome as it has been poorly studied and characterized. The mycobiome plays a significant role, similar to that of the gut microbiota, in maintaining a balanced enteric microbial ecosystem,[12,13] and has consequently been implicated in a number of gut-associated neurological and psychiatric diseases.[14] It is also increasingly being acknowledged that some individual species of fungi may have beneficial therapeutic effects. For example, *Saccharomyces boulardii* is well established as a potential probiotic.[15,16] Increased production of immunoglobulin A has been observed in mice fed *S. boulardii* following exposure to *C. difficile* toxin.[17] Furthermore, supernatants from *S. boulardii* cultures have been shown to inhibit the activation of T and dendritic cells in patients with inflammatory bowel disease (IBD).[18] It is possible that fungal strains could extensively modulate the immune system in a variety of ways, including interaction with C-type lectin receptors such as Dectin-1.[19] Overgrowth of enteric fungi may occur as a result of antibiotic therapy, and diets high in carbohydrates also influence fungal abundance and diversity.[20] Changes in mycobiome have also been associated with the development of human metabolic diseases including obesity and diabetes[21,22] psychiatric conditions[23] and eating disorders[24]. Whether these described changes are involved in, or simply associated with, the modulation of these conditions is unclear at present.

ARCHAEA

The human gut archaea have been poorly studied and characterized in both healthy and diseased individuals. Unfortunately, our understanding of their potential role in influencing the MGBA is therefore limited. However, studies have shown that their abundance and distribution is distinctly affected by diet.[25,26] Although evidence detailing the role of archaea in the MGBA is limited, it is undeniable that the human gastrointestinal tract contains a highly diverse population of archaea, specifically methanobacteriaceae,[27] which exist as commensal and mutualistic organisms. These archaea synthesize methane in the gut, which is a gasotransmitter and has been shown to possess stimulatory effects on the enteric nervous system and ileal motor contractions.[28]

GUT BACTERIA

Numerous large-scale research projects, including the Metagenomics of the Human Intestinal Tract (MetaHIT), have extensively characterized the composition of the gut bacterial microbiome.[29,30,31] As is often stated, the total estimated mass of bacteria in the human body is 1–2 kg, constituted of more than 1,500 genera and 40,000 species that collectively possess 10–100 times more genes than the human genome. The ecological state of the microbiome changes in response to age, diet and nutrition, health status, host genome, illness and disease, and medication and supplementation. The realization that gut microbiota has a constant effect on the maturation and development of many host cells has led to this flora being described as the "forgotten organ."[32] Exploration of the potential role and influence of these bacteria on the peripheral and central nervous systems has led to the general concept of the MGBA. The MGBA has now been shown to play an active role in the process of speciation in drosophila (mating preference),[33] behavior in zebrafish[34] and the aggregation phenomenon (swarming in locusts).[35]

The animal models used to explore the MGBA frequently employ the use of gnotobiotic (germ-free) animals, specifically mice. It has become clear that, at least in rodents, the timing of bacterial colonization is of crucial importance in determining whether or not the effects of bacterial communities have long-term effects.[36,37] Presumably, this is the result of bacteria–host interactions occurring at a susceptible developmental age. Gut bacteria are involved in the maturation and functional development of the enteric neurons and enteric as well as brain microglia. The number and 5-HT content of enterochromaffin cells are influenced to a large degree by the gut microbiota,[38] as is synaptogenesis, hippocampal neurogenesis, and brain-derived neurotrophic factor (BDNF).[39,40,41] Similarly, after treatment with commensal bacteria, previously exaggerated HPA axis stress responses in germ-free animals are returned to normal,[42] as is over-myelination in the pre-frontal cortex[43] and blood–brain barrier integrity.[44] These examples illuminate the importance of timing the exposure to bacteria during fetal, and even postnatal, development since colonization with individual bacteria after a certain time point, like weaning, do not normalize the targeted function. However, the host microbiota has been shown to constantly influence the maturation function of microglia in the brain, suggesting that other brain functions may continue to be capable of bacterial modulation during adulthood.[45] Therefore, the presence of indigenous gut bacteria is sufficient and necessary for the normal development and functioning of numerous pathways and structures of the central and peripheral nervous systems.

Another approach to investigating the MGBA is the use of antibiotics. This type of exploration is often performed using high doses of largely non-absorbed antibiotics supplemented with soluble antibiotics like penicillin.[46] Although these experiments have resulted in significant behavioral alterations, specific and reproducible metagenomic analyses to identify which microbiota are involved have achieved only limited success. Recently, use of a low-dose single soluble antibiotic (penicillin) in early life has been shown to render the host, in the presence of a high-fat diet, susceptible to obesity.[47] It was also shown to produce long-term behavioral deficits, as well as inflammatory changes in the brain.[48]

How Do Bacteria Influence Human Behavior?

There are multiple pathways through which bacteria may induce behavioral changes, such as those described above. They synthesize many molecules, which individually and collectively may promote behavioral effects in the host. Several neuroactive peptides, including many of the known neurotransmitters (e.g., gamma-aminobutyric acid [GABA], serotonin, catecholamines, and acetylcholine) are produced by bacteria within the human gut.[49,50] Even the gaseous neurotransmitters—carbon monoxide (CO), nitric oxide (NO), and hydrogen sulfide (H2S)—which are involved in neuronal communication in all tissues of the body, including the brain, and have profound immunological and neuroactive effects are synthesized by bacteria in considerable amounts in the gut lumen.[51,52] The field of study concerned with examining the ability of bacteria to influence behavior via neurochemical signaling with the host nervous system has been termed *Microbial Endocrinology*.[53]

One of the primary functions of gut bacteria is the digestion of food and the fermentation of otherwise indigestible glycans and fibers, primarily in the colon. This digestion results in the production of long and short-chain fatty acids (SCFA), the latter of which have been associated with modulations in brain function and behavior via several mechanisms in both normal, healthy animals and those in diseased states. For example, SCFAs, like butyrate, are involved in the maintenance and survival of the colonic epithelium. They have been shown to directly influence the immunoregulatory functioning of the immune system,[54] and also act as a potent antidepressant.[55] It has also been suggested that SCFAs—in particular, propionic acid—may deleteriously affect behavior in autistic models[56] and in Parkinson's disease.[57]

Individual components of bacteria are also capable of inducing significant host effects. These include exopolysaccharides such as polysaccharide adhesion (PSA), a structural membrane component of the Gram-negative pathobiont, *Bacteroides fragilis*. Oral administration of PSA has been shown to reproduce the significant immunoregulatory activity of the parent bacteria[58] and also activate the enteric nervous system.[59] The exopolysaccharides of *Bifidobacterium longum*[60] and *Bifidobacterium breve* UCC2003[61] both have significant immune down-regulatory functions, which may depend on Toll receptor (TLR) and C-type lectin receptors on host cells. *Lactobacillus rhamnosus* JB-1 similarly modulates the gut immune system through host TLR and C-type lectin receptors.[62] However, the extent to which exopolysaccharides are directly involved in the regulation of the MGBA is currently unknown.

MICROVESICLES

All bacteria, fungi, and archaea shed microvesicles (MV), a type of extracellular vesicle between 100 and 150 nm nanometers in diameter, on a continual basis.[63,64,65,66] These microvesicles carry varying cargos comprising membrane components, random DNA and RNA, and secreted products such as toxins. They are specifically called outer membrane vesicles (OMV) in gram-negative bacteria and membrane microvesicles (MV) in gram-positive bacteria. MV promote communication between bacteria and host and are responsible for horizontal gene transfer. OMV, on the other hand, have been successfully used as vaccines against infectious diseases and are capable of reproducing the beneficial immune effects of the parent bacteria. For example, *B. fragilis* organisms have been shown to release a capsular PSA, which induces regulatory T cells and mucosal tolerance and prevents experimental colitis, via OMVs.[67] We have similarly demonstrated that MV from *L. rhamnosus* JB-1 mimic immune and neuronal effects of JB-1 and are involved in the MGBA via activation of vagal afferent fibers in the gut.[68] OMV from the probiotic *E. coli* strain Nissle 1917 are taken up by columnar epithelial cells in the intestinal crypts and are therefore believed to be involved in major bacteria-host communication pathways.[69,70] Because they are nanoparticulate, any approach to fecal microbiota transplantation (FMT), however filtered, will unavoidably contain a broad bacterial microvesicular representation.

NEURONAL INTERACTION

The development of both the peripheral and central nervous system is influenced by the microbiome.[71,72,73] Most of the pathways listed above play some role in the maturation of the nervous system and the maintenance of its homeostasis. Gut bacteria may directly or indirectly influence these pathways. For example, one of the SCFAs, butyrate, is an extremely potent antidepressant agent,[74] and propionate, another SCFA, promotes stereotypic behavior in mice.[75] Bacteria–host interactions are bi-directional; by way of example, the enteric nervous system may in itself be responsible for the maintenance of a normal, balanced microbiome.[76] Recent exploration of bacteria–host interactions has shown significant effects on several different ion channels, including cannabinoid,[77] calcium-activated potassium channels (KCa 3.1),[78] and vanilloid receptors (TRVP1).[79] Furthermore, luminal commensal bacteria may influence gut motility through neuronal activation[80,81] and modulate vagal and spinal afferent signaling. The subdiaphragmatic section of the vagus nerve prevents bacterial afferent signaling to the brain and disrupts behavioral effects of the administration of commensal bacteria such as *L. rhamnosus* JB-1 and *B. longum*.[82,83] However, the role of the vagus nerve in transmitting bacterial signals to the brain thereby affecting behavior is not all encompassing. For example, the surgical removal of part of the vagus nerve, termed vagotomy, did not prevent the transfer, by FMT, of behavioral phenotypes from anxiolytic or anxiogenic mice to each other.[84]

Bacteria are also responsible for their own ecology through the production of factors, which render their environment conducive or noxious to other bacteria. They may provide molecules that act as specific energy substrates to certain bacteria, thereby regulating the gut microbiome. Alternatively, they also contain and promote the reproduction of phages, which may destroy certain bacteria or produce bacteriocins, which may target specific bacterial strains. An example of this is the production of the bacteriocin Abp118 by *Lactobacillus salivarius* UCC118, which specifically kills *Listeria monocytogenes* and protects mice from a fatal infection brought on by the organism.[85]

FECAL MICROBIOTA TRANSPLANTATION ISSUES

Experimental

Given the accumulating evidence that the gut microbiome can significantly influence the peripheral and central nervous systems, it is not surprising that investigators across disciplines have turned their attention to exploring the role of the gut microbiota in various models of neurological and psychiatric diseases. For example, evidence now exists for the role of intestinal dysbiosis in ischemic stroke[86] and spinal cord injury,[87] as both experimental conditions achieved beneficial outcomes following manipulation of the gut microbiome. The role of gut bacteria was also examined in two separate models of multiple sclerosis, each referred to as experimental allergic encephalomyelitis [EAE]. In the first study, treatment with *B. fragilis* or its exopolysaccharide, PSA, was found to protect against central nervous system demyelination and inflammation through Toll-like receptor 2.[88] In the second study, mice that developed a severe secondary form of EAE were found to harbor a dysbiotic gut microbiome compared with healthy control mice.[89] Further, reduced mortality and clinical disease severity were observed in mice treated with a cocktail of broad-spectrum antibiotics, supporting the reciprocal effects between experimental CNS inflammatory demyelination and modification of the microbiome. Recently, specific gut microbial metabolites have been identified which negatively or positively modulate astrocyte functioning in the brain.[90] Induction of inflammation in pregnancy with a viral mimic polyinosinic–polycytidilic acid (Poly[I:C]) produces offspring with immune and behavioral deficits that may mimic autism, which can be ameliorated by *B. fragilis*.[91,92] A wealth of literature now exists on the various potential roles and pathways involved in alleviating the effects of stress and abnormal behavior, which have been extensively reviewed elsewhere.[93]

Studies examining the effects of individual or communities of bacteria on different physiological systems have generally used germ-free mice to "normalize" the gut microbiome. In essence, this approach simplifies FMT from one mouse to another.

The seminal experiments of Bercik et al. showed that a behavioral phenotype is capable of being transferred in this model.[94] One extension of this experiment is the transfer of fecal material or bacteria derived from feces from patients with specific documented diseases into gnotobiotic mice.[95] These mice are loosely termed "humanized mice, in much the same way as immunodeficient mice engrafted with functional human cells and tissues. Recently, gut bacteria from patients with multiple sclerosis have been shown to exacerbate symptoms in the mouse model of multiple sclerosis, EAE.[96,97] This finding offers the opportunity to isolate the strain/s of bacteria which may be protective or potentially pathogenic in the human disease. Similar approaches have also been adopted using gut microbiota from patients with Parkinson's disease.[98] Oral administration of specific microbial metabolites to germ-free mice resulted in the transfer of motor deficits and overexpression of α-synuclein, a neuronal protein critical to the pathogenesis of Parkinson's. The link was further supported by the observation that antibiotic treatment of the humanized Parkinson's mice subsequently abolished Parkinson's-related motor symptoms.

Another recent study also reported the approach of humanized germ-free mice colonized with the fecal microbiota from individuals with disease, this time from patients with diarrhea-predominant irritable bowel syndrome (IBS) and co-morbid anxiety.[99] Mice inoculated with the fecal flora from patients with diarrhea-predominant IBS were found to exhibit faster gastrointestinal transit time, intestinal barrier dysfunction, innate immune activation, and anxiety-like behavior compared with healthy controls. These findings add to a growing body of credible evidence in the literature supporting the hypothesis that, to at least some extent, many neurodegenerative disorders are causally related to dysbiosis of the gut.

CLINICAL USE OF FECAL MICROBIOTA TRANSPLANTATION IN NEUROLOGICAL DISORDERS

The Gut

The gastrointestinal microbiome comprises the largest collection of organisms in the human body. It is well-positioned to influence the environment both locally and systemically via locally manufactured molecules, such as fermentation products, and secreted neuroactive molecules like neurotransmitters. In addition, the microbiome can directly influence its host by promoting the synthesis and secretion of potentially beneficial molecules and is capable of producing circulating molecules able to interact with neural tissues. Given the fact that the gastrointestinal microbiome is made up of living organisms and their byproducts and is housed within the human body, we will consider it an "organ" for the purposes of this chapter. Furthermore, in this clinical section the context of the "brain" includes all of its extensions (i.e., the spinal cord and distal nerves) so as to encompass all of the conditions that affect any part of the "extended brain," including neuropathy, pruritus, hyperesthesia, and other conditions.

In recent years, scientific research, clinical observations, animal studies, and commercial interest in the gut microbiome has increased exponentially. Use of FMT greatly increased in response to the emergence of the *Clostridium difficile* infection (CDI) epidemic in the early 2000s and the high mortality rate associated with the infection. Today, nearly 500,000 new *C. difficile* infections occur each year in the United States alone, with approximately 30,000 deaths annually.[100] The increased use of FMT for CDI has resulted in many observations of serendipitous improvements in other co-morbidities. In Australia, where there are fewer restrictions on FMT use compared to the United States, various microbiome-related, non-CDI, conditions have been successfully treated with FMT.[101,102,103] We acknowledge that most of the evidence presented in this chapter, which focus on the brain–FMT topic, is the result of small case studies and occasional prospective data and not from robust, randomized controlled trials (RCT). Consequently, this data should only be considered preliminary, although we hope that these positive findings will encourage funding for planned trials and reporting of results in the immediate future. It is possible that the FMT successes reported to date reflect only a small subset of conditions for which FMT (in its various forms) could be effective, due to our current inability to identify potentially FMT-responsive phenotypes.

FMT has been offered at the Centre for Digestive Diseases for approximately 30 years as a viable treatment option for patients presenting with complicated gastrointestinal conditions. The process, which includes donor selection, fecal material preparation, and route of administration, has continued to evolve over the years as we continue to collect and collate observations. The current FMT protocol adheres to the recommendations put forward by Bakken et al. (2011)[104] and more recently updated by Finch Therapeutics.[105] Under the protocol, fecal matter is collected from an established bank of donors and undergoes regular testing and screening for communicable diseases. Stringent stool testing is conducted to exclude current infections from clostridial species, protozoal organisms, and parasites, and serologic tests are conducted to rule out any communicable diseases (e.g., human immunodeficiency virus [HIV], Hepatitis A, B, and C). Furthermore, FMT donors must follow strict guidelines regarding the intake of concomitant medication and alcohol. Finally, the established route of delivery used at our center involves a combination of colonoscopic administration directly to the target site, which is supplemented with fecal enemas. Although these steps are customary at our center, FMT procedures and guidelines are not yet standardized worldwide.

Discussed below are some preliminary summaries of the efficacy of FMT in treating neurologic disorders in a clinical setting.

Effects of Fecal Microbiota Transplantation on Hepatic Encephalopathy

The brain may be influenced by molecules formed by bacteria residing in the gut. These molecules are capable of traveling from the gastrointestinal microbiome into the bloodstream through portal vein blood or possibly via neuronal streaming through the vagus nerve. Certain molecules are able to pass through the liver using the "first pass" mechanism, which clears blood in the portal vein of most of the toxic molecules it carries. Ethanol is one example of an exogenous toxin that is first oxidized by bacterial alcohol dehydrogenase into acetaldehyde before being oxidized further by colonic mucosal or bacterial aldehyde dehydrogenase to acetate. Some of the intracolonic acetaldehyde may also be absorbed by the portal vein to be metabolized by the liver.

Since we know very little about the various toxic molecules manufactured by the gastrointestinal microbiome, our strongest evidence comes from observations of disease states caused by these mechanisms, like hepatic encephalopathy. In this condition, end-stage liver disease caused by either alcoholism or hepatitis increases intestinal permeability and permits greater passage of gut-derived "toxins" into general circulation. From there, the toxins reach the brain and a large portion of afflicted patients go on to develop hepatic encephalopathy (HE). In the early stages of hepatic encephalopathy, patients suffer from inverted sleep–wake patterns (e.g., sleeping during day and staying awake at night), followed by lethargy and personality changes. The latter stages are marked by worsening confusion and progression to coma with brain swelling and, ultimately, death. These symptoms provide us with valuable insights into the influence the gastrointestinal microbiome is capable of exerting on brain functions. Marked reversal of hepatic encephalopathy is possible with agents like rifaximin and lactulose, which reduce the production of gastrointestinal microbiome molecules and subsequently reverse hepatic encephalopathy in many patients. This indirect evidence can be accrued by studying the brain effects of hepatic encephalopathy in response to manipulation of the gut microbiome. Kao et al. (2016) reported a patient with grade 1–2 HE and liver cirrhosis secondary to alcoholism and hepatitis C who was treated with FMT.[106] Prior to treatment, the patient experienced lethargy, sleep–wake cycle reversal, slow reaction time, and intermittent disorientation of time. Within the first week of treatment, objective measures of reaction time, Stoop test, serum ammonia, and quality of life were all significantly improved. The patient also reported improved appetite, alertness, and overall well-being. After missing his second FMT, the patient experienced subsequent deterioration of parameters, which improved again once treatment was restarted, with continued improvements in alertness, concentration, and sleep–wake cycle. Bajaj et al. (2017) conducted an open-label randomized clinical trial of single infusion FMT following five days of broad-spectrum antibiotic treatment in outpatient men with cirrhosis and recurrent hepatic encephalopathy.[107] Following a single infusion of FMT after antibiotics, patients experienced a reduction in hepatic encephalopathy episodes, hospitalizations, and significant improvements in cognition, dysbiosis, and clinical outcomes (Figure 11.1).

Hepatic encephalopathy provides a clear model for demonstrating the capabilities of the gastrointestinal microbiome in influencing brain function.

Effects of Fecal Microbiota Transplantation on Epilepsy

To date, a single case report exists reporting the reversal of chronic, recurrent epilepsy following FMT in a 22-year-old female with long-standing epilepsy (17 years in duration) adequately controlled with medication. The patient initially presented with poorly controlled Crohn's disease (CD), defined by a CDAI score of 361, and was referred to us for FMT. She received the first administration of 200 mL fecal material via gastroscopy using donor stool obtained from a primary school aged female donor, which was followed by further infusions. Her convulsions ceased after the first mid-gut fecal infusion, at which time her use of sodium valproate was discontinued. Interestingly, in the absence of all epilepsy medications, no further convulsions occurred over the ensuing 20 months of observation. The patient also

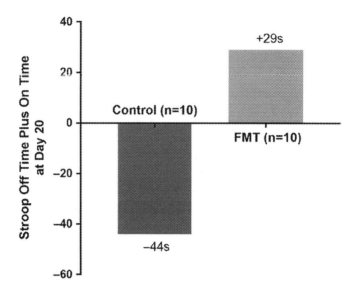

FIGURE 11.1 Improved clinical outcomes and cognitive function in patients administered FMT (n=10) compared with the control group (n=10) who received standard of care (Adapted from Bajaj JS et al. "T: A Randomized Clinical Trial" *Hepatology*. 2017 Dec;66(6):1727–1738, with permission)

experienced an improvement in Crohn's symptoms, with remission attained over the ensuing 20 months.[108]

We treated another patient with recurrent epilepsy in our clinic, who presented with a history of daily convulsions despite numerous guidelines-based treatments administered by consultant neurologists. Following vancomycin pre-treatment, the male patient received ten FMT colonic infusions of homogenized fresh human donor flora, followed immediately by three months of oral, lyophilized, encapsulated human FMT material at a dose of 4 x 10[11] colony forming units (CFUs) per day. Following rectal FMT, there was an almost total cessation of his grand mal seizures, which had been previously uncontrolled by numerous currently accepted pharmacological agents. This was followed by a total absence of seizures after six weeks of encapsulated FMT. If the findings from these small case reports are confirmed in larger, randomized clinical trials, we can foresee the utility of FMT not only as a treatment but also potentially as a diagnostic tool. FMT could identify the pathogenesis of epilepsy in some subset of patients, such as those arising in the gastrointestinal microbiome.

Relapsing-Remitting Multiple Sclerosis and Secondary Progressive MS

Our group has previously reported on three patients with concomitant multiple sclerosis who were treated at our clinic using repeated FMT for their chronic constipation. At presentation, one patient was unable to walk unassisted and required the use of crutches, while the two other patients had lost the ability to walk and were wheelchair-dependent. Unexpectedly, all three patients experienced complete reversal of their multiple sclerosis symptoms.[109] Following the preliminary success of

FMT, one may assume that a subset of patients with multiple sclerosis secrete molecules in their gastrointestinal microbiome that may affect the myelination process in the cortex, potentially as a result of molecular mimicry, and the FMT-mediated inhibition of the production of such substances could in fact reverse the condition by allowing myelin to regenerate and thereby re-establish normal function. All three of these patients achieved neurologic normality both functionally and on examination. Hence, fine movements and cortical behavior appear to have been restored in their entirety (Figure 11.2).

Hoban et al. (2016), using a genome-wide transcriptome profiling approach, reported significant upregulation of genes linked to myelination and myelin plasticity in germ-free mice.[110] These observed changes in myelin and activity-related gene expression could be reversed by colonization using a conventional microbiota following weaning, leading the authors to identify the microbiota as a potential therapeutic target for psychiatric disorders involving dynamic myelination in the prefrontal cortex. This was further explored by Makkawi *et al.* (2018),[111] who described a 61-year-old female patient with secondary progressive multiple sclerosis (SPMS) treated with FMT. She presented with seven relapses between 1998 and 2001, and her MRI showed numerous periventricular, juxtacortical, brainstem, and corpus callosum lesions confirming relapsing remitting multiple sclerosis. Despite an early positive response to glatiramer acetate treatment, her

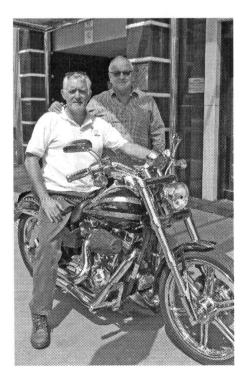

FIGURE 11.2   Patient with MS achieved near total reversal of MS symptoms allowing him to resume his previous activities such as riding motorcycles.

balance, ambulation, lower limb power, bladder function, and fatigue gradually worsened. Following several episodes of *C. difficile* enterocolitis in 2005 and 2006, which proved resistant to multiple courses of metronidazole and vancomycin, she received a single FMT from her partner. Following FMT, her Expanded Disability Status Scale immediately stabilized without other treatment or lifestyle changes. Over the next ten years, her Functional System scores minimally improved, as did her Modified Multiple Sclerosis Functional Composite scores, instead of worsening as expected. Taken together, the animal studies and otherwise unexplainable human observations following FMT again suggest that, as with hepatic encephalopathy, the gut microbiome likely plays an unexpected role in de- and re-myelination.

Parkinson's Disease

Parkinson's disease is a neurological condition characterized by abnormalities of movement including tremors, muscle stiffness, a mask-like facial appearance, micrographia, dysphagia, and a constellation of other symptoms. Based on autopsy evidence, Braak et al. (2003) and others postulated that Parkinson's begins in the gut with abnormal alpha-synuclein inclusions detectable in Meissner's (submucous) and Auerbach's (myenteric) plexus in the gut. This may be the cause or simply a marker of Parkinson's.[112] From here, alpha-synuclein is capable of traveling via neuronal streaming up the vagus nerve; interestingly, total vagotomy has been shown to be associated with a reduced incidence of Parkinson's disease.

In our practice, we have noted that treatment using certain antibiotics that exert influence on the gut microbiome (e.g., rifaximin, vancomycin, and metronidazole) has resulted in an improvement in Parkinson's disease symptoms in patients presenting for treatment of their co-morbid constipation, which is commonly seen with this disease.[113] A marked reduction in tremors was observed in a subset of these patients, reinforcing the involvement of the gastrointestinal microbiome as a possible contributor to the etiology of the disease. Near-complete disappearance of Parkinson's was seen in two out of five (40%) patients who underwent FMT for their constipation, and this was a durable effect. However, as these were the only patients to respond favorably to FMT, further research is required to determine the phenotype of Parkinson's patients who respond positively to FMT. This remarkable improvement in even a small subset of patients shows that there is an opportunity to reverse Parkinson's disease; however, a more complex protocol is likely required, perhaps with enhanced initial preparation of the gut prior to FMT using antimicrobial pre-treatment. In a mouse model of Parkinson's disease that overexpresses human alpha-synuclein, germ-free mice were found to move more freely and accumulate less alpha-synuclein in their brains than mice with gut microbes. Interestingly, when fecal material from patients with Parkinson's disease was transplanted into the guts of the mice, more movement dysfunction was observed compared with mice receiving bacteria from healthy humans. These findings link the abnormal neurological symptoms in mice overproducing alpha-synuclein to the presence of the gut microbiome. This link was subsequently confirmed by the observation that Parkinson's fecal material transplant into germ-free mice can, remarkably, cause development of Parkinson's-related motor symptoms.[114]

Autism Spectrum Disorder

Autism spectrum disorder (ASD) is a challenging and regressive disorder that affects young children typically aged two to five years and often develops after antibiotic usage. Although many observations have been made about the use of diet supplements, hyperbaric treatment, and antibiotics, only recently has data been amassed around the use of vancomycin to rapidly improve behavior in children with the condition. This improvement indicates that the gut microbiome is likely involved in the production of circulating substances, which may interfere with receptors in the brain, causing loss of language, abnormal movement behavior, and difficulty maintaining eye contact.[115]

Finegold (2008) demonstrated the presence of abnormal *Clostridia* and *Desulfovibrio* bacteria in the stool of ASD patients when compared with controls.[116] He postulated that neurotoxins manufactured by these pathogens are capable, either via circulation or by neuronal streaming, of crossing the blood–brain barrier and causing ASD-like symptoms. In our practice, we have noticed dramatic behavioral improvements in patients with ASD following vancomycin treatment, an effect which is even more potentiated when vancomycin is used in combination with rifaximin and a nitroimidazole. One group of patients was administered vancomycin and FMT orally within a chocolate-based drink on a daily basis for eight weeks. For these patients, both the gastrointestinal symptoms commonly seen in ASD and overall cognitive function improved before the end of the eight-week trial.[117] Although preliminary, these dramatic findings indicate that this is an area urgently requiring further research. Such a treatment may be able to more dramatically reverse symptoms if administered closer to the initiation of the disease (approximately 3–4 years of age).[118]

Tourette Syndrome

Tourette syndrome (TS) is a childhood-onset, neurological disorder defined by repetitive involuntary movements and vocalizations, which has a significantly negative impact on the patient's quality of life. Although evidence suggests that Tourette's is primarily an inherited disorder, the specific genetic abnormality has yet to be identified.[119] Previous studies have also implicated the involvement of dysfunctional cortico-basal ganglia-thalamo-cortical loops, which are responsible for movement execution and habit formation. However, these studies are limited by their small sample size and various deviating factors, which unfortunately preclude meaningful conclusions from being drawn from them.

Tourette's is notoriously difficult to treat and affected individuals are at an increased risk of developing other complicated concurrent conditions, including obsessive compulsive disorder, schizophrenia, and attention deficit hyperactivity disorder. Tourette's has no specific cure and treatment is largely focused on management of symptoms through behavioral modification and pharmacological therapy. The extent of influence the gut microbiota exercises over the brain and its effect on central physiology and function have been revisited in neurological conditions with the emergence of gut-brain axis communication.[120] As such, positive outcomes in case reports where FMT was administered for conditions such as Parkinson's disease and autism, coupled with the hypothesis that the gut microbiome may exert a large influence on the development or exacerbation of Tourette's, help position FMT as a viable therapeutic option.

One case of Tourette's being reversed by FMT has been reported in the literature.[121] A 9-year-old male presented with classic symptoms of Tourette's, including involuntary eye turning, headshaking, shrugging, and vocal tics, which he had experienced for two-and-a-half years. After receiving treatment with tiapride 100 mg three times daily and probiotics consisting of *Bacillus subtilis*, *Clostridium butyricum*, and an *Enterococcus*, the patient experienced an initial improvement in symptoms for two months before reporting a gradual recurrence of symptoms. The patient was subsequently offered FMT as a treatment for tic symptoms and was administered 100 ml dose FMT via gastroscopy into the small intestine and 300 ml via colonoscopy using stool from a healthy 14-year-old male donor. Following FMT, the patient experienced a dramatic improvement in symptoms, including a reduction in tic severity score from 31 to 5, motor severity score from 16 to 5, and vocal severity score from 15 to 0.

The central role of the gastrointestinal microbiota in certain neurological disorders, such as hepatic encephalopathy, Parkinson's disease, and autism spectrum disorders, suggests a complex relationship between the gut microbiota and the brain. Furthermore, the abovementioned case suggests an exciting new approach in the treatment of Tourette's, which unquestionably warrants further exploration of the long-term efficacy and safety of FMT in treating this condition.

CONCLUSIONS

Microbial therapy has a long history in the treatment of human disease and the maintenance of overall health.[122,123,124,125] The unquestionable success of FMT in recurrent, life-threatening, *Clostridium difficile* infections has now been well established in the scientific literature.[126,127] However, many aspects of this procedure and its efficacy remain unknown, both in experimental approaches to FMT and in the clinical setting. For instance, we do not know which components present in the transplanted material are responsible and/or essential for the success of the procedure. Although we believe that the microbes are responsible for the success of the treatment, appropriately designed and scaled clinical trials need to be performed to be certain.[128] We are also uncertain about the optimal route of administration for the material from the healthy donor (i.e., oral, endoscopic, via enema, etc.).[129] It is generally believed that more than one donor should provide material for transplantation therapy to increase the diversity of the final donor microbiome; however, clinical experience suggests that some individual donor samples yield greater success than others, for yet unknown reasons. Donor samples are screened for potential pathogens and any familial chronic disease incidence to minimize any potential long-term effects, including neurodegenerative disorders. At present, we lack high-quality, long-term studies of patients who have received FMT. Attempts are being made to minimize any possible long-term effects of the components of FMT other than bacteria in the donor material, but again, useful information with significant numbers of patients is not yet forthcoming.

NOTES

1. (Zilber-Rosenberg & Rosenberg, Role of microorganisms in the evolution of animals and plants: the hologenome theory of evolution, 2008;32(5)).
2. (Forsythe & Kunze, 2013;70(1)).
3. (Forsythe, Kunze, & Bienenstock, 2016;14(1)).
4. (Bienenstock, Kunze, & Forsythe, 2015;73(1)).
5. (Borre et al., 2014;20(9)).
6. (Sharon, Sampson, Geschwind, & Mazmanian, 2016).
7. (Tremlett, Bauer, Appel-Cresswell, Finlay, & Waubant, 2017).
8. (Ogilvie & Jones, 2015).
9. (Ma, You, Mai, Tokuyasi, & Liu, 2018).
10. (Kernbauer, Ding, & Cadwell, 2014).
11. (Cadwell, 2015).
12. (Huseyin, O'Toole, Cotter, & Scanlan, 2017).
13. (Jiang et al., 2017).
14. (Enaud et al., 2018).
15. (Jiang et al., 2017).
16. (Hatoum, Labrie, & Fliss, 2012).
17. (Qamar et al., 2001).
18. (Thomas, Metzke, Schmitz, Dorffel, & Baumgart, 2011).
19. (Iliev et al., 2012).
20. (Hoffmann et al., 2013).
21. (Mar Rodriguez et al., 2015).
22. (Kowalewska, Zorena, Szmigiero-kawko, Waz, & Mysliwiec, 2016).
23. (Severance et al., 2016).
24. (Gouba, Raoult, & Drancourt, 2014).
25. (Hoffmann et al., 2013).
26. (van de Pol et al., 2017).
27. (Koskinen et al., 2017).
28. (Park, Lee, Hussain, Lee, & Park, 2017).
29. (Gill et al., 2006).
30. (Zoetendal, Vaughan, & de Vos, 2006).
31. (Qin et al., 2010).
32. (O'Hara & Shanahan, 2006).
33. (Sharon et al., 2010).
34. (Borrelli et al., 2016).
35. (Dillon, Vennard, & Charnley, 2002).
36. (Borre et al., 2014;20(9)).
37. (Sudo et al., 2004).
38. (Yano et al., 2015; Borrelli et al., 2016).
39. (Sharon, Sampson, Geschwind, & Mazmanian, 2016).
40. (Borrelli et al., 2016).
41. (O'Leary, Ogbonnaya, Felice, Levone, & Fitzgerald, 2018).
42. (Sudo et al., 2004).
43. (Hoban et al., 2016).
44. (Braniste et al., 2014).
45. (Erny et al., 2015).
46. (Frohlich et al., 2016).
47. (Cox et al., 2014).
48. (Leclercq et al., 2017).
49. (Wang, 2014).

50. (Wall et al., 2014).
51. (Wang, 2014).
52. (Papapetropoulos, Foresti, & Ferdinandy, 2015).
53. (Lyte, 2013).
54. (Bienenstock, Kunze, & Forsythe, 2015;73(1)).
55. (Schroeder, Lin, Crusio, & Akbarian, 2007).
56. (Macfabe, 2012).
57. (Sampson et al., 2016).
58. (Mazmanian, Round, & Kasper, 2008).
59. (Mao et al., 2013).
60. (Schiavi et al., 2016).
61. (Fanning et al., 2012).
62. (Al-Nedawi et al., 2015).
63. (Al-Nedawi et al., 2015).
64. (Deatherage & Cookson, 2012).
65. (Ellis & Kuehn, 2010).
66. (Kuehn, 2012).
67. (Shen et al., 2012).
68. (Al-Nedawi et al., 2015).
69. (Canas et al., 2016).
70. (Fabrega et al., 2016).
71. (Forsythe, Kunze, & Bienenstock, 2016).
72. (Collins, Surette, & Bercik, 2012).
73. (Dinan & Cryan, 2017).
74. (Schroeder, Lin, Crusio, & Akbarian, 2007).
75. (Macfabe, 2012).
76. (Rolig et al., 2017).
77. (Rousseaux et al., 2007).
78. (Wang et al., 2010).
79. (Perez-Burgos et al., 2015).
80. (Perez-Burgos et al., 2013).
81. (Perez-Burgos, Mao, Bienenstock, & Kunze, 2014).
82. (Bravo et al., 2011).
83. (Bercik et al., 2011).
84. (Bercik et al., 2011).
85. (Corr et al., 2007).
86. (Benakis et al., 2016).
87. (Kigerl et al., 2016).
88. (Wang et al., 2014).
89. (Colpitts et al., 2017).
90. (Rothhammer et al., 2018).
91. (Garay, Hsiao, Patterson, & McAllister, 2013).
92. (Hsiao, McBride, Chow, Mazmanian, & Patterson, 2012 Jul 31).
93. (Dantzer, 2017).
94. (Bercik et al., 2011).
95. (Turnbaugh et al., 2009).
96. (Berer et al., 2017).
97. (Cekanaviciute et al., 2017).
98. (Sampson et al., 2016).
99. (De Palma et al., 2017).
100. (Lessa et al., 2015).

101. (Borody et al., 1989).
102. (Andrews & Borody, 1993).
103. (Borody, Warren, Leis, Surace, & Ashman, 2003).
104. (Bakken et al., 2011).
105. (Finch Therapeutics).
106. (Kao et al., 2016).
107. (Bajaj et al., 2017).
108. (He et al., 2017).
109. (Borody, Leis, Campbell, Torres, & Nowak, 2011).
110. (Hoban et al., Regulation of prefrontal cortex myelination by the microbiota., 2016).
111. (Makkawi, Camara-Lemarroy, & Metz, 2018).
112. (Braak, Rüb, Del Tredici, & Gai, 2003).
113. (Borody, Torres, Hills, & Ketheeswaran, 2009).
114. (Sampson et al., 2016).
115. (Sandler et al., 2000).
116. (Finegold, 2008).
117. (Kang et al., 2017).
118. (Kang et al., 2017).
119. (Felling & Singer, 2011).
120. (Sharon, Sampson, Geschwind, & Mazmanian, The Central Nervous System and the Gut microbiome., 2016).
121. (Zhao et al., 2017).
122. (Eiseman, Silen, Bascom, & Kauvar, 1958).
123. (Borody et al., 1989).
124. (Borody & Campbell, 2011).
125. (Brandt, Borody, & Campbell, 2011).
126. (van Nood et al., 2013).
127. (Kelly, 2013).
128. (Zuo et al., 2018).
129. (Kao et al., 2017).

BIBLIOGRAPHY

Al-Nedawi, K, M F Mian, N Hossain, K Karimi, Y K Mao, P Forsythe et al. 2015. "Gut commensal microvesicles reproduce parent bacterial signals to host immune and enteric nervous systems." *FASEB Journal* 29(2): 684–95.

Andrews, P J, and T J Borody. 1993. "Putting back the bugs: Bacterial treatment relieves chronic constipation and symptoms of irritable bowel syndrome." *The Medical Journal of Australia* 159(9): 633–4.

Bajaj, J, Z Kassam, A Fagan, E Gavis, E Liu, J Cox et al. 2017. "Fecal microbiota transplant from a rational stool donor improves hepatic encephalopathy: A randomized clinical trial." *Hepatology* 66(6): 1727–38.

Benakis, C, D Brea, S Caballero, G Faraco, J Moore, and M Murphy. 2016. "Commensal microbiota affects ischemic stroke outcome by regulating intestinal gammadelta T cells." *Nature Medicine* 28.

Bercik, P, A J Park, D Sinclair, A Khoshdel, J Lu, X Huang et al. 2011a. "The intestinal microbiota affect central levels of brain-derived neurotropic factor and behavior in mice." *Gastroenterology* 141(2): 599–609.

Bercik, P, A J Park, D Sinclair, A Khoshdel, J Lu, X Huang et al. 2011b. "The anxiolytic effect of *Bifidobacterium longum* NCC3001 involves vagal pathways for gut-brain communication." *Neurogastroenterology and Motility* 23(12): 1132–9.

Berer, K, L A Gerdes, E Cekanaviciute, X Jia, L Xiao, Z Xia et al. 2017. "Gut microbiota from multiple sclerosis patients enables spontaneous autoimmune encephalomyelitis in mice." *Proceedings of the National Academy of Sciences of the United States of America* 10719–24.

Bienenstock, J, W Kunze, and P Forsythe. 2015. "Microbiota and the gut-brain axis." *Nutrition Reviews* 73(1): 28–31.

Borody, T J, and J Campbell. 2011. "Fecal microbiota transplantation: Current status and future directions." *Expert Review of Gastroenterology & Hepatology* 5(6): 653–5.

Borody, T J, L George, P Andrews, S Brandl, S Noonan, P Cole et al. 1989. "Bowel-flora alteration: A potential cure for inflammatory bowel disease and irritable bowel syndrome?" *The Medical Journal of Australia* 150(10): 604.

Borody, T J, E F Warren, S Leis, R Surace, and O Ashman. 2003. "Treatment of ulcerative colitis using fecal bacteriotherapy." *Journal of Clinical Gastroenterology* 37(1): 42–7.

Borody, T, S Leis, J Campbell, M Torres, and A Nowak. 2011. "Fecal microbiota transplantation (FMT) in multiple sclerosis (MS)." *The American Journal of Gastroenterology* 106: S432–95.

Borre, Y E, G W O'Keeffe, G Clarke, C Stanton, T G Dinan, and J F Cryan. 2014. "Microbiota and neurodevelopmental window: Implications for brain disorders." *Trends in Molecular Medicine* 20(9): 509–18.

Borrelli, L, S Aceto, C Agnisola, S De Paolo, L Dipineto, R M Stilling et al. 2016. "Probiotic modulation of the microbiota-gut-brain axis and behaviour in zebrafish." *Scientific Reports* 6: 30046.

Braak, H, U Rüb, W P Del Tredici, and K Gai. 2003. "Idiopathic Parkinson's disease: Possible routes by which vulnerable neuronal types may be subject to neuroinvasion by an unknown pathogen." *Journal of Neural Transmission* 110(5): 517–36.

Brandt, L J, T J Borody, and J Campbell. 2011. "Endoscopic fecal microbiota transplantation: "first-line" treatment for severe clostridium difficile infection?" *Journal of Clinical Gastroenterology* 45(8): 655–7.

Braniste, V, M Al-Asmakh, C Kowal, F Anuar, A Abbaspour, and M Toth. 2014. "He gut microbiota influences blood-brain barrier permeability in mice." *Science Translational Medicine* 6(263): 158.

Bravo, J A, P Forsythe, M V Chew, E Escaravage, H M Savignac, T G Dinan et al. 2011. "Ingestion of Lactobacillus strain regulates emotional behavior and central GABA receptor expression in a mouse via the vagus nerve." *Proceedings of the National Academy of Sciences of the United States of America* 16050–5.

Cadwell, K. 2015. "Expanding the role of the virome: Commensalism in the gut." *Journal of Virology* 89(4): 1951–3.

Canas, M A, R Gimenez, M J Fabrega, L Toloza, L Baldoma, and J Badia. 2016. "Outer membrane vesicles from the probiotic *Escherichia coli* Nissle 1917 and the commensal ECOR12 enter intestinal epithelial cells via clathrin-dependent endocytosis and elicit differential effects on DNA damage." *PLOS ONE* 11(8): e0160374.

Cekanaviciute, E, B B Yoo, T F Runia, J W Debelius, S Singh, C A Nelson et al. 2017. "Gut bacteria from multiple sclerosis patients modulate human T cells and exacerbate symptoms in mouse models." *Proceedings of the National Academy of Sciences of the United States of America* 10713–8.

Collins, S M, M Surette, and P Bercik. 2012. "The interplay between the intestinal microbiota and the brain." *Nature Reviews in Microbiology* 10(11): 735–42.

Colpitts, S L, E J Kasper, A Keever, C Liljenberg, T Kirby, K Magori et al. 2017. "A bidirectional association between the gut microbiota and CNS disease in a biphasic murine model of multiple sclerosis." *Gut Microbes* 8(6): 561–73.

Corr, S C, Y Li, C U Riedel, P W O'Toole, C Hill, and C G Gahan. 2007. "Bacteriocin production as a mechanism for the antiinfective activity of *Lactobacillus salivarius* UCC118." *Proceedings of the National Academy of Sciences of the United States of America* 7617–21.

Cox, L M, S Yamanishi, J Sohn, A V Alekseyenko, J M Leung, I Cho et al. 2014. "Altering the intestinal microbiota during a critical developmental window has lasting metabolic consequences." *Cell* 158(4): 705–21.

Dantzer, R. 2017. *Inflammation-Associated Depression: Evidence, Mechanisms and Implications (Current Topics in Behavioral Neurosciences)*. Springer International Publishing AG.

Deatherage, B L, and B T Cookson. 2012. "Membrane vesicle release in bacteria, eukaryotes, and archaea: A conserved yet underappreciated aspect of microbial life." *Infection and Immunity* 80(6): 1948–57.

De Palma, G, M D Lynch, J Lu, V T Dang, Y Deng, J Jury et al. 2017. "Transplantation of fecal microbiota from patients with irritable bowel syndrome alters gut function and behavior in recipient mice." *Science Translational Medicine* 9(379).

Dillon, R J, C T Vennard, and A K Charnley. 2002. "A note: Gut bacteria produce components of a locust cohesion pheromone." *Journal of Applied Microbiology* 92(4): 759–63.

Dinan, T G, and J F Cryan. 2017. "Gut instincts: Microbiota as a key regulator of brain development, ageing and neurodegeneration." *Journal of Physiology* 595(2): 489–503.

Eiseman, B, W Silen, G S Bascom, and A J Kauvar. 1958. "Fecal enema as an adjunct in the treatment of pseudomembranous enterocolitis." *Surgery* 44(5): 854–9.

Ellis, T N, and M J Kuehn. 2010. "Virulence and immunomodulatory roles of bacterial outer membrane vesicles." *Microbiology and Molecular Biology Reviews* 74(1): 81–94.

Enaud, R, L E Vandenborght, N Coron, T Bazin, R Prevel, T Schaeverbeke et al. 2018. "The mycobiome: A neglected component in the microbiota-gut-brain axis." *Microorganisms* 6(1).

Erny, D, A L Hrabe de Angelis, D Jaitin, P Wieghofer, O Staszewski, E David et al. 2015. "Host microbiota constantly control maturation and function of microglia in the CNS." *Nature Neuroscience* 18(7): 965–77.

Fabrega, M J, L Aguilera, R Gimenez, E Varela, C M Alexandra, M Antolin, et al. 2016. "Activation of immune and defense responses in the intestinal mucosa by outer membrane vesicles of commensal and probiotic *Escherichia coli* strains." *Frontiers in Microbiology* 7: 705.

Fanning, S, L J Hall, M Cronin, A Zomer, J MacSharry, D Goulding, et al. 2012. "Bifidobacterial surface-exopolysaccharide facilitates commensal-host interaction through immune modulation and pathogen protection." *Proceedings of the National Academy of Sciences of the United States of America* 2108–13.

Felling, R J, and H S Singer. 2011. "Neurobiology of Tourette syndrome: Current Status and need for further investigation." *The Journal of Neuroscience* 31(35): 12387–95.

Finegold, S M. 2008. "Therapy and epidemiology of autism-clostridial spores as key elements." *Medical Hypotheses* 70(3): 508–11.

Forsythe, P, W Kunze, and J Bienenstock. 2016. "Moody microbes or fecal phrenology: What do we know about the microbiota-gut-brain axis?" *BMC Medicine* 14(1): 58.

Forsythe, P, and W A Kunze. 2013. "Voices from within:gut microbes and the CNS." *Cellular and Molecular Life Sciences* 70(1): 55–69.

Frohlich, E E, A Farzi, R Mayerhofer, F Reichmann, A Jacan, B Wagner et al. 2016. "Cognitive impairment by antibiotic-induced gut dysbiosis: Analysis of gut microbiota-brain communication." *Brain, Behaviour, and Immunity* 56: 140–55.

Garay, P A, E Y Hsiao, P H Patterson, and A K McAllister. 2013. "Maternal immune activation causes age- and region-specific changes in brain cytokines in offspring throughout development." *Brain, Behavior, and Immunity* 31: 54–68.

Gill, S R, M Pop, R T Deboy, P B Eckburg, P J Turnbaugh, B S Samuel et al. 2006. "Metagenomic analysis of the human distal gut microbiome." *Science* 312(5778): 1355–9.

Gouba, N, D Raoult, and M Drancourt. 2014. "Gut microeukaryotes during anorexia nervosa: A case report." *BMC Research Notes* 7: 33.

Hatoum, R, S Labrie, and I Fliss. 2012. "Antimicrobial and probiotic properties of yeasts: From fundamental to novel applications." *Frontiers in Microbiology* 3: 421.

He, Z, B-T Cui, T Zhang, P Li, C-Y Long, G-Z Ji, and F-M Zhang. 2017. "Fecal microbiota transplantation cured epilepsy in a case with Crohn's disease: The first report." *World Journal of Gastroenterology* 23(19): 3565.

Hoban, A E, R M Stilling, F J Ryan, F Shanahan, T G Dinan, M J Claesson et al. 2016. "Regulation of prefrontal cortex myelination by the microbiota." *Translational Psychiatry* 6(4): e774–9.

Hoffmann, C, S Dollive, S Grunberg, J Chen, H Li, G D Wu et al. 2013. "Archaea and fungi of the human gut microbiome: Correlations with diet and bacterial residents." *PLoS One* 8(6): e66019.

Hsiao, E Y, S W McBride, J Chow, S K Mazmanian, and P H Patterson. 2012. "Modeling an autism risk factor in mice leads to permanent immune dysregulation." *Proceedings of the National Academy of Sciences of the United States of America* 12776–81.

Huseyin, C E, P W O'Toole, P D Cotter, and P D Scanlan. 2017. "Forgotten fungi - the gut mycobiome in human health and disease." *FEMS Microbiology Reviews* 41(4): 479.

Iliev, I D, V A Funari, K D Taylor, Q Nguyen, C N Reyes, S P Strom et al. 2012. "Interactions between commensal fungi and the C-type lectin receptor Dectin-1 influence colitis." *Science* 336(6086): 1314–7.

Jiang, T T, T Y Shao, W X G Ang, J M Kinder, L H Turner, G Pham et al. 2017. "Commensal fungi recapitulate the protective benefits of intestinal bacteria." *Cell Host & Microbe* 22(6): 809–16.

Kang, D-W, J B Adams, A C Gregory, T Borody, L Chittick, A Fasano, R Krajmalnik-Brown et al. 2017. "Microbiota transfer therapy alters gut ecosystem and improves gastrointestinal and autism symptoms: An open-label study." *Microbiome* 5(1): 10.

Kao, D, B Roach, H Park, N Hotte, K Madsen, V Bain et al. 2016. "Fecal microbiota transplantation in the management of mild overt hepatic encephalopathy: A case report." *The American Journal of Gastroenterology* 110(Supplementary 1): 714.

Kao, D, B Roach, M Silva, P Beck, K Rioux, G G Kaplan et al. 2017. "Effect of oral capsule- vs colonoscopy-delivered fecal microbiota transplantation on recurrent *Clostridium difficile* infection: A randomized clinical trial." *JAMA* 318(20): 1985–93.

Kelly, C P. 2013. "Fecal microbiota transplantation – An old therapy comes of age." *New England Journal of Medicine* 368(5): 474–5.

Kernbauer, E, Y Ding, and K Cadwell. 2014. "An enteric virus can replace the beneficial function of commensal bacteria." *Nature* 516(7529): 94–8.

Kigerl, K A, J C Hall, L Wang, X Mo, Z Yu, and P G Popovich. 2016. "Gut dysbiosis impairs recovery after spinal cord injury." *The Journal of Experimental Medicine* 213(12): 2603–20.

Koskinen, K, M R Pausan, A K Perras, M Beck, C Bang, M Mora et al. 2017. "First insights into the diverse human archaeome: Specific detection of archaea in the gastrointestinal tract, lung, and nose and on skin." *mBio* 8(6).

Kowalewska, B, K Zorena, M Szmigiero-kawko, P Waz, and M Mysliwiec. 2016. "High inter-leukin-12 levels may prevent an increase in the amount of fungi in the gastrointestinal tract during the first years of diabetes mellitus type 1." *Disease Markers* 2016: 4685976.

Kuehn, M J. 2012. "Secreted bacterial vesicles as good samaritans." *Cell Host & Microbe* 12(4): 392–3.

Leclercq, S, F M Mian, A M Stanisz, L B Bindels, E Cambier, H Ben-Amram et al. 2017. "Low-dose penicillin in early life induces long-term changes in murine gut microbiota, brain cytokines and behavior." *Nature Communications* 8: 15062.

Lessa, F C, Y Mu, W M Bamberg, Z G Beldavs, G K Dumyati, J R Dunn et al. 2015. "Burden of *Clostridium difficile* infection in the United States." *New England Journal of Medicine* 372(9): 825–34.

Lyte, M. 2013. "Microbial endocrinology in the microbiome-gut-brain axis: How bacterial production and utilization of neurochemicals influence behavior." *PLOS Pathogens* 9(11): e1003726.

Ma, Y, X You, G Mai, T Tokuyasi, and C Liu. 2018. "A human gut phage catalog correlates the gut phageome with type 2 diabetes." *Microbiome* 6(1): 24.

Macfabe, D F. 2012. "Short-chain fatty acid fermentation products of the gut microbiome: Implications in autism spectrum disorders." *Microbial Ecology in Health and Disease* 23.

Makkawi, S, C Camara-Lemarroy, and L Metz. 2018. "Fecal microbiota transplantation associated with 10 years of stability in a patient with SPMS." *Neurology: Neuroimmunology and NeuroInflammation* 5: e459.

Mao, Y K, D L Kasper, B Wang, P Forsythe, J Bienenstock, and W A Kunze. 2013. "Bacteroides fragilis polysaccharide A is necessary and sufficient for acute activation of intestinal sensory neurons." *Nature Communications* 4: 1465.

Mar Rodriguez, M, D Perez, C F Javier, E Esteve, P Marin-Garcia, G Xifra et al. 2015. "Obesity changes the human gut mycobiome." *Scientific Reports* 5: 14600.

Mazmanian, S K, J L Round, and D L Kasper. 2008. "A microbial symbiosis factor prevents intestinal inflammatory disease." *Nature* 453(7195): 620–5.

O'Hara, A M, and F Shanahan. 2006. "The gut flora as a forgotten organ." *EMBO Reports* 7(7): 688–93.

O'Leary, O F, E S Ogbonnaya, D Felice, B R Levone, L C Conroy, P P Fitzgerald et al. 2018. "The vagus nerve modulates BDNF expression and neurogenesis in the hippocampus." *European Neuropsychopharmacology* 28(2): 307–16.

Ogilvie, L A, and B V Jones. 2015. "The human gut virome: A multifaceted majority." *Frontiers in Microbiology* 6: 918.

Papapetropoulos, A, R Foresti, and P Ferdinandy. 2015. "Pharmacology of the 'gasotransmitters' NO, CO and H2S: translational opportunities." *British Journal of Pharmacology* 172(6): 1395–6.

Park, Y M, Y J Lee, Z Hussain, Y H Lee, and H Park. 2017. "The effects and mechanism of action of methane on ileal motor function." *Neurogastroenterology and Motility* 29(9).

Perez-Burgos, A, Y K Mao, J Bienenstock, and W A Kunze. 2014. "The gut-brain axis rewired: Adding a functional vagal nicotinic "sensory synapse"." *FASEB Journal* 28(7): 3064–74.

Perez-Burgos, A, B Wang, Y K Mao, B Mistry, K Neufeld, A McVey, and J Bienenstock. 2013. "Psychoactive bacteria *Lactobacillus rhamnosus* (JB-1) elicits rapid frequency facilitation in vagal afferents." *American Journal of Physiology. Gastrointestinal and Liver Physiology* 304(2): G211–20.

Perez-Burgos, A, L Wang, K A McVey Neufeld, Y K Mao, M Ahmadzai, L J Janssen et al. 2015. "The TRPV1 channel in rodents is a major target for antinociceptive effect of the probiotic Lactobacillus reuteri DSM 17938." *Journal of Physiology* 593(17): 3943–57.

Rolig, A S, E K Mittge, J Ganz, J V Troll, E Melancon, T J Wiles, et al. 2017. "The enteric nervous system promotes intestinal health by constraining microbiota composition." *PLOS Biology* 15(2): e2000689.

Rothhammer, V, D M Borucki, E C Tjon, M C Takenaka, C C Chao, A Ardura-Fabregat et al. 2018. "Microglial control of astrocytes in response to microbial metabolites." *Nature* 16(7707).

Rousseaux, C, X Thuru, A Gelot, N Barnich, C Neut, L Dubuquoy, et al. 2007. "*Lactobacillus acidophilus* modulates intestinal pain and induces opioid and cannabinoid receptors." *Nature Medicine* 13(1): 35–7.

Sampson, T R, J W Debelius, T Thron, S Janssen, G G Shastri, Z E Ilhan, et al. 2016. "Gut microbiota regulate motor deficits and neuroinflammation in a model of Parkinson's disease." *Cell* 167(6): 1469–80.

Sandler, R H, S M Finegold, E R Bolte, C P Buchanan, A P Maxwell, M L Väisänen et al. 2000. "Short-term benefit from oral vancomycin treatment of regressive-onset autism." *Journal of Child Neurology* 15(7): 429–35.

Schiavi, E, M Gleinser, E Molloy, D Groeger, R Frei, R Ferstl et al. 2016. "The surface-associated exopolysaccharide of *Bifidobacterium longum* 35624 plays an essential role in dampening host proinflammatory responses and repressing local TH17 responses." *Applied and Environmental Microbiology* 82(24): 7185–96.

Schroeder, F A, C L Lin, W E Crusio, and S Akbarian. 2007. "Antidepressant-like effects of the histone deacetylase inhibitor, sodium butyrate, in the mouse." *Biological Psychiatry* 62(1): 55–64.

Severance, E G, K L Gressitt, C R Stallings, E Katsafanas, L A Schweinfurth, C L Savage et al. 2016. "*Candida albicans* exposures, sex specificity and cognitive deficits in schizophrenia and bipolar disorder." *NPJ Schizophrenia* 2: 16018.

Sharon, G, T R Sampson, D H Geschwind, and K Mazmanian. 2016. "The central nervous system and the gut microbiome." *Cell* 167(4): 915–32.

Sharon, G, D Segal, J M Ringo, A Hefetz, I Silber-Rosenberg, and E Rosenberg. 2010. "E. Commensal bacteria play a role in mating preference of *Drosophila melanogaster*." *Proceedings of the National Academy of Sciences of the United States of America* 107(46): 20.

Shen, Y, M L Giardino Torchia, G W Lawson, C L Karp, J D Ashwell, and S K Mazmanian. 2012. "Outer membrane vesicles of a human commensal mediate immune regulation and disease protection." *Cell Host & Microbe* 12(4): 509–20.

Sudo, N, Y Chida, Y Aiba, J Sonoda, N Oyama, X N Yu et al. 2004. "Postnatal microbial colonization programs the hypothalamic-pituitary-adrenal system for stress response in mice." *Journal of Physiology* 558(1): 263–75.

Tremlett, H, K C Bauer, S Appel-Cresswell, B B Finlay, and E Waubant. 2017. "The gut microbiomein human neurological disease: A review." *Annals of Neurology* 81(3): 369–82.

Turnbaugh, P J, V K Ridaura, J J Faith, F E Rey, R Knight, and J I Gordon. 2009. "The effect of diet on the human gut microbiome: A metagenomic analysis in humanized gnotobiotic mice." *Science Translational Medicine* 1(6): 6ra14.

van Nood, E, A Vrieze, M Nieuwdorp, S Fuentes, E G Zoetendal, W M de Vos et al. 2013. "Duodenal infusion of donor feces for recurrent *Clostridium difficile*." *New England Journal of Medicine* 368(5): 407–15.

Wang, B, Y K Mao, C Diorio, M Pasyk, R Y Wu, J Bienenstock, and W A Kunze. 2010a. "Luminal administration ex vivo of a live Lactobacillus species moderates mouse jejunal motility within minutes." *FASEB Journal* 24(10): 4078–88.

Wang, B, Y K Mao, C Diorio, L Wang, J D Huizinga, J Bienenstock, and W Kunze. 2010b. "*Lactobacillus reuteri* ingestion and IK(Ca) channel blockade have similar effects on rat colon motility and myenteric neurones." *Neurogastroenterology and Motility* 22(1): 98–107.

Wang, R. 2014. "Gasotransmitters: Growing pains and joys." *Trends in Biochemical Sciences* 39(5): 227–32.

Wang, Y, K M Telesford, J Ochoa-Repáraz, S Haque-Begum, M Christy, E J Kasper et al. 2014. "An intestinal commensal symbiosis factor controls neuroinflammation via TLR2-mediated CD39 signalling." *Nature Communications* 5: 4432.

Yano, J M, K Yu, G P Donaldson, G G Shastri, P Ann, L Ma et al. 2015. "Indigenous bacteria from the gut microbiota regulate host serotonin biosynthesis." *Cell* 161(2): 264–76.

Zhao, H, Y Shi, X Luo, L Peng, Y Yang, and L Zou. 2017. "The effect of fecal microbiota transplantation on a child with tourette syndrome." *Case Reports in Medicine* 2017: 6165239.

Zilber-Rosenberg, I, and E Rosenberg. 2008. "Role of microorganisms in the evolution of animals and plants: The hologenome theory of evolution." *FEMS Microbiology Reviews* 32(5): 723–35.

Zoetendal, E G, E E Vaughan, and W M de Vos. 2006. "A microbial world within us." *Molecular Microbiology* 59(6): 1639–50.

Zuo, T, S H Wong, K Lam, R Lui, K Cheung, W Tang, et al. 2018. "Bacteriophage transfer during faecal microbiota transplantation in *Clostridium difficile* infection is associated with treatment outcome." *Gut* 67(4): 634–43.

12 Lifestyle Influences on the Microbiome

Leo Galland

CONTENTS

INTRODUCTION

Human studies reveal substantial differences in gut microbial composition among individuals.[1,2,3] These differences have been attributed to age, host genetics, physiological or pathologic states, and lifestyle.[4,5,6] In this context, the concept of lifestyle describes habitual patterns of behavior among individuals and groups; factors like diet, physical activity, social interactions, sleep, hygiene, and the use of substances that include alcohol, tobacco, recreational drugs, and over-the-counter medications are all elements of an individual's lifestyle that have an influence on health. The importance of lifestyle factors in shaping the gut microbiome is evidenced by recent findings which show unrelated individuals sharing a household have far greater similarity in fecal microbiome composition than genetically related individuals living apart.[7] This result suggests that shared environment is more important than genetics in determining taxonomy of the gut microbiome.

DIETARY PATTERNS AND THE GUT MICROBIOME

Most studies have shown that good health is most often accompanied by increased diversity of species within the gut microbiome. Diversity of microbiome species is therefore considered a desirable outcome of dietary interventions. Reduced caloric intake[8] or high consumption of dietary fiber[9] increases gut bacterial diversity, whereas caloric overconsumption has the opposite effect.[10] Genetic sequence analysis of amplified microbial ribosomal RNA-encoding genes [16S ribosomal DNA (rDNA)], reveals that the human adult bacterial microbiome is comprised of five main phyla: *Firmicutes, Bacteroidetes, Actinobacteria, Proteobacteria,* and *Verrucomicrobia. Firmicutes* and *Bacteroidetes* are the most common phyla, while *Actinobacteria, Proteobacteria,* and *Verrucomicrobia* usually comprise 2% or less of organisms present in the microbiome. Most bacteria belong to the genera *Faecalibacterium, Bacteroides, Roseburia, Ruminococcus, Eubacterium, Coprabacillus,* and *Bifidobacterium.*[11] A diet high in animal protein and fat favors an abundance of *Bacteroides,* while a vegetarian diet or one high in monosaccharides favors abundance of *Prevotella,* another member of the *Bacteroidetes* phylum.[12] Most research has shown an inverse relationship between concentration of *Prevotella* and *Bacteroides* species, highlighting the impact of dietary patterns on these two abundant genera.[13] High consumption of oligosaccharides favors growth of *Bifidobacteria*[14] (the dominant genus of *Actinobacteria)* and *Faecalibacterium prausnitzii,* interdependent species usually associated with good health.[15,16,17]

The growth of Archea and fungi—non-bacterial components of the gut microbiome—may also be influenced by diet. Archea are primitive prokaryocytes, found in about half of human stool specimens. The dominant archeal genus in the human gut, *Methanobrevibacter,* contains the leading methane-producing organisms of the gut microbiome. Levels of *Methanobrevibacter* are positively associated with long-term consumption of carbohydrates. There are 16 fungal genera found in stool samples of healthy adults, with *Saccharomyces* and *Candida* being the most common. Although *Saccharomyces* colonization does not appear to show an association with diet, *Candida* responds very quickly to dietary changes. Candida levels increase with recent carbohydrate consumption but are not related to long-term dietary patterns.[18]

Dietary interventions tend to produce mild to moderate changes in microbiome taxonomy that vary from person to person and are quantitatively smaller than baseline inter-individual variability.[19,20] The ultimate goal of dietary interventions on gut microbiome composition is to produce both an abundance of bacteria associated with good health and to diversify the number of phyla present in the adult gut microbiome.

GUT MICROBIAL FOOD NETWORKS

The response of the gut microbiome to diet is in part determined by trophic interactions among unrelated members of the microbial community, so the success of dietary interventions may depend on the pre-existing microbial environment. Proteins and carbohydrates are broken down by primary fermenters, yielding short-chain fatty acids like acetate, propionate, and butyrate, and gases like hydrogen and carbon dioxide. These fermentation products supply carbon and energy for other community members.[21] The main challenge to microbial fermentation is the production of reducing equivalents that can disrupt oxidation-reduction (redox) balance and interfere with energy production. Species that trap hydrogen as methane (CH3), hydrogen sulfide (H2S), and ammonia (NH4) play critical roles in maintaining redox balance and enhancing the energy-extracting capacity of the microbiome.[22]

For example, by trapping hydrogen in CH3, Archea help *Ruminococcus* double ATP production.[22] The *Ruminoccus/Methanobrevibacter* syntrophic cluster also includes *Candida* and *Prevotella*. *Candida* species cooperate with host amylase to degrade starches to simpler carbohydrates that are fermented by *Prevotella* and *Ruminococcus*. Biofilms containing *Candida albicans* support increased colonization with *Prevotella* species.[23] Fermentation byproducts are then consumed by *Methanobrevibacter*, yielding carbon dioxide and/or methane. *Prevotella* degradation of starch produces small poly- and monosaccharides,[24] which provide *Candida* with additional substrate for fermentation. *Prevotella* can catabolize small polysaccharides to succinate, which is then consumed by *Ruminococcus,* yielding substrate for *Methanobrevibacter*.[25,26] Archeal methanogens play a key role in maintaining the robustness of this network in its response to dietary carbohydrate.

Sulfur-reducing bacteria (SRB) consume hydrogen in the generation of H2S, an autacoid with both pro-[27,28] and anti-inflammatory[29] signaling attributes. Like Archea, SRB are found in about half of human stool specimens[30] and attach directly to colonic mucosa.[30] Although sulfate-reducing activity is found in many phyla, the dominant SRB in the human colon are members of the genus *Desulfovibrio* in the phylum *Proteobacteria*.[31] Dietary sulfur is found in ingested protein and in sulfate and sulfite preservatives added to a variety of foods, like bread, preserved meat, dried fruit, and wine. Sulfate is also present in the common food additive carrageenan. Even without food, sulfur is present in sulfated glycans present in host-derived colonic mucus. Unlike Archaea, which through their syntrophism with *Ruminococcus* grow well in a carbohydrate-rich environment, *Desulfovibrio piger*, is syntrophic with *Bacteroides* species like *B. thetaiotamicron* and thrives when animals are fed a diet high in sugar and fat and low in complex polysaccharides.[32] When the diet lacks complex polysaccharides, *Bacteroides*-derived sulfatases liberate sulfates from mucosal glycans,[33] helping *D. piger* fill its appetite for sulfur.

The carbohydrate responsiveness of the *Prevotella–Ruminococcus–Methan obrevibacter–Candida* cluster and the growth-enhancing effects of *Bacteroides* on *Desulfovibrio* are adaptive. Organisms tend to grow well in environments enriched with their preferred metabolic substrates. Nonetheless, there are numerous human studies that show very different effects or no effect of diet on the taxonomy or the function of the gut microbiome, suggesting that other environmental influences may be stronger than diet. It should be noted that lab rats usually share the same environment.

HUMAN PARADOXES

There are a number of interesting paradoxes in the human microbiome. Vegans and omnivores living in an urban environment may have no significant differences in microbiome composition,[34] although metabolic products of the microbiome—the metabolome—differ markedly.[35] Furthermore, the difference in fecal microbiome composition between vegetarian and omnivore residents of a Slovenian village accounted for less than 4% of microbial variability.[36] These findings contrast sharply with the results of studies that compare people living in modern Western environments with those living in traditional agrarian societies.[37]

In clinical practice, the impact of diet on gut bacterial composition may yield results that are the opposite of what is expected. For Chinese infants with intractable epilepsy, treatment with a high fat, low carbohydrate ketogenic diet induces an increase in *Prevotella* and *Bifidobacteria*, despite the usual finding that growth of these genera is enhanced by carbohydrate feedings.[38] In patients with multiple sclerosis (MS), the impact of ketogenic diet was shown to be biphasic, initially decreasing the already reduced bacterial diversity and abundance of the gut microbiome and then after 12 weeks having the opposite effect by increasing bacterial diversity and abundance. Six months of ketogenic diet yielded a gut microbiome that was not significantly different from healthy controls eating a mixed diet, but it was significantly different from the baseline taxonomy of the MS microbiome.[39]

Clinical characteristics of the host may account for differing responses of the gut microbiome to dietary change. In mice with electrically induced or spontaneous tonic-clonic seizures, a ketogenic diet induces a rapid decrease in bacterial diversity and a marked increase in the growth of *Akkermansia muciniphila*, a strict anaerobe with complex metabolic effects. *Akkermansia* growth in these animals is associated with improved seizure control, apparently a result of elevation of the hippocampal GABA/glutamate ratio.[40] In contrast, BTBR(T+tf/j) (BTBR) mice who manifest a rodent model of autistic spectrum disorder (ASD), have a relative abundance of *Akkermansia* when fed a diet of laboratory chow. A ketogenic diet markedly reduces *Akkermansia* colonization in BTBR mice, with restoration of a normal behavior pattern.[41] Autism in humans may also respond to a ketogenic diet.[42] Magnetic resonance spectroscopy of humans with ASD demonstrates a relative elevation of the striatal GABA/glutamate ratio that correlates with severity of social disruption.[43] The evidence suggests that a ketogenic diet may exert therapeutic benefits in two very different disorders by altering the microbiome in opposite ways that are nonetheless therapeutic for the physiologic disturbance in each disorder.

Going further, these opposing disease-related associations for *Akkermansia muciniphila* have been found in human clinical studies, demonstrating that the relationship between intestinal microbes and health may be case-specific. *Akkermansia muciniphila* is the dominant human species in the phylum *Verrucomicrobia*, and typically accounts for less than 2% of the gut microbiome. *Akkermansia* colonization has been associated with protection against insulin resistance, obesity, and ulcerative colitis.[44] In a study of humans with post-traumatic stress disorder (PTSD), *Verrucomicrobia* and *Akkermansia* were significantly depleted from fecal samples when compared to a control population of individuals with similar trauma history who did not show evidence of PTSD.[45] People with PTSD demonstrate deficits in GABA functionality of specific brain areas when compared with trauma-matched controls.[46] It is possible that the GABA-enhancing effect of *Akkermansia*, which has been demonstrated in mice, exerts a protective effect on stress responses, so that loss of *Akkermansia* predisposes an individual to PTSD. Parkinson's disease, in contrast, is associated with an abundance of *Akkermansia* in stool samples[47,48] and with excessive GABA activity in the pons and putamen.[49]

These studies suggest that disease associations of gut microbes may be pathophysiologic and condition-specific. They also demonstrate the difficulties of translational research utilizing diet-driven microbiome interventions. In the author's clinical experience, dietary prescriptions intended to achieve clinical endpoints through the mediation of the microbiome must be individualized, have well-defined outcome goals, and be based on clinical characteristics of each patient rather than general notions of what constitutes "good" or "bad" bacteria.[50]

DIETARY ALTERATION OF GUT MICROBIAL METABOLISM

The impact of diet on the gut metabolome as it relates to health is presently at the forefront of microbiome research.[51] One prominent example of the focus of this research is the work being done to explore the role of trimethylamine oxide (TMAO) in cardiovascular disease and stroke. Plasma levels of TMAO are positively associated with the risk of major cardiovascular events.[52] One effect of TMAO is increased platelet adherence and promotion of thrombosis.[53] TMAO is the product of gut microbial metabolism of dietary choline to trimethylamine (TMA), followed by hepatic oxidation of TMA to TMAO. In mice, blocking TMAO production by feeding dimethylbutanol, a non-lethal inhibitor of TMA synthesis, prevents the development of choline-induced atherosclerosis, indicating that TMAO contributes to the pathogenesis of arterial disease in this model.[54] Resveratrol, a flavonoid found in red wine, reduces TMA production by the gut microbiome, which is one possible mechanism by which red wine consumption decreases the incidence of coronary heart disease.[55] High fat feeding, on the other hand, has been shown to produce a short-term increase in plasma TMAO among healthy young men.[56]

Researchers at the Cleveland Clinic demonstrated that the gut microbiome of human vegetarians produces significantly less TMA than the gut microbiome of omnivores.[57] A multi-center European study found that reduction of TMAO was associated with adherence to a Mediterranean dietary pattern among vegetarians and omnivores alike.[58] Paradoxically, a Chinese study found that individuals who had already suffered from stroke or transient ischemic attacks had decreased plasma levels of TMAO when compared to controls with asymptomatic atherosclerosis.[59] Clearly, the impact of TMAO reduction on primary or secondary prevention of cerebrovascular disease is uncertain.

The role of the SRB *Desulvovibrio piger* in autism demonstrates another paradox. *D. piger* fermentation produces propionic acid[60] and has been implicated in the etiology of autism spectrum disorders.[61] However, successful fecal transplantation in children with autism significantly improved behavioral abnormalities and at the same time increased the abundance of *Desulfovibrio* along with *Bifidobacteria* and *Prevotella*.[62] Microbial interactions may explain the paradox: *D. piger* alters the phenotype of the more prevalent *Bacteroides* species, reducing their synthesis of propionate,[63] so in a high *Bacteroides* milieu, *D. piger* might decrease total propionate synthesis and *Bifidobacteria* might convert propionate to acetate.[64]

There are three areas in which the impact of diet on the gut microbial metabolome has demonstrated a proven effect on human clinical outcomes: D -lactic acidosis, hyperammonemia, and gut fermentation/irritable bowel syndrome.

D-LACTIC ACIDOSIS

D-lactate, a neurotoxin, is one of the products of microbial fermentation of carbohydrates.[65] D-lactic acidosis is a well-known complication of short bowel syndrome, an
anatomical disorder which allows delivery of a high carbohydrate load to the colon.
Elevation of D-lactate in plasma may occur after various types of abdominal surgery,
as a result of increased intestinal permeability and bacterial translocation across the
intestinal mucosal barrier.[66]

Non-surgical causes of intestinal hyperpermeability also increase absorption
of D-lactate from the intestinal lumen.[67,68] Patients with chronic fatigue syndrome
(CFS) and neurocognitive dysfunction have increased levels of D-lactate producing bacteria in stool, raising the possibility that microbial D-lactate contributes
to symptoms of patients with CFS.[69] Although D-lactic acidosis is usually treated
with antibiotics, diet-induced microbiome alterations allow patients to overcome
neurotoxicity without antibiotics. Reducing consumption of monosaccharides
decreases microbial access to the principle substrates for lactic acid synthesis.[70]
Increasing consumption of oligosaccharides encourages the growth of organisms
like *Bifidobacteria* that produce acetate rather than lactate as the end product of
carbohydrate metabolism. Dietary supplementation with oligosaccharides and
selected probiotics has been shown to reduce neurotoxicity associated with D-lactic
acidosis.[71]

HYPERAMMONEMIA

Ammonia is another well-known neurotoxin, produced in the intestinal tract from
urea through the action of bacterial ureases.[72] Gut-derived ammonia is taken up by
the liver and consumed in the urea cycle. Urea cycle disorders and hepatic cirrhosis
are two major causes of hyperammonemia, but elevated blood ammonia may occur
without any known predisposing factors. Advanced glycation end products (AGE's)
are produced by cooking food, especially high protein foods, in the absence of water
(roasting, broiling, baking, as opposed to steaming or boiling). When rats are fed
chow heated to 125 degrees C, there is a marked increase in their consumption of
AGE's, associated with an increased abundance of *Bacteroides* and *Desulfovibrio*
species, increased protein fermentation and elevated ammonia production.[73] Studies
have illustrated the importance of blood ammonia levels in shaping behavior.
Chinese researchers compared blood ammonia levels of violent male prisoners with
non-prisoner controls who were matched for age and health status and were free
of liver disease. They found relatively high ammonia and relatively low hydrogen
sulfide among the prisoners and concluded that blood ammonia may be a biological
marker of behavioral disorders.[74]

By creating portosystemic shunts, cirrhosis allows absorbed ammonia to
escape hepatic metabolism, increasing blood ammonia, which contributes to the

pathogenesis of hepatic encephalopathy (HE). In addition to direct neurotoxic injury, ammonia alters the function of the blood–brain barrier, impairs intracerebral synthesis of serotonin and dopamine and produces abnormal neurotransmitters like octopamine.[75] Minimal hepatic encephalopathy (MHE) is a common neurocognitive disorder that occurs in 80% of cirrhotic patients[76] and often evades diagnosis.[77] It is characterized by subtle intellectual deficits and psychomotor abnormalities that have significant negative impact on health-related quality of life, impair motor vehicle operation and increase the incidence of vehicular accidents.[78] MHE is associated with altered composition of the gut microbiome, which differs between cirrhotics with or without HE.[79,80] Levels of urease-producing bacteria are positively associated with cognitive dysfunction in cirrhotic patients.[81]

The standard dietary treatment of patients with hyperammonemia due to urea cycle disorders is protein restriction. For patients with hepatic encephalopathy, however, protein restriction is not recommended, because cirrhosis produces malnutrition.[82,83] Instead, reduction of urease-producing bacteria by increasing sources of dietary fiber is successful. Consumption of chick peas, 200 grams per day for three weeks, reduced the level of ammonia-generating bacteria in stools of healthy human subjects.[84] Foods rich in resistant starch such as high amylase maize, peas, and potatoes reduce colonic ammonia generation.[85] Resistant starch has been used along with oligosaccharides and non-urease probiotics to reduce ammonia and improve cognitive dysfunction in people with MHE.[86,87]

GUT FERMENTATION: FRUCTOSE, FRUCTANS, AND IRRITABLE BOWEL SYNDROME

Humans have a limited ability to absorb fructose and what limited ability they do possess varies widely from person to person. When consumption of fructose or its fructan polymers exceeds absorptive capacity, the remaining sugars are fermented by colonic bacteria, producing uncomfortable symptoms like distension, flatulence, pain and altered bowel habits.[88] Many of these people will also experience neuropsychiatric symptoms like fatigue, depression, and anxiety.[89] Most people with these symptoms will ultimately be diagnosed with irritable bowel syndrome (IBS).

A diet low in fructose, fructans, and other fermentable carbohydrates (the low FODMAP diet) has been shown to help symptoms associated with IBS. Furthermore, adoption of a low FODMAP diet produces extensive changes in the gut bacterial microbiome, which occur in the opposite direction of an oligosaccharide-enriched diet: there is a significant decline in *Bifidobacteria* and *Faecalibacterium prausnitzii*, organisms that are ordinarily considered beneficial.[90] Despite depletion of these anti-inflammatory bacteria, cytokine profiles reveal decreased gut inflammation. The production of fecal short-chain fatty acids (SCFA), especially butyrate and acetate, is reduced, although there is no direct correlation between SCFA reduction and clinical improvement.[91]

When compared to a typical Australian diet, a low FODMAP diet reduces levels of *Akkermansia muciniphila* and *Clostridium* cluster XIVA, both considered important taxa in a health-promoting gut microbiome.[92] A study of US children treated with a low FODMAP diet for IBS found that a positive response to the diet was associated with pre-treatment abundance of *Faecalibacterium prausnitzii* and other saccharolytic organisms.[93] The paradox of the low FODMAP diet is that it achieves clinical benefits by reducing the growth of microbes considered to be beneficial. Therefore, the concept of dysbiosis may be relative when examining conditions like irritable bowel syndrome.

MINOR DIETARY COMPONENTS AND THE GUT MICROBIOME

Minor dietary components may have a greater impact on microbial growth and function than do macronutrients. Heating standard laboratory chow to produce AGE's, as mentioned above, increases protein fermentation and ammonia synthesis and reduces the diversity and richness of the microbiome, especially diminishing the *Ruminococcus/Prevotella* cluster.[94] Other minor dietary components with significant impact on the gut microbiome include polyphenols, emulsifiers, non-nutritive sweeteners, and contaminants.[95]

Polyphenols are bioactive non-nutrient plant compounds whose bioavailability and physiologic effects greatly depend on their transformation by components of the gut microbiota. Polyphenols, in return, alter microbial metabolism and growth. The impact of polyphenols on the gut microbiome is largely due to the ability of specific compounds to inhibit or enhance the growth of specific bacteria.[96] The reduction of TMA synthesis by resveratrol is one example that was mentioned above.[97] The benefits of polyphenol consumption for age-related cognitive decline may involve this bidirectional relationship: anti-inflammatory flavonoids need microbial enzymes to increase bioavailability and, in turn, flavonoids enhance the growth and metabolic activity of beneficial microbes.[98] In elderly adults, sleep quality and mental flexibility is positively associated with the abundance of *Verrucomicrobia/Akkermansia* species.[99] Enrichment of *Akkermansia* species is also a feature of the gut microbiome of healthy centenarians.[100] Flavonoids found in cranberries, black raspberries, blueberries, and pomegranate are prebiotic growth enhancers for *Akkermansia muciniphila* and may contribute to healthy aging in part through enhancement of *Akkermansia* carriage.[101,102,103,104,105]

Dietary emulsifiers like Polysorbate 80 and carboxymethylcellulose increase the inflammatory potential of the gut microbiome, in particular increasing the immunogenicity of the multi-species protein flagellin.[106] At the same time, they decrease the thickness of the gastrointestinal mucus layer and promote bacterial translocation.[107] Non-nutritive sweeteners like aspartame and sucralose are bacteriostatic. Their consumption by rats or mice alters the gut microbiome in ways that decrease insulin sensitivity.[108] The herbicide glyphosate is a common food contaminant, because of its widespread agricultural use. Glyphosate inhibits the Shikimate pathway for synthesis of aromatic amino acids. Even when dietary aromatic amino acids are abundant, exposing rats to glyphosate alters the function of their gut microbiome, decreasing synthesis of acetate and elevating fecal pH.[109] However, the impact of glyphosate may be age and sex-dependent. Female rats[110] and F1 pups[111] exposed to glyphosate at levels common in the North American diet demonstrate a significant decrease in *Lactobacillus* species, but this effect is not observed in adult males.

EFFECTS OF EXERCISE ON THE GUT MICROBIOME

The effects of exercise on the gut microbiome are hard to separate from changes in body weight or diet, which often accompany changes in physical activity. However, increasing cardiorespiratory fitness (CRF) is associated with increasing taxonomic diversity and richness of gut bacteria, and there is evidence to suggest that activity levels play a critical role in shaping the gut microbiome. For example, among Spanish women, an active, as opposed to a sedentary, lifestyle was associated with increased abundance of *Faecalibacterium prausnitzii, Roseburia hominis, and Akkermansia muciniphila*, species that are generally associated with better health.[112,113] Furthermore, Canadian researchers compared fecal bacteria of healthy individuals with varying CRF but similar body weight and dietary intakes.[114] CRF was positively associated with fecal butyrate concentration and the concentration of several butyrate-producing taxa: *Clostridiales, Roseburia, Lachnospiraceae,* and *Erysipelotrichaceae*. It is likely that regular exercise or high levels of CRF encourage the growth of gut bacteria that convert lactate to butyrate, enhancing energy harvest.[115]

A study of cyclists found enrichment of *Prevotella* and enhanced carbohydrate and amino acid catabolism by *Prevotella* species when compared to non-cyclist controls. Competitive cyclists (as opposed to amateurs) also showed an abundance of *Methanobrevibacter smithii* transcripts.[116] This organism consumes hydrogen ions to produce methane and, as described above, enhances the robustness of the *Prevotella–Ruminococcus* saccharolytic cluster. Among professional rugby players, serum levels of creatinine kinase, a marker of exercise intensity, are positively associated with taxonomic diversity and the abundance of *Akkermansia* species.[117] Finally, a study in mice found that voluntary wheel running affected the gut microbiome in a distinctly different fashion than forced treadmill running, indicating a modifying role of stress on exercise-induced changes of gut bacteria.[118]

HOW STRESS AND INFLAMMATION IMPACT THE GUT MICROBIOME

Bacteria both synthesize and respond to hormones and neurotransmitters: *Lactobacillus* species produce acetylcholine and gamma-aminobutyrate (GABA); *Bifidobacterium* species produce GABA; *Escherichia* produce norepinephrine, serotonin, and dopamine; *Streptococcus* and *Enterococcus* produce serotonin; *Bacillus* species produce norepinephrine and dopamine.[119] These organisms are clearly responsive to human hormones and neurotransmitters,[120] which have the potential to impact their growth and virulence.

Many studies illustrate the important role stress plays in shaping the gut microbiome. A study of college students undergoing the stress of final examinations found a decrease in the relative concentration of lactic acid bacteria in feces following the examination[121] (speciation was not performed). Lactic acid bacteria have immunomodulating effects[122,123] and may influence the broader composition of the gut microbiome.[124] In another study, Bailey and colleagues stressed mice with a process called social disruption (SDR), which significantly alters bacterial community structure in the cecum, especially when the microbiota are assessed immediately after exposure to the social stressor. SDR reduces the relative abundance of *Bacteroides*, while increasing the relative abundance of *Clostridium* species. SDR also increases circulating levels of inflammatory cytokines, IL-6 in particular. Cytokine changes correlate with stress-induced changes in microbiome composition.[125]

This impact can even be seen on a molecular level. The interbacterial communication system known as quorum sensing (QS) utilizes hormone-like compounds referred to as inducers to regulate bacterial gene expression. Enterohemorrhagic *Escherichia coli* (EHEC) serotype O157:H7 is responsible for outbreaks of bloody diarrhea. Sperandio and colleagues showed that exogenous epinephrine is an inducer of the 0157:H7 virulence factor.[126] EHEC growing in a stressed host may be more virulent than in a non-stressed host.

Physiologic concentrations of norepinephrine also enhance the growth of *E. coli* and other potentially pathogenic *Proteobacteria*.[127] These organisms are a major source of lipopolysaccharides (LPS) that provoke the release of inflammatory cytokines, interleukin18 (IL-18) in particular, by gut macrophages.[128] Bacterial peptides further induce intestinal macrophages and T-cells to produce the cytokines interleukin-1beta (IL-1b) and tumor necrosis factor-alpha (TNFa).[129] The adult human gut is believed to contain about one gram of LPS. Parenteral administration of LPS to humans in nanogram quantities (0.4 nanogram per kilogram body weight) increases plasma concentration of pro-inflammatory cytokines IL-6 and TNFa, along with salivary and plasma cortisol and plasma norepinephrine. These changes are accompanied by depressed mood, increased anxiety and impaired long-term memory for emotional stimuli.[130] In addition, visceral pain sensitivity thresholds are reduced and visceral pain (provoked by rectal distension) is rated as more unpleasant following administration of low dose LPS.[131] Increased LPS exposure, by increasing levels of inflammatory cytokines, creates a vicious cycle. Synthesis of nitric oxide, a universal corollary of inflammation, produces a nitrate-rich milieu, which encourages further growth of *Proteobacteria*.[132]

Elevated exposure to gut microbiome-derived LPS (endotoxemia) may occur in the elderly, in whom it is diminished by yogurt consumption,[133] and secondary to increased intestinal permeability resulting from extreme physiologic stress,[134] ethanol exposure[135] or a "fast-food style" Western diet, high in both carbohydrate and saturated fat.[136] Increased intestinal permeability has been described in patients with CFS,[137] fibromyalgia, and complex regional pain syndrome.[138]

Although stress-induced dysbiosis and its complications are well documented, there have been very few attempts to study the impact of stress management alone on the microbiome. Published papers used mindfulness and yoga as part of complex multimodal therapies.[139,140] Meditation by itself may interrupt the stress-inflammation cycle by reducing intestinal hyperpermeability,[141] which would help to alleviate endotoxemia in stressed individuals.

SUBSTANCE USE AND THE MICROBIOME

Exposure to substances that range from alcohol and tobacco to over-the-counter medications and personal hygiene and cleaning products may impact gut microbial taxonomy or function, sometimes in conjunction with a change in intestinal permeability.

ALCOHOL

Alcohol use and abuse have a definite impact on the diversity and health of the gut microbiome. Colon biopsies of patients with alcohol use disorder show a decrease in *Bacteroidites* and an increase in *Proteobacteria,* a pattern that is likely to be associated with inflammation. This dysbiosis is associated with increased levels of circulating endotoxin.[142] *Leclerq* and colleagues found that 30 to 50% of their subjects with alcohol use disorder had increased intestinal permeability, which was associated with changes in the fecal microbiome (primarily with loss of *Bifidobacteria* and *Faecalibacterium prausnitzii)* and with increased symptoms of withdrawal and alcohol cravings.[143] Cessation of drinking allowed *Bifidobacteria* to re-populate but provided no restoration of depleted *Faecalibacterium prausnitzii.*[144] They believe that chronic alcohol use produces dysbiosis, which in turn permits increased permeability, absorption of bacterial endotoxins and systemic inflammation. Those subjects for whom permeability did not improve after three weeks of abstention were more likely to have mood disorders and alcohol craving than others entering a rehabilitation program. Furthermore, Russian researchers found a decrease in butyrate-producing bacteria in association with alcohol dependence.[145]

TOBACCO

Observational studies in humans find that smoking tobacco, but not the use of electronic cigarettes, is associated with decreased diversity in the gut microbiome, accompanied by increased abundance of *Prevotella* and reduced abundance of *Bacteroides.*[146] This may reflect decreased diversity of the oral microbiome induced by cigarette smoking.[147] A small group of smokers was followed for several weeks after entering a smoking cessation program. Following abstention, there was an increase in microbial diversity with profound shifts in the fecal microbiome: an increase of *Firmicutes* and *Actinobacteria* and reduction of *Bacteroidetes* and *Proteobacteria.*[148] French scientists even speculate that the post-cessation microbial shifts enhance energy extraction from food and may explain the tendency to gain weight that occurs when tobacco is stopped.[149]

Animal experiments reveal a complex effect of tobacco smoke on the gut microbiome. Exposure of mice to cigarette smoke for 24 weeks produced a striking increase of *Lachnospiraceae* species in the colon. This family, a butyrate producer in the *Firmicutes* phylum, appears to have protective effects in the colon.[150] Its abundance in mice is associated with increased mRNA expression of genes regulating intestinal and colonic mucus (MUC2, MUC3, and MUC4). The colonic response to tobacco smoke in mice, mediated by *Lachnospiraceae,* might explain the protective effect of current cigarette smoking on ulcerative colitis, a disorder associated with a significant deficit in the activation of MUC2, MUC3, and MUC4 genes in humans.[151]

Interestingly, Parkinson's disease is another human disease in which cigarette smoking appears to have a protective effect. The gut microbiome of patients with early Parkinson's disease shows a significant decrease in abundance of several genera of *Lachnospiraceae*.[152] Some researchers attribute the preventive effect of cigarette smoking on the incidence of Parkinson disease to tobacco-induced alterations of gut bacteria.[153] Enhanced growth of *Lachnospiraceae* does not require tobacco smoke. It has also been demonstrated in response to feeding polyphenols: genistein, an isoflavonoid derived from soy,[154] and an extract of flavonoids derived from raspberry.[155]

MEDICATIONS

Almost one-quarter of non-antibiotic medications intended for human use impact the growth of at least one bacterial strain *in vitro*.[156] Dutch researchers have identified distinctive microbiome signatures associated with the use of several classes of drugs, including statins, antidepressants, and proton pump inhibitors (PPIs).[157] PPIs had the greatest impact on the microbiome, affecting 20% of taxa.

Self-administration of non-prescription drugs and/or dietary supplements can be viewed as a lifestyle choice. Omeprazole, esomeprazole, and lansoprazole are proton pump inhibitors (PPIs) available without prescription in the United States and used by millions of people for relief of dyspeptic symptoms like acid reflux and indigestion. Among British twins discordant for PPI use, regular use of PPIs is associated with decreased diversity and richness of the fecal microbiome and increased growth of *Streptococcus* species in the mouth and upper GI tract.[158] A prospective Japanese study found that four weeks of PPI use among patients with esophagitis increased fecal abundance of *Streptococcus* and *Lactobacillus* species when compared to pre-treatment levels.[159] *Streptococcal* overgrowth caused by PPI therapy has been implicated in the persistence of dyspepsia despite acid suppression.[160] Increased growth of *Enterococcus* induced by PPIs is associated with increased risk of steatohepatitis in humans and laboratory animals.[161] When duodenal or jejunenal aspirate is used as the diagnostic tool, PPI use is associated with an increased incidence of small intestinal bacterial overgrowth (SIBO).[162] In a Swiss study using duodenal aspirates obtained through endoscopy, omeprazole produced SIBO in 53% of patients and cimetidine, a histamine H2 antagonist that produces a less robust reduction of gastric acidity, produced SIBO in 17% of patients after four weeks. PPI-induced dysbiosis increases the incidence of *Clostridium difficile* colitis.[163]

CONCLUSION

Human physiology is strongly dependent on its interaction with gut microbial composition and function. Some important associations between lifestyle and health are mediated at least in part by the impact of lifestyle decisions on the gut microbiome. Although lifestyle changes can be effective in the treatment of disease, dietary interventions for changing the microbiome to improve clinical outcomes need to be tailored to the specific characteristics of individual patients. Furthermore, clinicians must recognize that any intervention may have multiple effects because of the interdependence of different microbial species on each other.

NOTES

1. Filippo C, Cavalieri D, Di Paola M, Ramazzotti M, Poullet JB, Massart S, Collini S, Pieraccini G, Lionetti P. Impact of diet in shaping gut microbiota revealed by a comparative study in children from Europe and rural Africa. *Proc Natl Acad Sci USA.* 2010;107:14691–6.

2. Eckburg PB, Bik EM, Bernstein CN, Purdom E, Dethlefsen L, Sargent M, Gill SR, Nelson KE, Relman DA. Diversity of the human intestinal microbial flora. *Science.* 2005;308:1635–8.

3. Turnbaugh PJ, Quince C, Faith JJ, McHardy AC, Yatsunenko T, Niazi F, Affourtit J, Egholm M, Henrissat B, Knight R, Gordon JI. Organismal, genetic, and transcriptional variation in the deeply sequenced gut microbiomes of identical twins. *Proc Natl Acad Sci USA.* 2010;107:7503–8.

4. Turnbaugh PJ, Gordon JI. The core gut microbiome, energy balance, and obesity. *J Physiol.* 2009;587:4153–8.

5. Rajilic-Stojanovic M, Heilig HG, Molenaar D, Kajander K, Surakka A, Smidt H, de Vos WM. Development and application of the human intestinal tract chip, a phylogenetic microarray: analysis of universally conserved phylotypes in the abundant microbiota of young and elderly adults. *Environ Microbiol.* 2009;11(7):1736–51.

6. Dethlefsen L, Eckburg PB, Bik EM, Relman DA. Assembly of the human intestinal microbiota. *Trends Ecol Evol.* 2006;21:517–23.

7. Daphna Rothschild D, Weisbrod O, Segal E, Environment dominates over host genetics in shaping human gut microbiota. *Nature.* 2018;555:210–5. doi: 10.1038/nature25973.

8. Remely M, Hippe B, Geretschlaeger I, Stegmayer S, Hoefinger I, Haslberger A. Increased gut microbiota diversity and abundance of *Faecalibacterium prausnitzii* and *Akkermansia* after fasting: a pilot study. *Wien Klin Wochenschr.* 2015;127(9–10): 394–8.

9. Han M, Wang C, Liu P, Li D, Li Y, Ma X. Dietary fiber gap and host gut microbiota. *Protein Pept Lett.* 2017;24(5):388–96. doi: 10.2174/0929866524666170220113312.

10. Joyce SA, Gahan CG. The gut microbiota and the metabolic health of the host. *Curr Opin Gastroenterol.* 2014;30(2):120–7.

11. Tap J, Mondot S, Levenez F, Pelletier E, Caron C, Furet JP, Ugarte E, Muñoz-Tamayo R, Paslier DL, Nalin R, Dore J, Leclerc M. Towards the human intestinal microbiota phylogenetic core. *Environ Microbiol.* 2009;11(10):2574–84.

12. Wu GD, Chen J, Hoffmann C, Bittinger K, Chen YY, Keilbaugh SA, Bewtra M, Knights D, Walters WA, Knight R, Sinha R, Gilroy E, Gupta K, Baldassano R, Nessel L, Li H, Bushman FD, Lewis JD. Linking long-term dietary patterns with gut microbial enterotypes. *Science.* 2011;334(6052):105–8.

13. Simpson HL, Campbell BJ. Dietary fibre-microbiota interactions. *Aliment Pharmacol Ther.* 2015;42(2):158–79. doi: 10.1111/apt.13248.

14. Walker WA. Initial intestinal colonization in the human infant and immune homeostasis. *Ann Nutr Metab.* 2013;63(Suppl 2):8–15.

15. El-Semman IE, Karlsson FH, Shoaie S, Nookaew I, Soliman TH, Nielsen J. Genome-scale metabolic reconstructions of *Bifidobacterium adolescentis* L2-32 and *Faecalibacterium prausnitzii* A2-165 and their interaction. *BMC Syst Biol.* 2014;8:41. doi: 10.1186/1752-0509-8-41.

16. Bottacini F, van Sinderen D, Ventura M. Omics of bifidobacteria: research and insights into their health-promoting activities. *Biochem J.* 2017;474(24):4137–52. doi: 10.1042/ BCJ20160756.

17. Claesson MJ, Jeffery IB, Conde S, Power SE, O/'Connor EM, Cusack S, Harris HMB, Coakley M, Lakshminarayanan B, O/'Sullivan O, Fitzgerald GF, Deane J, O/'Connor M, Harnedy N, O/'Connor K, O/'Mahony D, van Sinderen D, Wallace M, Brennan L,

Stanton C, Marchesi JR, Fitzgerald AP, Shanahan F, Hill C, Ross RP, O/'Toole PW. Gut microbiota composition correlates with diet and health in the elderly. *Nature.* 2012;488(7410):178–84. doi: 10.1038/nature11319.

18. Hoffmann C, Dollive S, Grunberg S, Chen J, Li H, Wu GD, Lewis JD, Bushman FD. Archaea and fungi of the human gut microbiome: correlations with diet and bacterial residents. *PLoS One.* 2013;8(6):e66019. doi: 10.1371/journal.pone.0066019.

19. Albenberg LG, Wu GD. Diet and the intestinal microbiome: associations, functions, and implications for health and disease. *Gastroenterology.* 2014;146(6):1564–72.

20. Healey GR, Murphy R, Brough L, Butts CA, Coad J. Interindividual variability in gut microbiota and host response to dietary interventions. *Nutr Rev.* 2017;75(12):1059–80. doi: 10.1093/nutrit/nux062.

21. Fischbach MA, Sonnenburg JL. Eating for two: how metabolism establishes interspecies interactions in the gut. *Cell Host Microbe.* 2011;10(4):336–47.

22. Stams AJ, Plugge CM. Electron transfer in syntrophic communities of anaerobic bacteria and archaea. *Nat Rev Microbiol.* 2009;7(8):568–77.

23. Janus MM, Crielaard W, Volgenant CM, van der Veen MH, Brandt BW, Krom BP. *Candida albicans* alters the bacterial microbiome of early in vitro oral biofilms. *J Oral Microbiol.* 2017;9(1):1270613. doi: 10.1080/20002297.2016.1270613. eCollection 2017.

24. Downes J, Tanner AC, Dewhirst FE, Wade WG. *Prevotella saccharolytica* sp. nov., isolated from the human oral cavity. *Int J Syst Evol Microbiol.* 2010;60:2458–61.

25. Kovatcheva-Datchary P, Egert M, Maathuis A, Rajilic-Stojanovic M, de Graaf AA, Smidt H, de Vos WM, Venema K. Linking phylogenetic identities of bacteria to starch fermentation in an in vitro model of the large intestine by RNA-based stable isotope probing. *Environ Microbiol.* 2009;11:914–26.

26. Purushe J, Fouts DE, Morrison M, White BA, Mackie RI; North American Consortium for Rumen Bacteria, Coutinho PM, Henrissat B, Nelson KE. Comparative genome analysis of *Prevotella ruminicola* and *Prevotella bryantii*: insights into their environmental niche. *Microb Ecol.* 2010;60:721–9.

27. Pitcher MC, Beatty ER, Cummings JH. The contribution of sulphate reducing bacteria and 5-aminosalicylic acid to faecal sulphide in patients with ulcerative colitis. *Gut.* 2000;46(1):64–72.

28. Levine J, Ellis CJ, Furne JK, Springfield J, Levitt MD. Fecal hydrogen sulfide production in ulcerative colitis. *Am J Gastroenterol.* 1998;93(1):83–7.

29. Wallace JL, Vong L, McKnight W, Dicay M, Martin GR. Endogenous and exogenous hydrogen sulfide promotes resolution of colitis in rats. *Gastroenterology.* 2009;137(2):569–78, e1.

30. Stewart JA, Chadwick VS, Murray A. Carriage, quantification, and predominance of methanogens and sulfate-reducing bacteria in faecal samples. *Lett Appl Microbiol.* 2006;43(1):58–63.

31. Scanlan PD, Shanahan F, Marchesi JR. Culture-independent analysis of desulfovibrios in the human distal colon of healthy, colorectal cancer and polypectomized individuals. *FEMS Microbiol Ecol.* 2009;69(2):213–21.

32. Rey FE, Gonzalez MD, Cheng J, Wu M, Ahern PP, Gordon JI. Metabolic niche of a prominent sulfate-reducing human gut bacterium. *Proc Natl Acad Sci USA.* 2013;110(33):13582–7. doi: 10.1073/pnas.1312524110.

33. Benjdia A, Martens EC, Gordon JI, Berteau O. Sulfatases and a radical S-adenosyl-L-methionine (AdoMet) enzyme are key for mucosal foraging and fitness of the prominent human gut symbiont, *Bacteroides thetaiotaomicron. J Biol Chem.* 2011;286(29):25973–82.

34. Federici E, Prete R, Lazzi C, Pellegrini N, Moretti M, Corsetti A, Cenci G. Bacterial composition, genotoxicity, and cytotoxicity of fecal samples from individuals consuming omnivorous or vegetarian diets. *Front Microbiol.* 2017;8:300. doi: 10.3389/fmicb.2017.00300. eCollection 2017.

35. Wu GD, Compher C, Chen EZ, Smith SA, Shah RD, Bittinger K, Chehoud C, Albenberg LG, Nessel L, Gilroy E, Star J, Weljie AM, Flint HJ, Metz DC, Bennett MJ, Li H, Bushman FD, Lewis JD. Comparative metabolomics in vegans and omnivores reveal constraints on diet-dependent gut microbiota metabolite production. *Gut.* 2016;65(1):63–72. doi: 10.1136/gutjnl-2014-308209. Epub 2014 Nov 26.

36. Matijašić BB, Obermajer T, Lipoglavšek L, Grabnar I, Avguštin G, Rogelj I. Association of dietary type with fecal microbiota in vegetarians and omnivores in Slovenia. *Eur J Nutr.* 2014;53(4):1051–64. doi: 10.1007/s00394-013-0607-6. Epub 2013 Oct 31.

37. Simpson HL, Campbell BJ. Review article: dietary fibre-microbiota interactions. *Aliment Pharmacol Ther.* 2015;42(2):158–79. doi: 10.1111/apt.13248.

38. Xie G, Zhou Q, Qiu CZ, Dai WK, Wang HP, Li YH, Liao JX, Lu XG, Lin SF, Ye JH, Ma ZY, Wang WJ. Ketogenic diet poses a significant effect on imbalanced gut microbiota in infants with refractory epilepsy. *World J Gastroenterol.* 2017;23(33):6164–71. doi: 10.3748/wjg.v23.i33.6164.

39. Swidsinski A, Dörffel Y, Loening-Baucke V, Gille C, Göktas Ö, Reißhauer A, Neuhaus J, Weylandt KH, Guschin A, Bock M. Reduced mass and diversity of the colonic microbiome in patients with multiple sclerosis and their improvement with ketogenic diet. *Front Microbiol.* 2017;8:1141. doi: 10.3389/fmicb.2017.01141. eCollection 2017.

40. Olson CA, Vuong HE, Yano JM, Liang QY, Nusbaum DJ, Hsiao EY. The gut microbiota mediates the anti-seizure effects of the ketogenic diet. *Cell.* 2018;173(7):1728–41. e13. doi: 10.1016/j.cell.2018.04.027.

41. Newell C, Bomhof MR, Reimer RA, Hittel DS, Rho JM, Shearer J. Ketogenic diet modifies the gut microbiota in a murine model of autism spectrum disorder. *Mol Autism.* 2016;7(1):37. doi: 10.1186/s13229-016-0099-3.

42. El-Rashidy O, El-Baz F, El-Gendy Y, Khalaf R, Reda D, Saad K. Ketogenic diet versus gluten free casein free diet in autistic children: a case-control study. *Metab Brain Dis.* 2017;32(6):1935–41. doi: 10.1007/s11011-017-0088-z.

43. Horder J, Petrinovic MM, Mendez MA, Bruns A, Takumi T, Spooren W, Barker GJ, Künnecke B, Murphy DG. Glutamate and GABA in autism spectrum disorder – a translational magnetic resonance spectroscopy study in man and rodent models. *Transl Psychiatry.* 2018;8(1):106. doi: 10.1038/s41398-018-0155-1.

44. Derrien M, Belzer C, de Vos WM. Akkermansia muciniphila and its role in regulating host functions. *Microb Pathog.* 2017;106:171–81. doi: 10.1016/j.micpath.2016.02.005.

45. Hemmings SMJ, Malan-Müller S, van den Heuvel LL, Demmitt BA, Stanislawski MA, Smith DG, Bohr AD, Stamper CE, Hyde ER, Morton JT, Marotz CA, Siebler PH, Braspenning M, Van Criekinge W, Hoisington AJ, Brenner LA, Postolache TT, McQueen MB, Krauter KS, Knight R, Seedat S, Lowry CA. The microbiome in posttraumatic stress disorder and trauma-exposed controls: an exploratory study. *Psychosom Med.* 2017;79(8):936–46. doi: 10.1097/PSY.0000000000000512.

46. Averill LA, Purohit P, Averill CL, Boesl MA, Krystal JH, Abdallah CG. Glutamate dysregulation and glutamatergic therapeutics for PTSD: evidence from human studies. *Neurosci Lett.* 2017;649:147–55. doi: 10.1016/j.neulet.2016.11.064.

47. Heintz-Buschart A, Pandey U, Wicke T, Sixel-Döring F, Janzen A, Sittig-Wiegand E, Trenkwalder C, Oertel WH[3], Mollenhauer B[2,5], Wilmes P[1]. The nasal and gut microbiome in Parkinson's disease and idiopathic rapid eye movement sleep behavior disorder. *Mov Disord.* 2018;33(1):88–98. doi: 10.1002/mds.27105.

48. Gerhardt S, Mohajeri MH. Changes of colonic bacterial composition in Parkinson's disease and other neurodegenerative diseases. *Nutrients*. 2018;10(6). pii: E708. doi: 10.3390/nu10060708.

49. Emir UE, Tuite PJ, Öz G. Elevated pontine and putamenal GABA levels in mild-moderate Parkinson disease detected by 7 tesla proton MRS. *PLoS One*. 2012;7(1):e30918.

50. Galland L. The gut microbiome and the brain. *J Med Food*. 2014;17(12):1261–72. doi: 10.1089/jmf.2014.7000.

51. Kinross J, Li JV, Muirhead LJ, Nicholson J. Nutritional modulation of the metabonome: applications of metabolic phenotyping in translational nutritional research. *Curr Opin Gastroenterol*. 2014;30(2):196–207. doi: 10.1097/MOG.

52. Tang WH, Wang Z, Levison BS, Koeth RA, Britt EB, Fu X, Wu Y, Hazen SL. Intestinal microbial metabolism of phosphatidylcholine and cardiovascular risk. *N Engl J Med*. 2013;368(17):1575–84. doi: 10.1056/NEJMoa1109400.

53. Zhu W, Gregory JC, Org E, Buffa JA, Gupta N, Wang Z, Li L, Fu X, Wu Y, Mehrabian M, Sartor RB, McIntyre TM, Silverstein RL, Tang WHW, DiDonato JA, Brown JM, Lusis AJ, Hazen SL. Gut microbial metabolite TMAO enhances platelet hyperreactivity and thrombosis risk. *Cell*. 2016;165(1):111–24. doi: 10.1016/j.cell.2016.02.011.

54. Wang Z, Roberts AB, Buffa JA, Levison BS, Zhu W, Org E, Gu X, Huang Y, Zamanian-Daryoush M, Culley MK, DiDonato AJ, Fu X, Hazen JE, Krajcik D, DiDonato JA, Lusis AJ, Hazen SL. Non-lethal inhibition of gut microbial trimethylamine production for the treatment of atherosclerosis. *Cell*. 2015;163(7):1585–95. doi: 10.1016/j.cell.2015.11.055.

55. Lyu M, Wang YF, Fan GW, Wang XY, Xu SY, Zhu Y. Balancing herbal medicine and functional food for prevention and treatment of cardiometabolic diseases through modulating gut microbiota. *Front Microbiol*. 2017;8:2146. doi: 10.3389/fmicb.2017.02146.

56. Boutagy NE, Neilson AP, Osterberg KL, Smithson AT, Englund TR, Davy BM, Hulver MW, Davy KP. Short-term high-fat diet increases postprandial trimethylamine-N-oxide in humans. *Nutr Res*. 2015;35(10):858–64. doi: 10.1016/j.nutres.2015.07.002.

57. Koeth RA, Wang Z, Levison BS, Buffa JA, Org E, Sheehy BT, Britt EB, Fu X, Wu Y, Li L, Smith JD, DiDonato JA, Chen J, Li H, Wu GD, Lewis JD, Warrier M, Brown JM, Krauss RM, Tang WH, Bushman FD, Lusis AJ, Hazen SL. Intestinal microbiota metabolism of L-carnitine, a nutrient in red meat, promotes atherosclerosis. *Nat Med*. 2013;19(5):576–85. doi: 10.1038/nm.3145.

58. De Filippis F, Pellegrini N, Vannini L, Jeffery IB, La Storia A, Laghi L, Serrazanetti DI, Di Cagno R, Ferrocino I, Lazzi C, Turroni S, Cocolin L, Brigidi P, Neviani E, Gobbetti M, O'Toole PW, Ercolini D. High-level adherence to a Mediterranean diet beneficially impacts the gut microbiota and associated metabolome. *Gut*. 2016;65(11):1812–21. doi: 10.1136/gutjnl-2015-309957.

59. Yin J, Liao SX, He Y, Wang S, Xia GH, Liu FT, Zhu JJ, You C, Chen Q, Zhou L, Pan SY, Zhou HW. Dysbiosis of gut microbiota with reduced trimethylamine-N-oxide level in patients with large-artery atherosclerotic stroke or transient ischemic attack. *J Am Heart Assoc*. 2015;4(11). pii: e002699. doi: 10.1161/JAHA.115.002699.

60. MacFabe DF. Enteric short-chain fatty acids: microbial messengers of metabolism, mitochondria, and mind: implications in autism spectrum disorders. *Microb Ecol Health Dis*. 2015;26:28177.

61. Finegold SM, Downes J, Summanen PH. Microbiology of regressive autism. *Anaerobe*. 2012;18(2):260–2. doi: 10.1016/j.anaerobe.2011.12.018.

62. Kang DW, Adams JB, Gregory AC, Borody T, Chittick L, Fasano A, Khoruts A, Geis E, Maldonado J, McDonough-Means S, Pollard EL, Roux S, Sadowsky MJ, Lipson KS, Sullivan MB, Caporaso JG, Krajmalnik-Brown R. Microbiota transfer therapy alters gut ecosystem and improves gastrointestinal and autism symptoms: an open-label study. *Microbiome*. 2017;5(1):10. doi: 10.1186/s40168-016-0225-7.

63. Rey FE, Gonzalez MD, Cheng J, Wu M, Ahern PP, Gordon JI. Metabolic niche of a prominent sulfate-reducing human gut bacterium. *Proc Natl Acad Sci USA*. 2013;110(33):13582–7. doi: 10.1073/pnas.1312524110.

64. Kaneko T, Mori H, Iwata M, Meguro S. Growth stimulator for bifidobacteria produced by *Propionibacterium freudenreichii* and several intestinal bacteria. *J Dairy Sci*. 1994;77(2):393–404.

65. Thurn JR, Pierpont GL, Ludvigsen CW, Eckfeldt JH. D-lactate encephalopathy. *Am J Med*. 1985;79(6):717–21.

66. Qiao Z, Li Z, Li J, Lu L, Lv Y, Li J. Bacterial translocation and change in intestinal permeability in patients after abdominal surgery. *J Huazhong Univ Sci Technolog Med Sci*. 2009;29(4):486–91.

67. Zhao Y, Qin G, Sun Z, Che D, Bao N, Zhang X. Effects of soybean agglutinin on intestinal barrier permeability and tight junction protein expression in weaned piglets. *Int J Mol Sci*. 2011;12(12):8502–12.

68. Ying C, Chunmin Y, Qingsen L, Mingzhou G, Yunsheng Y, Gaoping M, Ping W. Effects of simulated weightlessness on tight junction protein occludin and Zonula Occluden-1 expression levels in the intestinal mucosa of rats. *J Huazhong Univ Sci Technolog Med Sci*. 2011;31(1):26–32.

69. Sheedy JR, Wettenhall RE, Scanlon D, Gooley PR, Lewis DP, McGregor N, Stapleton DI, Butt HL, De Meirleir KL. Increased d-lactic acid intestinal bacteria in patients with chronic fatigue syndrome. *In Vivo*. 2009;23(4):621–8.

70. Mayne AJ, Handy DJ, Preece MA, George RH, Booth IW. Dietary management of D-lacticacidosis in short bowel syndrome. *Arch Dis Child*. 1990;65(2):229–31.

71. Takahashi K, Terashima H, Kohno K, Ohkohchi N. A stand-alone synbiotic treatment for the prevention of D-lactic acidosis in short bowel syndrome. *Int Surg*. 2013;98(2):110–3.

72. Qureshi MO, Khokhar N, Shafqat F. Ammonia levels and the severity of hepatic encephalopathy. *J Coll Physicians Surg Pak*. 2014;24(3):160–3.

73. Qu W, Yuan X, Zhao J, Zhang Y, Hu J, Wang J, Li J. Dietary advanced glycation end products modify gut microbial composition and partially increase colon permeability in rats. *Mol Nutr Food Res*. 2017;61(10). doi: 10.1002/mnfr.201700118.

74. Duan Y, Wu X, Liang S, Jin F. Elevated blood ammonia level is a potential biological risk factor of behavioral disorders in prisoners. *Behav Neurol*. 2015;2015:797862. doi: 10.1155/2015/797862.

75. Skowrońska M, Albrecht J. Alterations of blood brain barrier function in hyperammonemia: an overview. *Neurotox Res*. 2012;21(2):236–44.

76. Kawaguchi T, Taniguchi E, Sata M. Effects of oral branched-chain amino acids on hepatic encephalopathy and outcome in patients with liver cirrhosis. *Nutr Clin Pract*. 2013;28(5):580–8.

77. Irimia R, Stanciu C, Cojocariu C, Sfarti C, Trifan A. Oral glutamine challenge improves the performance of psychometric tests for the diagnosis of minimal hepatic encephalopathy in patients with liver cirrhosis. *J Gastrointestin Liver Dis*. 2013;22(3): 277–81.

78. Montgomery JY, Bajaj JS. Advances in the evaluation and management of minimal hepatic encephalopathy. *Curr Gastroenterol Rep*. 2011;13(1):26–33.

79. Bajaj JS, Ridlon JM, Hylemon PB, Thacker LR, Heuman DM, Smith S, Sikaroodi M, Gillevet PM. Linkage of gut microbiome with cognition in hepatic encephalopathy. *Am J Physiol Gastrointest Liver Physiol*. 2012;302(1):G168–75.

80. Bajaj JS, Hylemon PB, Ridlon JM, Heuman DM, Daita K, White MB, Monteith P, Noble NA, Sikaroodi M, Gillevet PM. Colonic mucosal microbiome differs from stool microbiome in cirrhosis and hepatic encephalopathy and is linked to cognition and inflammation. *Am J Physiol Gastrointest Liver Physiol*. 2012;303(6):G675–85.

81. Zhang Z, Zhai H, Geng J, Yu R, Ren H, Fan H, Shi P. Large-scale survey of gut microbiota associated with MHE via 16S rRNA-based pyrosequencing. *Am J Gastroenterol.* 2013;108(10):1601–11.
82. Singh RH. Nutritional management of patients with urea cycle disorders. *J Inherit Metab Dis.* 2007;30(6):880–7.
83. Cabral CM, Burns DL. Low-protein diets for hepatic encephalopathy debunked: let them eat steak. *Nutr Clin Pract.* 2011;26(2):155–9. doi: 10.1177/0884533611400086.
84. Fernando WM, Hill JE, Zello GA, Tyler RT, Dahl WJ, Van Kessel AG. Diets supplemented with chickpea or its main oligosaccharide component raffinose modify faecal microbial composition in healthy adults. *Benef Microbes.* 2010;1(2):197–207. doi: 10.3920/BM2009.0027.
85. Wutzke KD, Tisztl M, Salewski B, Glass Ä. Dietary fibre-rich resistant starches promote ammonia detoxification in the human colon as measured by lactose-[^{15}N$_2$]ureide. *Isotopes Environ Health Stud.* 2015;51(4):488–96. doi: 10.1080/10256016.2015.1092967.
86. Malaguarnera M, Greco F, Barone G, Gargante MP, Malaguarnera M, Toscano MA. *Bifidobacterium longum* with fructo-oligosaccharide (FOS) treatment in minimal hepatic encephalopathy: a randomized, double-blind, placebo-controlled study. *Dig Dis Sci.* 2007;52(11):3259–65.
87. Liu Q, Duan ZP, Ha DK, Bengmark S, Kurtovic J, Riordan SM. Synbiotic modulation of gut flora: effect on minimal hepatic encephalopathy in patients with cirrhosis. *Hepatology.* 2004;39(5):1441–9.
88. Putkonen L, Yao CK, Gibson PR. Fructose malabsorption syndrome. *Curr Opin Clin Nutr Metab Care.* 2013;16(4):473–7. doi: 10.1097/MCO.0b013e328361c556
89. Eaton KK. Gut fermentation: a reappraisal of an old clinical condition with diagnostic tests and management: discussion paper. *J R Soc Med.* 1991;84(11):669–71.
90. Hustoft TN, Hausken T, Ystad SO, Valeur J, Brokstad K, Hatlebakk JG, Lied GA. Effects of varying dietary content of fermentable short-chain carbohydrates on symptoms, fecal microenvironment, and cytokine profiles in patients with irritable bowel syndrome. *Neurogastroenterol Motil.* 2017;29(4). doi: 10.1111/nmo.12969.
91. Valeur J, Røseth AG, Knudsen T, Malmstrøm GH, Fiennes JT, Midtvedt T, Berstad A. Fecal fermentation in irritable bowel syndrome: influence of dietary restriction of fermentable oligosaccharides, disaccharides, monosaccharides and polyols. *Digestion.* 2016;94(1):50–6. doi: 10.1159/000448280.
92. Halmos EP, Christophersen CT, Bird AR, Shepherd SJ, Gibson PR, Muir JG. Diets that differ in their FODMAP content alter the colonic luminal microenvironment. *Gut.* 2015;64(1):93–100. doi: 10.1136/gutjnl-2014-307264.
93. Chumpitazi BP, Cope JL, Hollister EB, Tsai CM, McMeans AR, Luna RA, Versalovic J, Shulman RJ. Randomised clinical trial: gut microbiome biomarkers are associated with clinical response to a low FODMAP diet in children with the irritable bowel syndrome. *Aliment Pharmacol Ther.* 2015;42(4):418–27. doi: 10.1111/apt.13286.
94. Qu W, Yuan X, Zhao J, Zhang Y, Hu J, Wang J, Li J. Dietary advanced glycation end products modify gut microbial composition and partially increase colon permeability in rats. *Mol Nutr Food Res.* 2017;61(10). doi: 10.1002/mnfr.201700118.
95. Roca-Saavedra P, Mendez-Vilabrille V, Miranda JM, Nebot C, Cardelle-Cobas A, Franco CM, Cepeda A. Food additives, contaminants and other minor components: effects on human gut microbiota – a review. *J Physiol Biochem.* 2018;74(1):69–83. doi: 10.1007/s13105-017-0564-2.
96. Etxeberria U, Fernández-Quintela A, Milagro FI, Aguirre L, Martínez JA, Portillo MP. Impact of polyphenols and polyphenol-rich dietary sources on gut microbiota composition. *J Agric Food Chem.* 2013;61(40):9517–33. doi: 10.1021/jf402506c.
97. Laparra JM, Sanz Y. Interactions of gut microbiota with functional food components and nutraceuticals. *Pharmacol Res.* 2010;61(3):219–25.

98. Flanagan E, Müller M, Hornberger M, Vauzour D. impact of flavonoids on cellular and molecular mechanisms underlying age-related cognitive decline and neurodegeneration. *Curr Nutr Rep.* 2018;7(2):49–57. doi: 10.1007/s13668-018-0226-1.

99. Anderson JR, Carroll I, Azcarate-Peril MA, Rochette AD, Heinberg LJ, Peat C, Steffen K, Manderino LM, Mitchell J, Gunstad J. A preliminary examination of gut microbiota, sleep, and cognitive flexibility in healthy older adults. *Sleep Med.* 2017;38:104–7. doi: 10.1016/j.sleep.2017.07.018.

100. Biagi E, Franceschi C, Rampelli S, Severgnini M, Ostan R, Turroni S, Consolandi C, Quercia S, Scurti M, Monti D, Capri M, Brigidi P, Candela M. Gut microbiota and extreme longevity. *Curr Biol.* 2016;26(11):1480–5. doi: 10.1016/j.cub.2016.04.016.

101. Pan P, Lam V, Salzman N, Huang YW, Yu J, Zhang J, Wang LS. Black raspberries and their anthocyanin and fiber fractions alter the composition and diversity of gut microbiota in F-344 rats. *Nutr Cancer.* 2017;69(6):943–51. doi: 10.1080/01635581.2017.1340491.

102. Anhê FF, Pilon G, Roy D, Desjardins Y, Levy E, Marette A. Triggering Akkermansia with dietary polyphenols: a new weapon to combat the metabolic syndrome? *Gut Microbes.* 2016;7(2):146–53. doi: 10.1080/19490976.2016.1142036.

103. Anhê FF, Nachbar RT, Varin TV, Vilela V, Dudonné S, Pilon G, Fournier M, Lecours MA, Desjardins Y, Roy D, Levy E, Marette A. A polyphenol-rich cranberry extract reverses insulin resistance and hepatic steatosis independently of body weight loss. *Mol Metab.* 2017;6(12):1563–73. doi: 10.1016/j.molmet.2017.10.003.

104. Roopchand DE, Carmody RN, Kuhn P, Moskal K, Rojas-Silva P, Turnbaugh PJ, Raskin I. Dietary polyphenols promote growth of the gut bacterium *Akkermansia muciniphila* and attenuate high-fat diet-induced metabolic syndrome. *Diabetes.* 2015;64(8):2847–58. doi: 10.2337/db14-1916.

105. Anhê FF, Nachbar RT, Varin TV, Vilela V, Dudonné S, Pilon G, Fournier M, Lecours MA, Desjardins Y, Roy D, Levy E, Marette A. A polyphenol-rich cranberry extract reverses insulin resistance and hepatic steatosis independently of body weight loss. *Mol Metab.* 2017;6(12):1563–73. doi: 10.1016/j.molmet.2017.10.003.

106. Chassaing B, Van de Wiele T, De Bodt J, Marzorati M, Gewirtz AT. Dietary emulsifiers directly alter human microbiota composition and gene expression ex vivo potentiating intestinal inflammation. *Gut.* 2017;66(8):1414–27. doi: 10.1136/gutjnl-2016-313099.

107. Chassaing B, Koren O, Goodrich JK, Poole AC, Srinivasan S, Ley RE, Gewirtz AT. Dietary emulsifiers impact the mouse gut microbiota promoting colitis and metabolic syndrome. *Nature.* 2015;519(7541):92–6. doi: 10.1038/nature14232.

108. Nettleton JE, Reimer RA, Shearer J. Reshaping the gut microbiota: impact of low calorie sweeteners and the link to insulin resistance? *Physiol Behav.* 2016;164(Pt B):488–93. doi: 10.1016/j.physbeh.2016.04.029.

109. Nielsen LN, Roager HM, Casas ME, Frandsen HL, Gosewinkel U, Bester K, Licht TR, Hendriksen NB, Bahl MI. Glyphosate has limited short-term effects on commensal bacterial community composition in the gut environment due to sufficient aromatic amino acid levels. *Environ Pollut.* 2018;233:364–76. doi: 10.1016/j.envpol.2017.

110. Lozano VL, Defarge N, Rocque LM, Mesnage R, Hennequin D, Cassier R, de Vendômois JS, Panoff JM, Séralini GE, Amiel C. Sex-dependent impact of Roundup on the rat gut microbiome. *Toxicol Rep.* 2017;5:96–107. doi: 10.1016/j.toxrep.2017.12.005.

111. Mao Q, Manservisi F, Panzacchi S, Mandrioli D, Menghetti I, Vornoli A, Bua L, Falcioni L, Lesseur C, Chen J, Belpoggi F, Hu J. The Ramazzini Institute 13-week pilot study on glyphosate and Roundup administered at human-equivalent dose to Sprague Dawley rats: effects on the microbiome. *Environ Health.* 2018;17(1):50. doi: 10.1186/s12940-018-0394-x.

112. Bressa C, Bailén-Andrino M, Pérez-Santiago J, González-Soltero R, Pérez M, Montalvo-Lominchar MG, Maté-Muñoz JL, Domínguez R, Moreno D, Larrosa M. Differences in gut microbiota profile between women with active lifestyle and sedentary women. *PLoS One.* 2017;12(2):e0171352. doi: 10.1371/journal.pone.0171352.

113. Codella R, Luzi L, Terruzzi I. Exercise has the guts: how physical activity may positively modulate gut microbiota in chronic and immune-based diseases. *Dig Liver Dis.* 2018;50(4):331–41. doi: 10.1016/j.dld.2017.11.016.
114. Estaki M, Pither J, Baumeister P, Little JP, Gill SK, Ghosh S, Ahmadi-Vand Z, Marsden KR, Gibson DL. Cardiorespiratory fitness as a predictor of intestinal microbial diversity and distinct metagenomic functions. *Microbiome.* 2016;4(1):42. doi: 10.1186/s40168-016-0189-7.
115. Monda V, Villano I, Messina A, Valenzano A, Esposito T, Moscatelli F, Viggiano A, Cibelli G, Chieffi S, Monda M, Messina G. Exercise modifies the gut microbiota with positive health effects. *Oxid Med Cell Longev.* 2017;2017:3831972. doi: 10.1155/2017/3831972.
116. Petersen LM, Bautista EJ, Nguyen H, Hanson BM, Chen L, Lek SH, Sodergren E, Weinstock GM. Community characteristics of the gut microbiomes of competitive cyclists. *Microbiome.* 2017;5(1):98. doi: 10.1186/s40168-017-0320-4.
117. O'Sullivan O, Cronin O, Clarke SF, Murphy EF, Molloy MG, Shanahan F, Cotter PD. Exercise and the microbiota. *Gut Microbes.* 2015;6(2):131–6. doi: 10.1080/19490976.2015.1011875.
118. Allen JM, Berg Miller ME, Pence BD, Whitlock K, Nehra V, Gaskins HR, White BA, Fryer JD, Woods JA. Voluntary and forced exercise differentially alters the gut microbiome in C57BL/6J mice. *J Appl Physiol.* 2015;118(8):1059–66. doi: 10.1152/japplphysiol.01077.2014.
119. Cryan JF, Dinan TG. Mind-altering microorganisms: the impact of the gut microbiota on brain and behaviour. *Nat Rev Neurosci.* 2012;13(10):701–12.
120. Freestone PP, Sandrini SM, Haigh RD, Lyte M. Microbialendocrinology: how stress influences susceptibility to infection. *Trends Microbiol.* 2008;16(2):55–64.
121. Knowles SR, Nelson EA, Palombo EA. Investigating the role of perceived stress on bacterial flora activity and salivary cortisol secretion: a possible mechanism underlying susceptibility to illness. *Biol Psychol.* 2008;77(2):132–7.
122. Elmadfa I, Klein P, Meyer AL. Immune-stimulating effects of lactic acidbacteria in vivo and in vitro. *Proc Nutr Soc.* 2010;69(3):416–20.
123. Li CY, Lin HC, Lai CH, Lu JJ, Wu SF, Fang SH. Immunomodulatory effects of lactobacillus and Bifidobacterium on both murine and human mitogen-activated T cells. *Int Arch Allergy Immunol.* 2011;156(2):128–36.
124. Charlier C, Cretenet M, Even S, Le Loir Y. Interactions between *Staphylococcus aureus* and lactic acid bacteria: an old story with new perspectives. *Int J Food Microbiol.* 2009;131(1):30–9.
125. Bailey MT, Dowd SE, Galley JD, Hufnagle AR, Allen RG, Lyte M. Exposure to a social stressor alters the structure of the intestinal microbiota: implications for stressor-induced immunomodulation. *Brain Behav Immun.* 2011;25(3):397–407.
126. Sperandio V, Torres AG, Jarvis B, Nataro JP, Kaper JB. Bacteria-host communication: the language of hormones. *Proc Natl Acad Sci USA.* 2003;100(15):8951–6.
127. Lyte M. Microbialendocrinology and infectious disease in the 21st century. *Trends Microbiol.* 2004;12(1):14–20.
128. Ulevitch RJ, Tobias PS. Receptor-dependent mechanisms of cell stimulation by bacterial endotoxin. *Annu Rev Immunol.* 1995;13:437–57.
129. Heumann D, Barras C, SeverinA, Glauser MP, Tomasz A. Gram-positive cell walls stimulate synthesis of tumor necrosis factor alpha and interleukin-6 by human monocytes. *Infect Immun.* 1994;62:2715–21.
130. Grigoleit JS, Kullmann JS, Wolf OT, Hammes F, Wegner A, Jablonowski S, Engler H, Gizewski E, Oberbeck R, Schedlowski M. Dose-dependent effects of endotoxin on neurobehavioral functions in humans. *PLoS One.* 2011;6(12):e28330.

131. Benson S, Kattoor J, Wegner A, Hammes F, Reidick D, Grigoleit JS, Engler H, Oberbeck R, Schedlowski M, Elsenbruch S. Acute experimental endotoxemia induces visceral hypersensitivity and altered pain evaluation in healthy humans. *Pain*. 2012;153(4):794–9.

132. Winter SE, Bäumler AJ. Dysbiosis in the inflamed intestine: chance favors the prepared microbe. *Gut Microbes*. 2014;5(1):71–3. doi: 10.4161/gmic.27129.

133. Schiffrin EJ, Parlesak A, Bode C, Bode JC, van't Hof MA, Grathwohl D, Guigoz Y. Probiotic yogurt in the elderly with intestinal bacterial over growth: endotoxaemia and innate immune functions. *Br J Nutr*. 2009;101(7):961–6.

134. Grimaldi D, Guivarch E, Neveux N, Fichet J, Pène F, Marx JS, Chiche JD, Cynober L, Mira JP, Cariou A. Markers of intestinal injury are associated with endotoxemia in successfully resuscitated patients. *Resuscitation*. 2013;84(1):60–5.

135. Elamin E, Masclee A, Dekker J, Jonkers D. Ethanol disrupts intestinal epithelial tight junction integrity through intracellular calcium-mediated Rho/ROCK activation. *Am J Physiol Gastrointest Liver Physiol*. 2014;306(8):G677–85.

136. Neves AL, Coelho J, Couto L, Leite-Moreira A, Roncon-Albuquerque R Jr. Metabolic endotoxemia: a molecular link between obesity and cardiovascular risk. *J Mol Endocrinol*. 2013;51(2):R51–64.

137. Maes M, Mihaylova I, Leunis JC. Increased serum IgA and IgM against LPS of entero-bacteria in chronicfatiguesyndrome (CFS): indication for the involvement of gram-negative enterobacteria in the etiology of CFS and for the presence of an increased gut-intestinalpermeability. *J Affect Disord*. 2007;99(1–3):237–40.

138. Goebel A, Buhner S, Schedel R, Lochs H, Sprotte G. Altered intestinal permeability in patients with primary fibromyalgia and in patients with complex regional pain syn-drome. *Rheumatology*. 2008;47(8):1223–7.

139. Peterson CT, Lucas J, John-Williams LS, Thompson JW, Moseley MA, Patel S, Peterson SN, Porter V, Schadt EE, Mills PJ, Tanzi RE, Doraiswamy PM, Chopra D. Identification of altered metabolomic profiles following a panchakarma-based ayurvedic intervention in healthy subjects: the self-directed biological transformation initiative (SBTI). *Sci Rep*. 2016;6:32609. doi: 10.1038/srep32609.

140. Schnorr SL, Bachner HA. Integrative therapies in anxiety treatment with special emphasis on the gut microbiome. *Yale J Biol Med*. 2016;89(3):397–42.

141. Househam AM, Peterson CT, Mills PJ, Chopra D. The effects of stress and medita-tion on the immune system, human microbiota, and epigenetics. *Adv Mind Body Med*. 2017;31(4):10–25.

142. Mutlu EA, Gillevet PM, Rangwala H, Sikaroodi M, Naqvi A, Engen PA, Kwasny M, Lau CK, Keshavarzian A. Colonic microbiome is altered in alcoholism. *Am J Physiol Gastrointest Liver Physiol*. 2012;302(9):G966–78. doi: 10.1152/ajpgi.00380.2011.

143. Leclercq S, Matamoros S, Cani PD, Neyrinck AM, Jamar F, Stärkel P, Windey K, Tremaroli V, Bäckhed F, Verbeke K, de Timary P, Delzenne NM. Intestinal permeability, gut-bacterial dysbiosis, and behavioral markers of alcohol-dependence severity. *Proc Natl Acad Sci USA*. 2014;111(42):E4485–93. doi: 10.1073/pnas.1415174111. Epub 2014 Oct 6.

144. de Timary P, Leclercq S, Stärkel P, Delzenne N. A dysbiotic subpopula-tion of alcohol-dependent subjects. *Gut Microbes*. 2015;6(6):388–91. doi: 10.1080/19490976.2015.1107696.

145. Dubinkina VB, Tyakht AV, Odintsova VY, Yarygin KS, Kovarsky BA, Pavlenko AV, Ischenko DS, Popenko AS, Alexeev DG, Taraskina AY, Nasyrova RF, Krupitsky EM, Shalikiani NV, Bakulin IG, Shcherbakov PL, Skorodumova LO, Larin AK, Kostryukova ES, Abdulkhakov RA, Abdulkhakov SR, Malanin SY, Ismagilova RK, Grigoryeva TV, Ilina EN, Govorun VM. Links of gut microbiota composition with alcohol dependence syndrome and alcoholic liver disease. *Microbiome*. 2017;5(1):141. doi: 10.1186/s40168-017-0359-2.

146. Stewart CJ, Auchtung TA, Ajami NJ, Velasquez K, Smith DP, De La Garza R 2nd, Salas R, Petrosino JF. Effects of tobacco smoke and electronic cigarette vapor exposure on the oral and gut microbiota in humans: a pilot study. *Peer J.* 2018;6:e4693. doi: 10.7717/peerj.4693. eCollection 2018.

147. Yu G, Phillips S, Gail MH, Goedert JJ, Humphrys MS, Ravel J, Ren Y, Caporaso NE. The effect of cigarette smoking on the oral and nasal microbiota. *Microbiome.* 2017;5(1):3. doi: 10.1186/s40168-016-0226-6.

148. Biedermann L, Zeitz J, Mwinyi J, Sutter-Minder E, Rehman A, Ott SJ, Steurer-Stey C, Frei A, Frei P, Scharl M, Loessner MJ, Vavricka SR, Fried M, Schreiber S, Schuppler M, Rogler G. Smoking cessation induces profound changes in the composition of the intestinal microbiota in humans. *PLoS One.* 2013;8(3):e59260.

149. Begon J, Juillerat P, Cornuz J, Clair C. [Smoking and digestive tract: a complex relationship. Part 2: Intestinal microblota and cigarette smoking]. Rev Med Suisse. 2015 Jun 10;11(478):1304-6.

150. Angelberger S, Reinisch W, Makristathis A, Lichtenberger C, Dejaco C, Papay P, Novacek G, Trauner M, Loy A, Berry D. Temporal bacterial community dynamics vary among ulcerativecolitis patients after fecal microbiota transplantation. *Am J Gastroenterol.* 2013;108(10):1620–30. doi: 10.1038/ajg.2013.257.

151. Allais L, Kerckhof FM, Verschuere S, Bracke KR, De Smet R, Laukens D, Van den Abbeele P, De Vos M, Boon N, Brusselle GG, Cuvelier CA, Van de Wiele T. Chronic cigarette smoke exposure induces microbial and inflammatory shifts and mucin changes in the murine gut. *Environ Microbiol.* 2016;18(5):1352–63. doi: 10.1111/1462-2920.12934.

152. Hill-Burns EM, Debelius JW, Morton JT, Wissemann WT, Lewis MR, Wallen ZD, Peddada SD, Factor SA, Molho E, Zabetian CP, Knight R, Payami H. Parkinson's disease and Parkinson's disease medications have distinct signatures of the gut microbiome. *Mov Disord.* 2017;32(5):739–49. doi: 10.1002/mds.26942. Epub 2017 Feb 14.

153. Derkinderen P, Shannon KM, Brundin P. Gut feelings about smoking and coffee in Parkinson's disease. *Mov Disord.* 2014;29(8):976–9. doi: 10.1002/mds.25882.

154. Paul B, Royston KJ, Li Y, Stoll ML, Skibola CF, Wilson LS, Barnes S, Morrow CD, Tollefsbol TO. Impact of genistein on the gut microbiome of humanized mice and its role in breast tumor inhibition. *PLoS One.* 2017;12(12):e0189756. doi: 10.1371/journal.pone.0189756.

155. Garcia-Mazcorro JF, Pedreschi R, Chew B, Dowd SE, Kawas JR, Noratto G. Dietary supplementation with raspberry extracts modifies the fecal microbiota in obese diabetic db/db mice. *J Microbiol Biotechnol.* 2018;28:1247–59. doi: 10.4014/jmb.1803.03020.

156. Maier L, Pruteanu M, Kuhn M, Zeller G, Telzerow A, Anderson EE, Brochado AR, Fernandez KC, Dose H, Mori H, Patil KR, Bork P, Typas A. Extensive impact of nonantibiotic drugs on human gut bacteria. *Nature.* 2018;555(7698):623–28. doi: 10.1038/nature25979.

157. Imhann F, Vich Vila A, Bonder MJ, Lopez Manosalva AG, Koonen DPY, Fu J, Wijmenga C, Zhernakova A, Weersma RK. The influence of proton pump inhibitors and other commonly used medication on the gut microbiota. *Gut Microbes.* 2017;8(4):351–8. doi: 10.1080/19490976.2017.1284732.

158. Jackson MA, Goodrich JK, Maxan ME, Freedberg DE, Abrams JA, Poole AC, Sutter JL, Welter D, Ley RE, Bell JT, Spector TD, Steves CJ. Proton pump inhibitors alter the composition of the gut microbiota. *Gut.* 2015. 2016;65(5):749–56. doi: 10.1136/gutjnl-2015-310861.

159. Hojo M, Asahara T, Nagahara A, Takeda T, Matsumoto K, Ueyama H, Matsumoto K, Asaoka D, Takahashi T, Nomoto K, Yamashiro Y, Watanabe S. Gut microbiota composition before and after use of proton pump inhibitors. *Dig Dis Sci.* 2018;63:2940–9. doi: 10.1007/s10620-018-5122-4.

160. Minalyan A, Gabrielyan L, Scott D, Jacobs J, Pisegna JR. The gastric and intestinal microbiome: role of proton pump inhibitors. *Curr Gastroenterol Rep.* 2017;19(8):42. doi: 10.1007/s11894-017-0577-6.

161. Llorente C, Jepsen P, Inamine T, Wang L, Bluemel S, Wang HJ, Loomba R, Bajaj JS, Schubert ML, Sikaroodi M, Gillevet PM, Xu J, Kisseleva T, Ho SB, DePew J, Du X, Sørensen HT, Vilstrup H, Nelson KE, Brenner DA, Fouts DE, Schnabl B. Gastric acid suppression promotes alcoholic liver disease by inducing overgrowth of intestinal Enterococcus. *Nat Commun.* 2017;8(1):837. doi: 10.1038/s41467-017-00796-x.

162. Lo WK, Chan WW. Proton pump inhibitor use and the risk of small intestinal bacterial overgrowth: a meta-analysis. *Clin Gastroenterol Hepatol.* 2013;11(5):483–90. doi: 10.1016/j.cgh.2012.12.011.

163. Naito Y, Kashiwagi K, Takagi T, Andoh A, Inoue R. Intestinal dysbiosis secondary to proton-pump inhibitor use. *Digestion.* 2018;97(2):195–204. doi: 10.1159/000481813.

Index

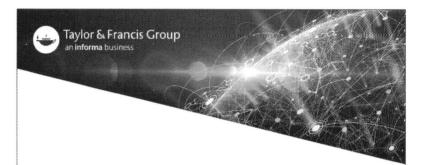

Printed in the United States
by Baker & Taylor Publisher Services